Tim Higgins

Chemistry Dept.

1997.

New Perspectives in Drug Design

New Perspectives in Drug Design

edited by

P.M. DEAN
Department of Pharmacology
University of Cambridge
UK

G. JOLLES
Rhône-Poulenc Rorer
Antony
France

and
C.G. NEWTON
Rhône-Poulenc Rorer
Dagenham
UK

ACADEMIC PRESS
Harcourt Brace & Company
London San Diego New York
Boston Sydney Tokyo Toronto

ACADEMIC PRESS LIMITED
24–28 Oval Road,
London NW1 7DX

United States Edition published by
ACADEMIC PRESS INC.
San Diego, CA 92101

This book is printed on acid-free paper

A catalogue record of this book is
available from the British Library

ISBN 0–12–208070–X

Based on the Proceedings of the Ninth International Round Table of the Rhône-Poulenc Rorer Foundation, Turnberry, Scotland, 1994

Cover illustration: X-ray structure of the anti-cancer drug Taxotere® (docetaxel) with superimposed solvent-accessible (Connolly) surface. X-ray coordinates taken from Gueritte-Voegelein, F., Guenard, D., Mangatel, L., Potier, P., Guilhem, J., Cesario, M. and Pascard, C., (1990). *Acta Crystallogr*. **C46**, 781–784. Photograph taken from a display on a Silicon Graphics IRIS 4000 workstation, generated with the programme Insight® (Biosym Inc.).

Typeset by J&L Composition Ltd, Filey, North Yorkshire and
Printed and bound in Great Britain by Hartnolls Ltd, Bodmin, Cornwall

Contributors

Barakat, M.T. Drug Design Group, Department of Pharmacology, University of Cambridge, Tennis Court Road, Cambridge CB1 2QJ, UK.

Bartlett, P.A. Department of Chemistry, University of California, Berkeley, CA 94720, USA.

Clementi, S. Laborotorio di Chemiometrica, Dipartimento di Chimica, Università di Perugia, Via Elce di Sotto, 10; 06123 Perugia, Italy.

Cruciani, G. Laboratorio di Chemiometria, Dipartimento di Chimica, Università di Perugia, Via Elce di Sotto, 10; 06123 Perugia, Italy.

Dean, P.M. Drug Design Group, Department of Pharmacology, University of Cambridge, Tennis Court Road, Cambridge CB2 1QJ, UK.

Gigonzac, O. Rhône-Poulenc Rorer Central Research, CRVA, 13 quai Jules Guesde, BP 14, 94403 Vitry-sur-Seine Cedex, France.

Guitton, J.D. Rhône-Poulenc Rorer Central Research, CRVA, 13 quai Jules Guesde, BP 14, 94403 Vitry-sur-Seine Cedex, France.

Guy, R.K. Department of Chemistry, The Scripps Research Institute, 10666 North Torrey Pines Road, La Jolla, CA 92037, USA.

Hirschmann, R. Department of Chemistry, University of Pennsylvania, Philadelphia PA 19104, USA.

IJzerman, A.P. Leiden/Amsterdam Center for Drug Research, Division of Medicinal Chemistry, PO Box 9502, 2300RA Leiden, The Netherlands.

James-Surcouf, E. Rhône-Poulenc Rorer Central Research, CRVA, 13 quai Jules Guesde, BP 14, 94403 Vitry-sur-Seine Cedex, France.

Kuntz, I.D. Department of Pharmaceutical Chemistry, University of California, San Francisco, CA 94143–0446, USA.

Laoui, A. Rhône-Poulenc Rorer Central Research, CRVA, 13 quai Jules Guesde, BP 14, 94403 Vitry-sur-Seine Cedex, France.

Laroche, V. Rhône-Poulenc Rorer Central Research, CRVA, 13 quai Jules Guesde, BP 14, 94403 Vitry-sur-Seine Cedex, France.

Lauri, G. Department of Chemistry, University of California, Berkeley, CA 94720, USA.

Leach, A.R. Department of Chemistry, University of Southampton, Southampton, Hampshire SO9 5NH, UK.

Lewis, R.A. Rhône-Poulenc Rorer Central Research, Dagenham Research Centre, Rainham Road South, Dagenham, Essex RM10 7XS, UK.

Luttmann, C. Rhône-Poulenc Rorer Central Research, CRVA, 13 quai Jules Guesde, BP 14, 94403 Vitry-sur-Seine Cedex, France.

Mark, A.E. Department of Physical Chemistry, Swiss Federal Institute of Technology, ETH Zentrum, CH 8092, Zurich, Switzerland.

McLay, I.M. Rhône-Poulenc Rorer Central Research, Dagenham Research Centre, Rainham Road South, Dagenham, Essex RM10 7XS, UK.

Mason, J.S. Rhône-Poulenc Rorer Central Research, 500 Arcola Road, PO Box 1200, Collegeville, PA 19426–0107, USA.

Meng, E.C. Department of Pharmaceutical Chemistry, University of California, San Francisco, CA 94143–0446, USA.

Morgan, B.P. Department of Chemistry, University of California, Berkeley, CA 94720, USA.

Morgat, A. Rhône-Poulenc Rorer Central Research, CRVA, 13 quai Jules Guesde, BP 14, 94403 Vitry-sur-Seine Cedex, France.

Morize, I. Rhône-Poulenc Rorer Central Research, CRVA, 13 quai Jules Guesde, BP 14, 94403 Vitry-sur-Seine Cedex, France.

Nicolaou, K.C. The Scripps Research Institute 10666 North Torrey Pines Road, La Jolla, CA 92037, USA, and Department of Chemistry, University of California, San Diego, CA 92037, USA.

Pantel, G. Rhône-Poulenc Rorer Central Research, CRVA, 13 quai Jules Guesde, BP 14, 94403 Vitry-sur-Seine Cedex, France.

Petsko, G.A. Departments of Biochemistry and Chemistry and Rosenstiel Basic Medical Sciences Research Center, Brandeis University, Waltham, MA 02254–9110, USA.

Pyun, H.-J. Department of Chemistry, University of California, Berkeley, CA 94720, USA.

Riganelli, D. Laboratorio di Chemiometria, Dipartimento di Chimica, Università di Perugia, Via Elce di Sotto, 10; 06123 Perugia, Italy.

Ringe, D. Departments of Biochemistry and Chemistry and Rosenstiel Basic Medical Sciences Research Center, Brandeis University, Waltham, MA 02254–9110, USA.

Roques, B.P. Département de Pharmacochimie Moléculaire et Structurale, U266 INSERM-URA D1500 CNRS, Faculté de Pharmacie, 4 avenue de l'Observatoire, 75270 Paris Cedex 06, France.

Rubin-Carrez, C. Rhône-Poulenc Rorer Central Research, CRVA, 13 quai Jules Guesde, BP 14, 94403 Vitry-sur-Seine Cedex, France.

Shoichet, B.K. Department of Pharmaceutical Chemistry, University of California, San Francisco, CA 94143–0446, USA.

Smith III, A.B. Department of Chemistry, University of Pennsylvania, Philadelphia, PA 19104, USA.

Sprengeler, P.A. Department of Chemistry, University of Pennsylvania, Philadelphia, PA 19104, USA.

Todorov, N.P. Drug Design Group, Department of Pharmacology, University of Cambridge, Tennis Court Road, Cambridge CB2 1QJ, UK.

Valigi, R. Laboratorio di Chemiometria, Dipartimento di Chimica, Università di Perugia, Via Elce di Sotto, 10; 06123 Perugia, Italy.

van der Wenden, E.M. Leiden/Amsterdam Center for Drug Research, Division of Medicinal Chemistry, PO Box 9502, 2300RA Leiden, The Netherlands.

van Galen, P.J.M. Leiden/Amsterdam Center for Drug Research, Division of Medicinal Chemistry, PO Box 9502, 2300RA Leiden, The Netherlands.

van Gunsteren, W.F. Department of Physical Chemistry, Swiss Federal Institute of Technology, ETH Zentrum, CH 8092 Zurich, Switzerland.

Wong, C.-H. Department of Chemistry, The Scripps Research Institute, 10666 North Torrey Pines Road, La Jolla, CA 92037, USA.

Participants

Ashton, M.J. Rhône-Poulenc Rorer Central Research, Dagenham Research Centre, Rainham Road South, Dagenham, Essex RM10 7XS, UK.

Barreau, M. Rhône-Poulenc Rorer Central Research, CRVA, 13 quai Jules Guesde, 94403 Vitry-sur-Seine Cedex, France.

Barton, J.N. Rhône-Poulenc Rorer Central Research, 500 Arcola Road, PO Box 1200, Collegeville, PA 19426–0107, USA.

Boumendil, G. Rhône-Poulenc Foundation, 20 avenue Raymond Aron, 92165 Antony Cedex, France.

Burns, C. Rhône-Poulenc Rorer Central Research, CRVA, 13 quai Jules Guesde, 94403 Vitry-sur-Seine Cedex, France.

Campbell, H.F. Rhône-Poulenc Rorer Central Research, 500 Arcola Road, PO Box 1200, Collegeville, PA 19426–0107, USA.

Campbell, M.M. School of Chemistry, University of Bath, Claverton Down, Bath, Avon BA2 7AY, UK.

Cheney, D.L. Rhône-Poulenc Rorer Central Research, 500 Arcola Road, PO Box 1200, Collegeville, PA 19426–0107, USA.

Commerçon, A. Rhône-Poulenc Rorer Central Research, CRVA, 13 quai Jules Guesde, 94403 Vitry-sur-Seine Cedex, France.

Dauber-Osguthorpe, P. School of Chemistry, University of Bath, Claverton Down, Bath BA2 7AY, UK.

Dereu, N. Rhône-Poulenc Rorer Central Research, CRVA, 13 quai Jules Guesde, 94403 Vitry-sur-Seine Cedex, France.

Djuric, S.W. Rhône-Poulenc Rorer Central Research, 500 Arcola Road, PO Box 1200, Collegeville, PA 19426–0107, USA.

Dubroeucq, M.-C. Rhône-Poulenc Rorer Central Research, CRVA, 13 quai Jules Guesde, 94403 Vitry-sur-Seine Cedex, France.

Freyssinet, G. Rhône-Poulenc SA, 25 quai Paul Doumer, 92408 Courbevoie Cedex, France.

Garrett, C. Rhône-Poulenc Rorer Central Research, CRVA, 13 quai Jules Guesde, 94403 Vitry-sur-Seine Cedex, France.

Good, A. UCSF School of Pharmacy, 513 Parnassus Avenue, Room S-926, San Francisco, CA 94143–0446, USA.

Goodman, J. University Chemical Laboratory, University of Cambridge, Lensfield Road, Cambridge CB2 1EW, UK.

Harris, N.V. Rhône-Poulenc Rorer Central Research, Dagenham Research Centre, Rainham Road South, Dagenham, Essex RM10 7XS, UK.

He, W. Rhône-Poulenc Rorer Central Research, 500 Arcola Road, PO Box 1200, Collegeville, PA 19426–0107, USA.

Husson, H.-P. Laboratoire de Chimie Thérapeutique, Faculté des Sciences, Pharmaceutiques et Biologiques, Université René Descartes, 4 avenue de l'Observatoire, 75270 Paris Cedex 06, France.

Johnson, A.P. School of Chemistry, University of Leeds, Leeds LS2 9JT, UK.

Jolles, G. Rhône-Poulenc Rorer, 20 avenue Raymond Aron, 92165 Antony Cedex, France.

Klein, S.I. Rhône-Poulenc Rorer Central Research, 500 Arcola Road, PO Box 1200, Collegeville, PA 19426–0107, USA.

Le Goas, R. Agrochemical Research Centre, Rhône-Poulenc Agro, La Dargoire, 14 à 20 Rue Pierre Baizet, 69263 Lyon Cedex 09, France.

Le Pecq, J.-B. Rhône-Poulenc Rorer Central Research, CRVA, 13 quai Jules Guesde, 94403 Vitry-sur-Seine Cedex, France.

Mayaux, J.-F. Rhône-Poulenc Rorer Central Research, CRVA, 13 quai Jules Guesde, 94403 Vitry-sur-Seine Cedex, France.

McCarthy, C. Rhône-Poulenc Rorer Central Research, Dagenham Research Centre, Rainham Road South, Dagenham, Essex RM10 7XS, UK.

Menard, P.R. Rhône-Poulenc Rorer Central Research, 500 Arcola Road, PO Box 1200, Collegeville, PA 19426–0107, USA.

Mignani, S. Rhône-Poulenc Rorer Central Research, CRVA, 13 quai Jules Guesde, 94403 Vitry-sur-Seine Cedex, France.

Molino, B.F. Rhône-Poulenc Rorer Central Research, 500 Arcola Road, PO Box 1200, Collegeville, PA 91426–0107, USA.

Mornon, J.-P. Laboratoire de Minéralogie-Cristallographie, CNRS URA09, Université P. et M. Curie, 4 Place Jussieu, 75252 Paris Cedex 05, France.

Myers, M.R. Rhône-Poulenc Rorer Central Research, 500 Arcola Road, PO Box 1200, Collegeville, PA 19426–0107, USA.

Newton, C.G. Rhône-Poulenc Rorer Central Research, Dagenham Research Centre, Rainham Road South, Dagenham, Essex RM10 7XS, UK.

Osguthorpe, D. School of Chemistry, University of Bath, Claverton Down, Bath BA2 7AY, UK.

Palfreyman, M.N. Rhône-Poulenc Rorer Central Research, Dagenham Research Centre, Rainham Road South, Dagenham, Essex RM10 7XS, UK.

Paris, J.-M. Rhône-Poulenc Rorer Central Research, CRVA, 13 quai Jules Guesde, 94403 Vitry-sur-Seine Cedex, France.

Perez, S. INRA, Laboratoire de Physicochimie de Macromolécules, Rue de la Géraudière, 44072 Nantes Cedex 03, France.

Perkins, T.D.J. Department of Pharmacology, University of Cambridge, Tennis Court Road, Cambridge CB2 1QJ, UK.

Peyronel, J.-F. Rhône-Poulenc Rorer Central Research, CRVA, 13 quai Jules Guesde, 94403 Vitry-sur-Seine Cedex, France.

Pickett, S. Rhône-Poulenc Rorer Central Research, Dagenham Research Centre, Rainham Road South, Dagenham, Essex RM10 7XS, UK.

Pinder, S. Rhône-Poulenc Rorer Central Research, Dagenham Research Centre, Rainham Road South, Dagenham, Essex RM10 7XS, UK.

Porter, B. Rhône-Poulenc Rorer Central Research, Dagenham Research Centre, Rainham Road South, Dagenham, Essex RM10 7XS, UK.

Potier, P. Institut de Chimie des Substances Naturelles, Centre National de la Recherche Scientifique, Avenue de la Terrasse, 91198 Gif-sur-Yvette Cedex, France.

Randle, J.C.R. Rhône-Poulenc Rorer Central Research, CRVA, 13 quai Jules Guesde, 94403 Vitry-sur-Seine Cedex, France.

Ratcliffe, A.J. Rhône-Poulenc Rorer Central Research, Dagenham Research Centre, Rainham Road South, Dagenham, Essex RM10 7XS, UK.

Spada, A.P. Rhône-Poulenc Rorer Central Research, 500 Arcola Road, PO Box 1200, Collegeville, PA 19426–0107, USA.

Taylor, J.B. Rhône-Poulenc Rorer Central Research, Dagenham Research Centre, Rainham Road South, Dagenham, Essex RM10 7XS, UK.

Thomas, E.J. Department of Chemistry, University of Manchester, Brunswick Street, Manchester M13 9PL, UK.

Vovelle, F. Centre de Biologie Moléculaire du CNRS, 1A, avenue de la Recherche Scientifique, 45071 Orleans Cedex 2, France.

Vuilhorgne, M. Rhône-Poulenc Rorer Central Research, CRVA, 13 quai Jules Guesde, 94403 Vitry-sur-Seine, France.

Wermuth, C.G. Faculté de Pharmacie, Laboratoire de Chimie Organique, Université Louis Pasteur, 74 route du Rhin, BP 24, 67401 Illkirch Cedex, France.

Westhof, E. Laboratoire de Cristallographie Biologique, Institut de Biologie Moléculaire et Cellulaire, CNRS, 15 rue René Descartes, 67084 Strasbourg Cedex, France.

Zakrzewska, K. Laboratoire de Biochimie Théorique, Institut de Biologie Physico-Chimique, CNRS, 13 rue Pierre et Marie Curie, 75005 Paris Cedex, France.

Contents

A colour plate section appears between pages 144–145

Preface

Drug design is the aesthetic goal of every practising medicinal chemist. The design element may be found in many aspects of the discovery of a new drug: it can be incorporated into the identification of a lead compound by intelligent screening; it is involved when a new molecule for synthesis is created by computer, or by intuition, based upon an intelligent understanding of the protein target and the molecular dynamics of docking ligands therein. Drug design can be found in converting lead compounds – which are not drugs for pharmacokinetic or other reasons, such as peptides and carbohydrates – into molecules which fulfil the same role but which are more feasible as pharmaceuticals. The identification of such peptidomimetics or carbohydrate mimetics is a key element in future drug design.

The understanding of structure–activity relationships has developed extensively over the last decade, with very powerful statistical techniques available to predict activities of designed, yet hitherto unsynthesized, compounds. Here again, the design element is found in the discovery of new medicines.

And, yet, drug design is not just the identification of lead compounds, target compounds or the prediction of activity of drugs. It must still, necessarily, encompass the synthesis of such molecules. As quoted in this work, organic synthesis remains in the stone age, compared to what nature can do, both in terms of the structural complexity of the products and efficiency of the reactions – and this from the author of one of the finest total syntheses of new medicinal agents yet reported (Chapter 5).

The conference which underlies this book was held at Turnberry, Scotland, in April 1994, and was sponsored by a grant from the Rhône-Poulenc Rorer Foundation; researchers from that company together with leading academic research workers discussed over three days all aspects of drug design. The sessions ranged from the practicalities of synthetic organic chemistry to the potential pitfalls in the mathematics of free-energy calculations. Many overlaps were produced between these two extremes and what began as a mosaic of themes, became obviously intertwined as the conference progressed.

Twelve years ago, the Foundation sponsored a first meeting on the same topic under the deliberately provocative title: 'Drug Design, Fact or Fantasy? ' At the end of the recent Round Table, a manichean answer to that question is still not obvious: major steps forward have indeed been accomplished over the last years to favour 'fact', but a long way has certainly to be covered before the medicinal chemist will be able to rely totally upon rational and mathematical approaches to reach directly the objective: innovative, active, bioavailable and well-tolerated drugs. We hope that the present contributions and discussions will help to appreciate where we now stand on this long journey.

We trust that this volume will be a thought-provoking ensemble of these perspectives in drug design and will provoke readers from all continents to continue this great work which has done so much to improve human health in the twentieth century, into the twenty-first century.

P.M. Dean, G. Jolles and C.G. Newton

Acknowledgements

It is our pleasure to thank all the contributors, as well as all the participants, who agreed to come to Scotland to attend the International Round Table, the ninth in the Rhône-Poulenc Rorer Foundation series, on 'New Perspectives in Drug Design'. Their stimulating presence made this conference a highly successful scientific event, and enabled preparation of this volume.

We are most grateful to all the discussants for their valuable contributions and to our colleagues from Rhône-Poulenc Rorer for their generous advice and kind help, especially to Drs M.J. Ashton and E. James-Surcouf who acted very efficiently as session moderators.

We wish to acknowledge the financial support of the Rhône-Poulenc Rorer Foundation, who acted as sponsor to the Round Table, according to its objective of fostering exchanges on scientific topics of current interest to both the pharmaceutical industry and academia, and to provide the international scientific community with the results of these conferences.

We are indebted to the expert assistance of Mrs Y. Raindle and Mrs B. Taylor, for diligently assisting in the organization and execution of the meeting. Tape transcription of the discussions was performed by Dr Mary Firth; her professionalism and competence were highly appreciated.

Finally, we wish to thank the staff at Academic Press Ltd (London) for their expert and kind assistance in producing this volume.

1

Some Interactions of Macromolecules with Low Molecular Weight Ligands. Recent Advances in Peptidomimetic Research

R. HIRSCHMANN, A.B. SMITH, III and P.A. SPRENGELER

Department of Chemistry, University of Pennsylvania, Philadelphia, PA 19104, USA

Introduction

Peptidomimetic research is a rapidly advancing area of medicinal chemistry (Hirschmann, 1991) which had its beginning with the recognition that potential peptidal drug candidates are susceptible to rapid cleavage by proteolytic enzymes in the gastrointestinal tract and in circulation. As a result, they generally lack oral bioavailability and possess unacceptably short biological half-lives even after parenteral administration. It was, therefore, logical to seek to overcome these shortcomings by replacing the peptidal amide backbone with isosteric substitutions. This approach led to the synthesis of so-called pseudopeptides by many laboratories, generating analogues which displayed improved biostability. The pseudopeptide approach is still, however, beset by limitations, notably lack of oral bioavailability. The field was reviewed by Spatola (1983) and more recent developments are described by Sherman and Spatola (1990). The synthesis of small cyclic peptides constituted an alternate approach toward improved biostability, since such

New Perspectives in Drug Design
ISBN 0–12–208070–X

compounds were expected to be resistant to cleavage by proteases. An example of such a peptide prepared by Veber *et al.* (1981) and its limitations will be discussed below.

The Discovery of the Enkephalins

If we exclude pseudopeptides from consideration, peptidomimetic research can be said to have begun with the discovery, by Hughes *et al.* (1975), of the enkephalins, two endogenous pentapeptides, whose receptor also binds the non-peptide morphine. Since all three compounds are opiate agonists, it is now widely assumed that the enkephalin receptor has much in common with the morphine receptor. The significance of the fact that morphine is a peptidomimetic was not, however, fully appreciated by many of us who were interested in finding a path from peptides to orally active drugs. On the other hand, Furukawa and co-workers (1982) represent a laboratory that had chosen early on to screen non-peptidal chemical libraries for angiotensin II antagonists. This effort was rewarded with the discovery that the tetrasubstituted imidazole (**1**) displayed an IC_{50} of 43 μM for the angiotensin II receptor. This lead was subsequently developed into nanomolar antagonists with good pharmacokinetic properties at both DuPont and SmithKline Beecham. These peptidomimetics, like morphine, have no obvious atom-for-atom overlap with their peptidal counterpart. Later on, Evans *et al.* (1986) and Bock *et al.* (1989), having recognized both diazepam and D-tryptophan-like components in asperlicin (**2**), successfully exploited this fungal screening lead to generate orally bioavailable peripheral as well as central cholecystokinin antagonists.

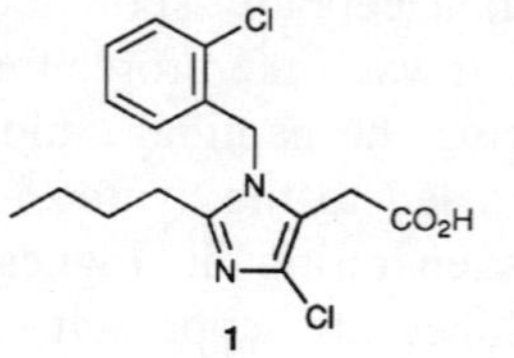

1

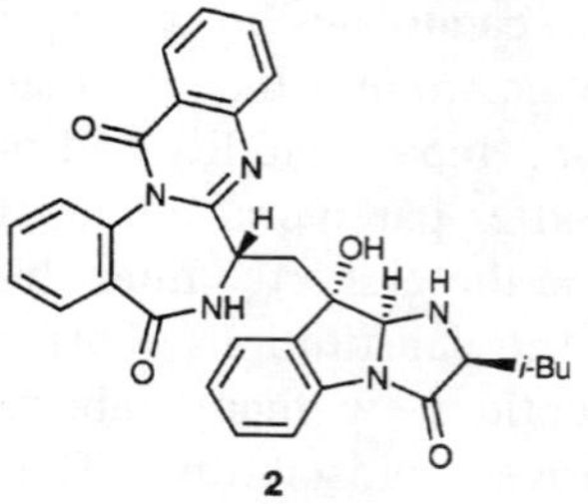

2

Peptidomimetics with Designed New Scaffolds

Background

Our work bridges the gap between pseudopeptides and morphine-type peptidomimetics (Hirschmann, 1992). The compounds which we designed and synthesized with our colleagues at the University of Pennsylvania (Penn) are not amide isosteres; they do, however, retain readily discernible mimics of peptide side chains. The purpose of this review is to show that such research, in addition to generating compounds with desirable chemical and biological properties, can broaden our understanding of the interaction of small molecules with receptors, and that in addition it can generate concepts broadly applicable to medicinal chemistry.

Farmer (1980) insightfully proposed the use of rigid scaffolds to generate peptidomimetics, but he did not explore this idea experimentally. Bélanger and Dufresne (1986) were the first to do so. They designed ligand **3** for the opiate receptor with a bicyclo[2.2.2]octane scaffold, building on a model for the bioactive conformation of methionine enkephalin. This paper was overlooked by many of us. More recently, Olson *et al.* (1989) described the synthesis of the thyrotropin-releasing hormone (TRH) mimic **4**, which bound to the low-affinity, but not to the endocrine TRH receptor. It is very encouraging that **4** has good oral bioavailability.

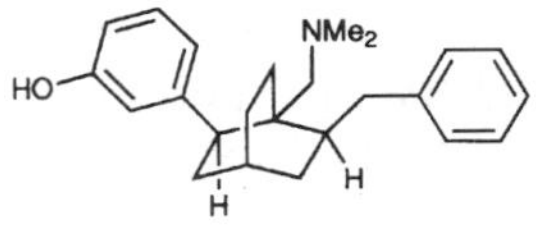

3

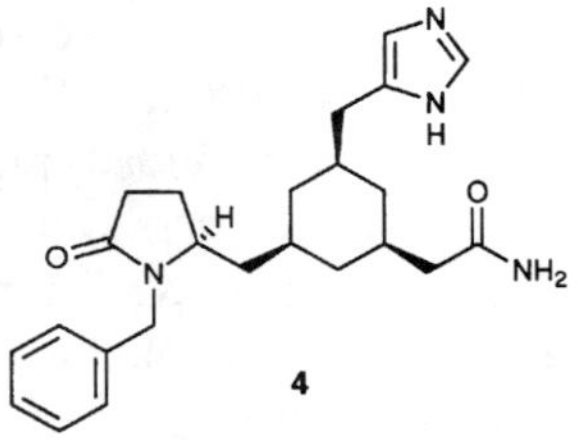

4

β-D-Glucose: A Novel Scaffold for β-Turn Mimetics

Previous work

At about the same time, we at Penn[1] reported a conceptually similar program (Nicolaou *et al.*, 1990), generating mimetics of the tetradecapeptide somatostatin (SRIF). The point of departure for this project was the cyclic hexapeptide L-363,301 (**5**), which had been designed and synthesized by Veber *et al.* (1981). As expected, this potent SRIF analogue was stable to proteases.

[1] This project was initiated by R. Hirschmann and K.C. Nicolaou in 1988. When the latter left the University of Pennsylvania in 1989, A.B. Smith, III became involved in this research.

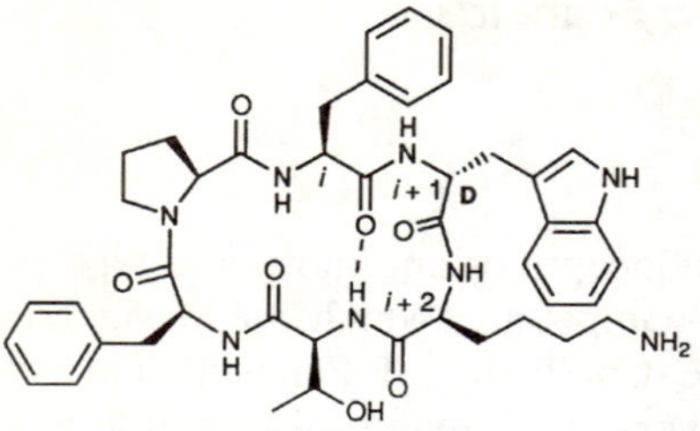

5 (L-363,301)

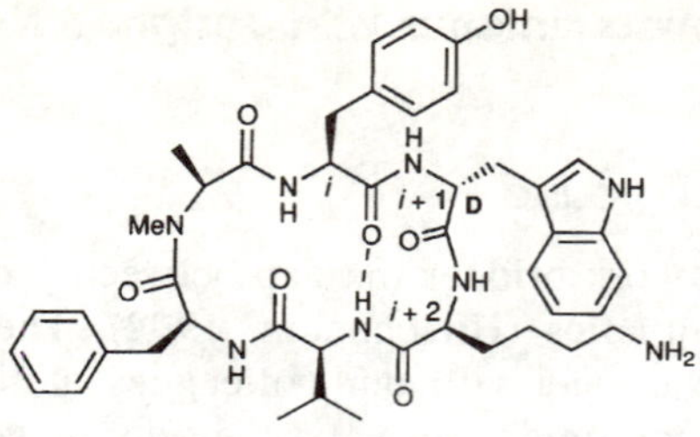

6 (MK-678)

Later, Veber *et al.* (1984) reported the chemically closely related analogue MK-678 (**6**), which was also stable to proteases but which was, nevertheless, found around 1980 to have poor oral bioavailability in human subjects (less than 5%). This led one of us (R.H., then at Merck) to realize that stability of even small peptides to proteases does not assure oral bioavailability. It occurred to us that the secondary amide bonds of **6** might interfere with its transport into the portal vein. This suggested dispensing with the peptidal amide backbone entirely and the need to find a scaffold such as benzene or cyclohexane which would correctly orient the requisite peptide side chains of the β-turns of SRIF and **5**; these are known to be principally responsible for receptor binding and activation.[2]

At Penn, because of the expertise in carbohydrate chemistry of our former collaborator K.C. Nicolaou and for other reasons which we listed elsewhere (Hirschmann *et al.*, 1993a), we selected β-D-glucose as the scaffold. Our colleagues, J. Salvino, S. Pietranico, E.M. Leahy, and later C.A. Cichy and P.G. Spoors synthesized compounds typified by **7a** and **7b** which had *in vitro* binding affinities for SRIF receptors of about 5.5 μM in experiments carried out initially by T. Reisine and K. Raynor (Penn) and later confirmed and extended by L. Maechler (Panlabs). Two lines of evidence indicate that these glycosides are indeed recognized by an SRIF receptor as mimics of **5**. First, representative compounds were shown by C. Donaldson and W. Vale (Salk) and later by K. Cheng and R. Smith (Merck) in functional assays to inhibit GRF-induced growth hormone release by cultured rat anterior pituitary cells (i.e. to display SRIF agonism). Second, the structure–activity relationships of the cyclic hexapeptides strikingly parallel those of the corresponding sugars as reported by Hirschmann *et al.* (1993a). It is particularly encouraging that L. Maechler (Panlabs) was able to show that the activity-enhancing substitution in the peptide series, resulting from the replacement of Phe^7 by His^7, is strikingly mimicked when the 2-benzyl group in a sugar is replaced by the imidazole counterpart, to give **8**; the latter was synthesized by W.C. Shake-

[2] The side chains of Phe^7, Trp^8 and Lys^9 in the *i,i+1*, and *i+2* positions, respectively of the β-turn of SRIF had been shown to suffice for binding and activation of the SRIF receptor (Veber *et al.*, 1981).

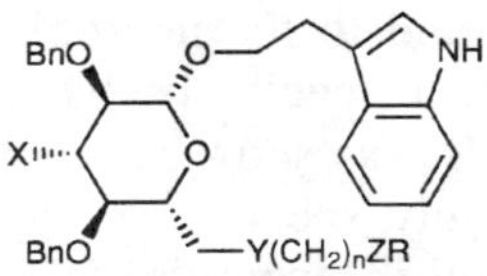

7a n = 6, X = H, Y = NH, Z = O, R =H
7b n = 6, X = OBn, Y = O, Z = NH, R = H
7c n = 5, X = OBn, Y = NH, Z = O, R = H
7d n = 5, X = H, Y = NH, Z = O, R = H
7e n = 5, X = OBn, Y = O, Z = NH, R = Ac
7f n = 5, X = OBn, Y = O, Z = NH, R = H

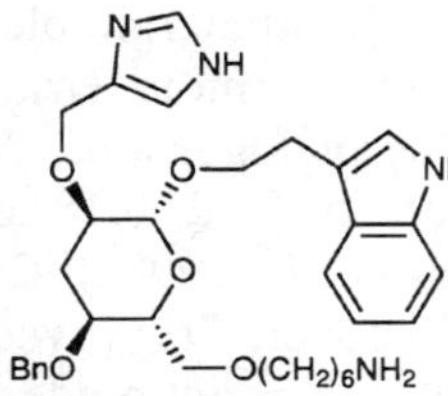

8

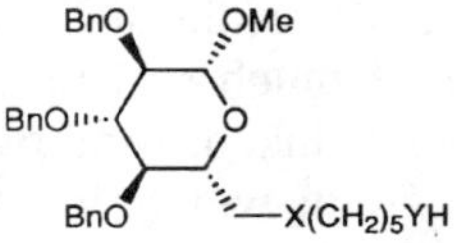

9a X = O, Y = NH
9b X = NH, Y = O

speare. Indeed, we had predicted correctly the affinities of all of our sugars from the potencies of the corresponding peptides except for compounds **9a** and **9b**.

Unexpected findings

Chemistry

Given the extensive prior art in sugar chemistry, we expected to encounter little difficulty in the synthesis of our target compounds. In fact some of the transformations were not trivial or gave unexpected results. These include the need to introduce indole and imidazole functionalized side chains, the chemoselectivity between *O*- and *N*-alkylation, and the synthesis of the 4-deoxy analogue. We are pleased to acknowledge B. Arison's (Merck) valuable contribution to structural assignment.

Biology

The binding of **9a,b** to the SRIF receptor was a completely unexpected result, which has become central to the current research by M. Cichy and J. Hynes at Penn. If our current interpretations are valid, ongoing syntheses could afford significant enhancement in both affinity and potency.

One of the most important results that has emerged from our studies is the discovery, initially by K. Raynor and T. Reisine (Penn), and later confirmed by M.R. Cascieri and C.D. Strader (Merck), that compounds such as **7c** bind also to the β_2-adrenergic receptor. The latter investigators were also able to show **7c** to be a β-adrenergic blocking agent, albeit a weak one (IC_{50} 3 mM). This result, and the more striking discovery by M.R. Cascieri and C.D. Strader that the analogues **7c**, **7d** and **7e** bind to the neurokinin-1 receptor with IC_{50} values of 0.12, 0.18 and 0.06 μM, respectively, has been reported by Hirschmann *et al.* (1992a). Compound **7e** was shown to be a substance P antagonist. Moreover, **7e** proved to be highly specific for the substance P receptor in that it does not bind to some 50 other receptors including the SRIF receptor. That the subtle modification involving *N*-acetylation (i.e. **7f** → **7e**) produced a profound switch in receptor affinity from the SRIF to the neurokinin-1 (NK-1) receptor is of great interest. Conversely, the glycoside **8**, which showed enhanced affinity for the SRIF receptor, had no affinity for the NK-1 receptor. Taken together, our results suggest that the SRIF, β_2-adrenergic, and the NK-1 receptors have much structural similarity beyond the fact that these receptors are G-protein linked. Moreover, our results indicate that simple glycosides represent scaffolds which, like the benzodiazepines, tricyclics, steroids, c-hexapeptides and others have been described as 'promiscuous' or 'privileged' platforms. These observations also suggest that simple sugars represent attractive targets for combinatorial chemical libraries.

An additional unexpected result of our work, not presently understood, is the observation that in the glycosides an ε-amino nitrogen mimic is not required in the C-6 side chain for SRIF receptor binding or activation, since compounds such as **7c** and **7d** bound to the SRIF receptor, and **7b** was an agonist in a functional assay.

Finally, the high affinity of **7e** for the NK-1 receptor led us to acetylate the primary amino group of MK-678 to learn whether the resulting compound would bind to the NK-1 receptor. This proved not to be the case, but *N*-acetyl MK-678 unexpectedly proved to be an SRIF agonist, although its affinity for the SRIF receptor was only 1/20 that of MK-678. This result runs counter to the widely accepted impression that the free ε-amino group of lysine is required in peptidal SRIF agonists, and thus changes our understanding of the interaction of the SRIF receptor with its ligands.

For details of our efforts with T. Kawasaki, J.W. Leahy and W.C. Shakespeare to exploit other scaffolds (steroids) in non-peptide peptidomimetic research see Hirschmann (1992) and Hirschmann *et al.* (1992b, 1993b).

The Pyrrolinones: Mimics of β-Strands and β-Pleated Sheets

State of the art

Our pyrrolinone program had inhibition of proteases as its initial goal. We began this project, like the above peptide hormone/neurotransmitter mimetic research, in the spring of 1988. It had become clear to us as a result of a conversation of R.H. with Daniel Rich (University of Wisconsin) that hydrogen bonding between the amide backbones of proteolytic enzymes and their substrates/inhibitors, both organized as β-strands, plays a critical role in binding of the ligands to the macromolecules. This fact profoundly influenced our design of a new scaffold for the attachment of critical side chains. The design of protease inhibitors with novel scaffolding therefore represents a considerably more challenging task than hormone mimetic design, because hydrogen bonding capability must be retained in the scaffold of the enzyme inhibitors while still discarding the secondary amide backbone. The implementation of this concept is discussed below.

Design and conformation of the pyrrolinones

Early endeavours by J.L. Wood, and one of us (P.A.S.) based on the then fragmentary published information with known peptidal renin inhibitors, led us to synthesize initially a 1-acyl-2-amino cyclopentene as a first generation enaminone scaffold (Wood *et al.*, 1990; Smith *et al.*, 1995). This approach, however, failed to generate renin inhibition. M.K. Holloway (Merck) showed in subsequent docking experiments with the Merck renin model that this failure was probably due to the fact that the cyclopentene ring exceeds the available space in the active site of renin.

At this juncture, one of us (A.B.S.) recommended that prior to further efforts to design specific protease inhibitors, we seek a scaffold for the peptide backbone, capable of iterative construction, that would mimic the extended β-strand/sheet conformation of peptides. Interactive computer modelling led us to explore 3,5-linked pyrrolin-4-ones as inhibitors of proteases. Modelling suggested excellent overlap between the enaminone (**10**) and peptide (**11**), in several critical respects as shown in Fig. 1.1 (Smith *et al.*, 1992). Peptide **11**, a crystalline methyl ester of an equine angiotensinogen fragment (Precigoux *et al.*, 1987), is known to pack as a parallel β-pleated sheet in the solid state. Computer modelling indicated that the dihedral angles ψ and ω, as well as the ϕ angles of the pyrrolinone provide excellent overlap with the tetrapeptide methyl ester. Finally it seemed reasonable to assume that intramolecular hydrogen bonding between pyrrolinone carbonyls and the NH of a neighbouring pyrrolinone ring would stabilize the desired planar β-strand conformation. A second, equally important function of this intramolecular hydrogen bond will be discussed below.

Synthetic methodology developed by R.C. Holcomb, T.P. Keenan, and M.C. Guzman (Smith *et al.*, 1992, 1993) made possible the synthesis of **10** by T.P. Keenan and M.C. Guzman. It was subsequently crystallized and converted into the corresponding amine which was also obtained as a crystalline solid. Least-squares comparisons of the X-ray structures of **10** and of the free amino analogue of **10**, and that of **11** confirmed the expected overlap of carbonyl groups and side chains, and suggested a 2.5 Å intramolecular hydrogen bond between the NH and the neighbouring carbonyl oxygen atom.

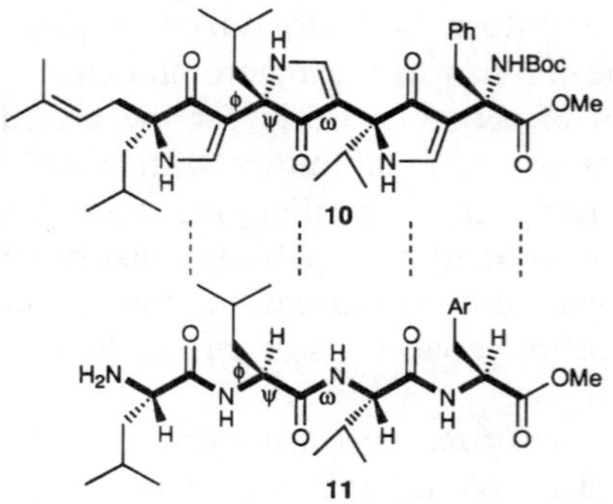

Fig. 1.1 Correspondence between carbonyls and side chains of pyrrolinone **10** and peptide **11**.

The potential of 3,5-linked pyrrolinones to generate β-pleated sheets
The above results, which support the rationale for the design and are therefore pleasing, do not, however, answer one of the critical questions: will the vinylogous nitrogen of the pyrrolinone, displaced from its position in peptides, be able to participate in interstrand hydrogen bonding and β-pleated sheet formation? Examination of the unit cells of the above pyrrolinones by P.J. Carroll (Penn) clearly demonstrated interstrand hydrogen bonding. Consequently we were now confident that the pyrrolinone scaffold would permit β-pleated sheet formation not only with neighbouring strands, but also with proteolytic enzymes, and that the successful design of pyrrolinone-based inhibitors was all but assured.

Protease inhibitors and initial evaluation of their transport properties
The sustained efforts of R. Akaishi, D.R. Jones, T.P. Keenan, M.C. Guzman and R.C. Holcomb permitted the synthesis of four pyrrolinone targets, three of which were found by P.K.S. Siegal and J.A. Zugay (Merck) to have IC_{50} values against renin in the 0.6–18 μM range (Smith *et al.*, 1994b). These compounds did not inhibit HIV-1 protease, another aspartate protease. By contrast, the fourth pyrrolinone inhibited only the viral enzyme for reasons that are presently not understood. Having thus demonstrated the relevance of the pyrrolinone design for protease inhibition, we concentrated our efforts on the medically more important viral enzyme. In doing so we patterned the selection of side chains, N- and C-termini, and transition state isosteres on prior art. Using the known Merck peptidal inhibitor **12** as a model (Vacca *et al.*, 1991), we designed (Fig. 1.2) and synthesized **13** to permit side-by-side biological evaluation of these two compounds (A. Pasternak). The preliminary results obtained by P.L. Darke, E.A. Emini, M.K. Holloway and W.A. Schleif (Merck) proved interesting (Smith *et al.*, 1994a). Peptide **12** was more potent (IC_{50} 0.6 nM) in inhibiting the isolated HIV-1 protease than the pyrrolinone (**13**) (IC_{50} 10 nM), suggesting that the latter is an excellent, but not perfect

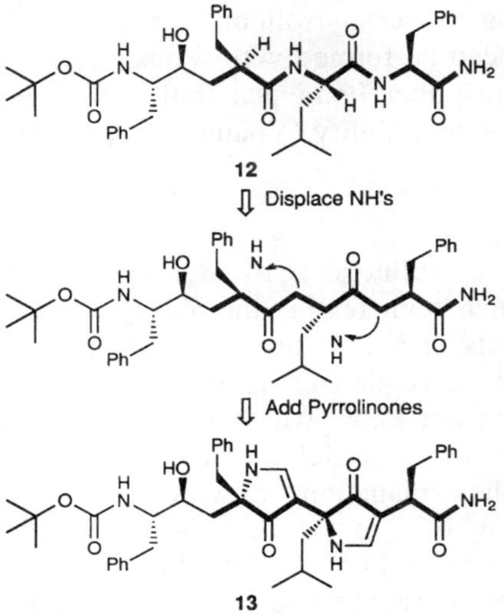

Fig. 1.2 Design of enaminone-based protease inhibitor **13**.

peptidomimetic. The more remarkable observation, however, was the fact that in a cellular assay the pyrrolinone (**13**) was the more potent compound (CIC [cellular inhibitory concentration]$_{95}$ 1.5 μM vs. 6.0 μM), implying that **13** is more readily transported into the cell[3] than the peptide **12**. If these results can be confirmed and extended, we will have achieved a principal goal: the design of protease inhibitors which are stable to proteases and in addition possess improved transport properties.

A proposed explanation for improved transport into cells

Encouraged to do so by P.S. Anderson (Merck), we sought a molecular explanation for the above improved transport properties. It occurred to one of us (R.H.) that recent publications from the drug metabolism group at Upjohn are relevant. Conradi *et al.* (1992), demonstrated that *N*-methylation of the secondary amide bond of a tetrapeptide increases passive transport across CaCo-2 cell monolayers, results that nicely support the underlying hypothesis for our peptidomimetic research, that the secondary amide bonds interfere with transport. Importantly, the publications by Conradi *et al.* (1991) and Karls *et al.* (1991) cited earlier studies by Stein (1967) and Diamond and Wright (1969). Taken altogether, the latter two publications point out that for diverse solutes, transport into plant and animal cells correlates inversely with the number of hydrogen bonds with water, since transport must be preceded by desolvation, an energy-requiring process. Because intramolecular hydro-

[3] The assay involved MT-4 cells, a human lymphoid cell line.

gen bonds, like those in our pyrrolinones, reduce by two the number of hydrogen bonds that can be formed with water, such bonds increase permeability. It is of interest that brain penetration may also be improved by reducing hydrogen bonding ability (Young *et al.*, 1988).

Summary of results

We believe that the pyrrolinone scaffold represents the first mimic of a peptidal β-strand which both retains the ability to participate in β-pleated sheet formation and is stable to proteases. In a preliminary experiment, however, **13** failed to give desired plasma levels in two dogs after oral administration. We do not know whether this observation is the result of, for example, its inappropriately high molecular weight (735 Da) and/or rapid excretion. Whatever the explanation, our work shows that two concepts can be incorporated into drug design: (1) decreasing the number of primary or secondary amide bonds and/or (2) introducing functionality capable of replacing solvation by intramolecular hydrogen bonding. Both enable the medicinal chemist to influence favourably the transport properties of a compound by decreasing solvation.

Concluding Comments

It is well known that the immunoregulant cyclosporin (**14**) has good oral bioavailability, especially when administered in oil. The two concepts that have been discussed above serve nicely to explain the favourable transport properties of **14**. As can be seen in Fig. 1.3, 7 of the 11 amide bonds of **14** are tertiary rather than secondary. Three of the remaining secondary amide bonds are cross-ring intramolecularly hydrogen bonded and even the fourth, a solvent exposed secondary amide bond, is capable of intramolecular hydrogen bonding. These observations are consistent with the idea that reducing the

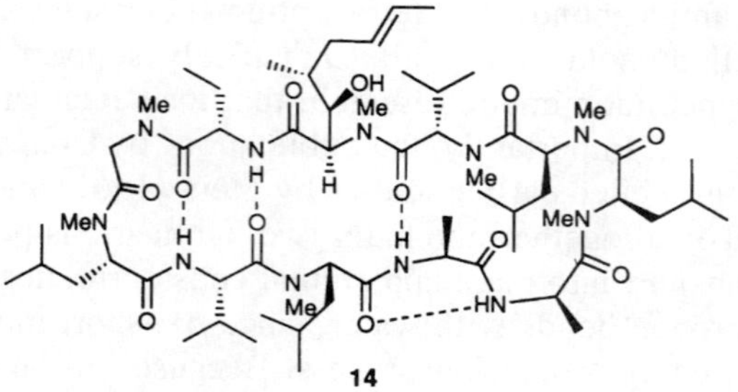

14

Fig. 1.3 Rationalization of the oral bioavailability of cyclosporin A (**14**) (see text).

number of solvent exposed secondary amide bonds and/or involving them in intramolecular hydrogen bonding can improve transport properties.

Acknowledgements

The authors are indebted to all of our collaborators mentioned herein for their contributions and are pleased to acknowledge support of this investigation by the National Institutes of Health (Institute of General Medical Sciences) through grant GM-41821 and by Bachem, Inc. (Torrance, CA), the Merck Research Laboratories, Sterling Winthrop, and ICI.

References

Bélanger, P.C. and Dufresne, C. (1986). *Can. J. Chem.* **64**, 1514–1520.

Bock, M.G., Di Pardo, R., Evans, B.E., Rittle, K.E., Whitter, W.L., Veber, D.F., Anderson, P.S. and Freidinger, R.M. (1989). *J. Med. Chem.* **32**, 16–23.

Conradi, R.A., Hilgers, A.R., Ho, N.F.H. and Burton, P.S. (1991). *Pharmac. Res.* **8**, 1453–1460.

Conradi, R.A., Hilgers, A.R., Ho, N.F.H. and Burton, P.S. (1992). *Pharmac. Res.* **9**, 435–439.

Diamond, J.M. and Wright, E.M. (1969) *Proc. R. Soc. Lond. B* **172**, 273–316.

Evans, B.E., Bock, M.G., Rittle, K.E., Di Pardo, R.M., Whitter, W.L., Veber, D.F., Anderson, P.S. and Freidinger, R.M. (1986). *Proc. Natl. Acad. Sci. USA* **83**, 4918–4922.

Farmer, P.S. (1980). *In* 'Drug Design' (E.J. Ariens, ed.), vol. 10, pp. 119–143. Academic Press, New York.

Furukawa, Y., Kishimoto, S. and Nishikawa, K. (1982). US Patent 4,355,040.

Hirschmann, R. (1991). *Angew. Chem. Int. Ed. Engl.* **30**, 1728–1801.

Hirschmann, R. (1992). *In* 'Proceedings of the Second Japan Symposium on Peptide Chemistry. Peptide Chemistry 1992' (N. Yamaichara, ed.), pp. 466–470. ESCOM, Leiden.

Hirschmann, R., Nicolaou, K.C., Pietranico, S., Salvino, J., Leahy, E.M., Sprengeler, P.A., Furst, G., Smith, A.B. III, Strader, C.D., Cascieri, M.A., Candelore, M.R., Donaldson, C., Vale, W. and Maechler, L. (1992a). *J. Am. Chem. Soc.* **114** 9217–9218.

Hirschmann, R., Sprengeler, P.A., Kawasaki, T., Leahy, J.W., Shakespeare, W.C. and Smith, A.B., III (1992b). *J. Am. Chem. Soc.* **114**, 9699–9701.

Hirschmann, R., Nicolaou, K.C., Pietranico, S., Leahy, E.M., Salvino, J., Arison, B., Cichy, C., Spoors, P.G. Shakespeare, W.C., Sprengeler, P.A., Hamley, P., Smith, A.B., III, Reisine, T., Raynor, K., Maechler, L., Donaldson, C, Vale, W., Freidinger, R.M., Cascieri, M.R. and Strader, C.D. (1993a). *J. Am. Chem. Soc.* **115** 12550–12568.

Hirschmann, R., Sprengeler, P.A., Kawasaki, T., Leahy, J.W., Shakespeare, W.C. and Smith, A.B., III. (1993b). *Tetrahedron Symposia in Print* **49**, 3665–3676.

Hughes, J., Smith, T.W., Kosterliz, H.W., Fothergill, A., Morgan, B.A. and Morris, H.R. (1975). *Nature* **258**, 577–579.

Karls, M.S., Rush, B.D., Wilkinson, K.F., Vidmar, T.J., Burton, P.S. and Ruwart, M.J. (1991). *Pharmac. Res.* **8**, 1477–1481.

Nicolaou, K.C., Salvino, J.M., Raynor, K., Pietranico, S., Reisine, T., Freidinger, R.M. and Hirschmann, R. (1990). *In* 'Peptides – Chemistry Structure and Biology: Proceedings of the 11th American Peptide Symposium' (J.E. River and R.G. Marshall eds), pp. 881–884. ESCOM, Leiden.

Olson, G.L., Cheung, H.C., Voss, M.E., Hill, D.E., Kahn, M., Madison, V.S., Cook, C.M., Spinwall, J. and Vincout, G. (1989). *In* 'Biotechnology USA'. pp. 348–360. Conference Management Corporation, Norwalk.

Precigoux, G., Courseille, C., Geoffre, S. and Leroy, F. (1987). *J. Am. Chem Soc.* **109**, 7463–7465.

Sherman, D.B. and Spatola, A.F. (1990). *J. Am. Chem. Soc.* **112**, 433–441.

Smith, A.B., III, Keenan, T.P., Holcomb, R.C., Sprengeler, P.A., Guzman, M.C., Wood, J.L., Carroll, P.J. and Hirschmann, R. (1992). *J. Am. Chem. Soc.* **114**, 10672–10674.

Smith, A.B., III, Holcomb, R.C., Guzman, M.C., Keenan, T.P., Sprengeler, P.A. and Hirschmann, R. (1993). *Tetrahedron Lett.* **34**, 63–66.

Smith, A.B., III, Hirschmann, R., Pasternak, A., Ryouichi, A., Guzman, M.C., Jones, D.R., Keenan, T.P., Sprengeler, P.A., Darke, P.L., Emini, E.A., Holloway, M.K. and Schleif, W.A. (1994). *J. Med. Chem.* **37**, 215–218.

Smith, A.B., III, Hirschmann, R., Akaishi, R., Jones, D.R., Keenan, T.P., Guzman, M.C., Holcomb, R.C., Sprengeler, P.A. and Wood, J.L. (1995). *Peptide Sci.* **37**, 29–53.

Spatola, A.F. (1983). *In* 'Chemistry and Biochemistry of Amino Acids, Peptides and Proteins' (B. Weinstein ed.), pp. 267–357. Marcel Dekker, New York.

Stein, W.D. (1967). *In* 'The Movement of Molecules Across Cell Membranes', pp. 65–125. Academic Press, New York.

Vacca, J.P., Guare, J.P., deSolms, S.J., Sanders, W.M., Giuliani, E.A., Young, S.D., Darke, P.L., Zugay, J., Sigal, I.S., Schleif, W.A., Quintero, J.C., Emini, E.A., Anderson, P.S. and Huff, J.R. (1991). *J. Med. Chem.* **34**, 1225–1228.

Veber, D.F., Freidinger, R.M., Perlow, D.S., Palaveda, Jr. W.J., Holly, F.W., Strachan, R.G., Nutt, R.F., Arison, B.H., Homnick, C., Randall, W.C., Glitzer, M.S., Saperstein, R. and Hirschmann, R. (1981). *Nature* **292**, 55–58.

Veber, D.F., Saperstein, R., Nutt, R.F., Freidinger, R.M., Brady, S.F., Curley, P., Perlow, D.S., Paleveda, W.J., Colton, C.D., Zacchei, A.G., Tocco, D.J., Hoff, D.R., Vandlen, R.L., Gerich, J.E., Hall, L., Mandarino, L., Cordes, E.H., Anderson, P.S. and Hirschmann, R. (1984). *Life Sci.* **34**, 1371–1378.

Wood, J.L., Jones, D.R., Hirschmann, R. and Smith, A.B. III. (1990). *Tetrahedron Lett.* **31**, 6329–6330.

Young, R.C., Mitchell, R.C., Brown, T.H., Ganellin, C.R., Griffiths, R., Jones, M., Rana, K.K., Saunders, D., Smith, I.R., Sore, N.E., and Wilks, T.J. (1988). *J. Med. Chem.* **31**, 656–671.

Discussion

M.M. Campbell

With reference to the β-D-glucose systems, there is a subtle point here which I am sure was built into the planning: that the backbone is probably effectively buried relative to certain other scaffolds that have been introduced. I think, for example, of the spiro bicyclo scaffolding introduced by Glaxo, where parts of the scaffold are probably sticking out and could potentially interfere with the binding domain of the receptor. I suspect in your case, that the novel backbone is probably completely buried relative to certain other groups that have been introduced as β-turn mimetics. Have you any comments on that?

R.F. Hirschmann
This is, of course, a β-turn mimetic – it is meant only to be that. We knew that somatostatin had a β-turn, as I indicated, and the β-D-glucose was employed as a possible scaffold to mimic that turn. It is not meant to be presented here as an alternative to a peptide scaffolding in any situation other than the one mimicking a β-turn.

I.M. McLay
You showed a very nice result of how the somatostatin analogue **7e** based on the β-D-glucose system had antagonist activity to substance P, but you did not explain or give any theories about how you think it mimics substance P (which also has a β-turn). Have you any ideas about how the sugar (**7e**) binds to the substance P receptor, and what similarities it has with substance P itself? [*R.F. Hirschmann*: No.] Have you looked, though, to see if you can find the explanation?

R.F. Hirschmann
We have looked, and can speculate that the aromatic rings at the C-terminus of substance P have something in common with the aromatic rings in our sugar, but there is no evidence for it. We would like very much – and are hoping – to be able to get a still more potent substance P antagonist. As you know, substance P receptor subtypes have been discovered, and also several non-peptidal molecules have been discovered by screening. Catherine Strader has kindly offered to see which of these non-peptidal fermentation product substance P receptor antagonists can be displaced by our sugars. This may help answer the interesting question that you have asked, to which I certainly do not have an answer at the moment.

I.D. Kuntz
Given your broad experience in the pharmaceutical industry, what do you foresee for peptidomimetics? Will these be a 'way station' of some form, or will they be a legitimate pharmaceutical target that can sustain itself over a long period of time?

R.F. Hirschmann
I think they already are legitimate targets. The most striking examples so far come from the category that I described which involved screening of libraries,

of fermentation broths, and I think in the future the screening of combinatorial libraries. The example that I cited was the angiotensin II antagonist, for which the lead came from Japan, where there are compounds in the clinic or at least about to be in the clinic. Pfizer's substance P antagonist came out of screening fermentation broths.

In our enthusiasm for rational drug design, publications in the *Reader's Digest* and elsewhere led the public to believe that nowadays if we want to have a drug for a certain disease we just sit down in front of the computer – and out comes the drug. There has been so much over-emphasis on this that when somebody asked a marketing executive at Merck whether the company screened, he replied that they would not do that – but, if anything is being done to a great extent, it is to screen broths and so forth.

In a way, this is not so bad because this kind of operation shows how subtle the interactions are between a small molecule and a receptor – infinitely more subtle than our minds, in my opinion. One example that has always intrigued me is the work with the β_2-adrenergic receptor where it was shown that aspartate 113 of the receptor is required to bind not only compounds like adrenaline and noradrenaline but also all the β-blockers. Not surprisingly, a mutation in which aspartate 113 was replaced by serine 113 did not bind any of these ligands of the wild-type receptor.

Screening the catechol library, led to a molecule which did not have an amine and which was a potent β-agonist. Medicinal chemists are, of course, very good at explaining results after they know the outcome, so it was not difficult to draw suitable hydrogen bonds to explain this result.

If we think about it, the one amino acid in the receptor that absolutely has to be present was replaced with a natural ligand – the aspartate. The one basic amine in the agonist was replaced. The two critical components have been dispensed with – and, the product of the two was an agonist.

I think we can understand it, but we do not know how to predict it. A fair degree of humility in all this, and also perhaps a sense of humour, are the two important components in medicinal chemistry.

2

Drug Design Based on Structural Similarity and Molecular Biology

B.P. ROQUES

Département de Pharmacochimie Moléculaire et Structurale,
U266 INSERM-URA D1500 CNRS, Faculté de Pharmacie,
4, ave de l'Observatoire – 75270 Paris Cedex 06, France

The last conference organized by Rhône-Poulenc Rorer on the subject of Drug Design (Jolles and Wooldridge, 1984) led to a solid dose of scepticism about the ambitious challenge to design new chemical structures from direct investigation of the size, shape and electrostatic potential of the target receptor site. In contrast, the optimization of a lead compound discovered by serendipity using quantitative structure – activity relationships (QSAR) was underlined.

Twelve years after the conference, and ten years after the book, the field of structure-based drug design is becoming a standard method in medicinal chemistry. This is due, in part, to a better definition of the biological targets at the atomic level, resulting from a considerable progress in the three-dimensional determination of proteins alone or complexed with a ligand. As discussed in this book, the structure of a different protein is solved, on average, nearly every day either by X-ray crystallography or by ^{1}H NMR. The efficiency of the latter technique is impressive and proteins containing more than 200 amino acids can now be studied by multidimensional NMR techniques. Obviously, the use of these methodologies is dependent on the expression of large quantities of proteins by recombinant technologies. This offers, in addition, the possibility of labelling homogenously or selectively the constituent amino acids with stable isotopes such as ^{13}C, ^{15}N and ^{19}F to simplify the analysis of the ^{1}H NMR spectra of proteins. Nevertheless, solid phase synthesis is now replacing protein recombinant technology for proteins (or functional domains of proteins) containing no more than 150 residues, as

New Perspectives in Drug Design
ISBN 0–12–208070–X

discussed in this chapter. Even this limit should be overcome in the near future by coupling protein domains by a non-peptide bond (Rose, 1994).

Details of the 3D arrangement of the active site of a receptor or an enzyme could serve as a basis for the design of novel molecules (Roques, 1988). Nevertheless, at present, few examples of pharmacologically relevant protein or nucleic acid targets have been analysed in sufficient detail to allow the *de novo* design of lead compounds. Therefore, more of the examples of drug candidates now in clinical trials have been obtained by using structural analogies between protein targets and by conformational analysis of natural or screened ligands.

Modulation of Regulatory Peptide Functions: Antagonists versus Peptidase Inhibitors

Peptides are probably the most important group of intracellular messengers in living organisms. They are able to convey information both over short distances (e.g. neuropeptides in the central nervous system and trophic factors acting in autocrine or paracrine systems) and over longer distances (regulatory peptides and hormones). In all cases, these compounds interact with specific receptors and their physiological actions are interrupted mainly, but not exclusively, by ectopeptidases cleaving the native peptide into inactive fragments. Considerable interest in membrane-bound peptidases emerged at the end of the 1970s following the discovery that inhibition of angiotensin converting enzyme (ACE) (peptidyl-dipeptidase, EC 3.4.15.1), the enzyme involved in the formation of angiotensin II from angiotensin I, produced antihypertensive effects (Ondetti *et al.*, 1977). Three years later, the inhibition of another membrane-bound zinc metallopeptidase, neutral endopeptidase-24.11 (EC 3.4.24.11, NEP, neprilysin) (Kerr and Kenny, 1974a,b), involved in the inactivation of the opioid peptide enkephalins in the brain, was shown to induce analgesic responses (Roques *et al.*, 1980). Interest was further heightened when it was shown that NEP is involved in the inactivation of the atrial natriuretic peptide mainly in the kidney (Kenny and Stephenson, 1988).

The advantage of peptidase inhibitors over compounds able to stimulate or block peptide receptors is that these molecules are expected to modify only the extracellular levels of endogenous peptide messengers.

This approach should thus avoid overstimulation (in the case of agonists) or overblockade (in the case of antagonists) of receptors, which may be a cause of side-effects. Thus, the severe drawbacks of morphine (tolerance, physical and psychological dependence, respiratory depression, constipation) which are due to ubiquitous stimulation of opioid receptors are no longer found with inhibitors able to block the metabolism of the natural peptide messengers (enkephalins) by both neutral endopeptidase 24.11 (NEP) and aminopeptidase

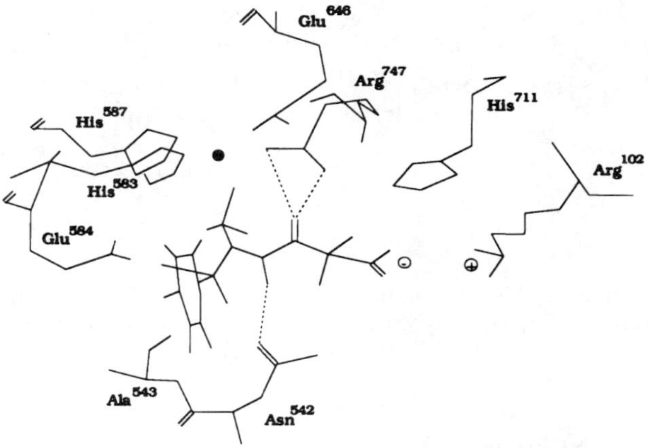

Fig. 2.1 Schematic representation of the binding of the NEP inhibitor, retrothiorphan, to the active site of the enzyme, with the sulphydryl group of the inhibitor pointing toward the zinc atom. Site-directed mutagenesis studies have confirmed the proposed roles of Glu584 in catalysis (Devault *et al.*, 1988b), His583, His587 (Devault *et al.*, 1988a), and Glu646 (Le Moual *et al.*, 1991) in zinc binding, Arg747 and Arg102 (Bateman *et al.*, 1989; Beaumont *et al.*, 1991, 1992) in ligand binding, and His711 (Bateman *et al.*, 1990) which may be involved in transition state binding. Asn542 and Ala543 are probably involved in substrate binding (Benchetrit *et al.*, 1988). All of these residues, except Arg102, have their homologues in the active site of TLN, and the binding mode of retrothiorphan is taken from data obtained by co-crystallization of the inhibitor with this enzyme (Roderick *et al.*, 1989).

N (APN) (Roques *et al.*, 1993). The concept of mixed inhibitors has been developed by taking into account that the two metabolizing ectoenzymes belong to the group of zinc metallopeptidases (Fournié-Zaluski *et al.*, 1984a; Roques and Fournié-Zaluski, 1986). NEP was the first physiologically relevant zinc metallopeptidase to be cloned (Devault *et al.*, 1987). The enzyme contains 749 amino acids with a small N-terminal intracytoplasmic domain followed by a short hydrophobic helix anchoring the enzyme in the plasma membrane. The large hydrophilic extracellular domain is *N*-glycosylated and contains the active site, characterized by a consensus sequence VxxHExxH found in endo- and aminopeptidases but not in carboxypeptidases (Roques, 1993). The histidines in the sequence act as two of the three zinc ligands and the glutamate residue is involved in substrate hydrolysis.

All the critical amino acids present in the active site of thermolysin (TLN), a zinc-metalloendopeptidase that has been crystallized alone and with various inhibitors (Matthews, 1988), have also been found in NEP (Fig. 2.1). This was established by using both a new method of sequence comparison called hydrophobic cluster analysis (HCA) (Benchetrit *et al.*, 1988) and site-directed mutagenesis (Devault *et al.*, 1988a,b; Le Moual *et al.*, 1991). Unlike

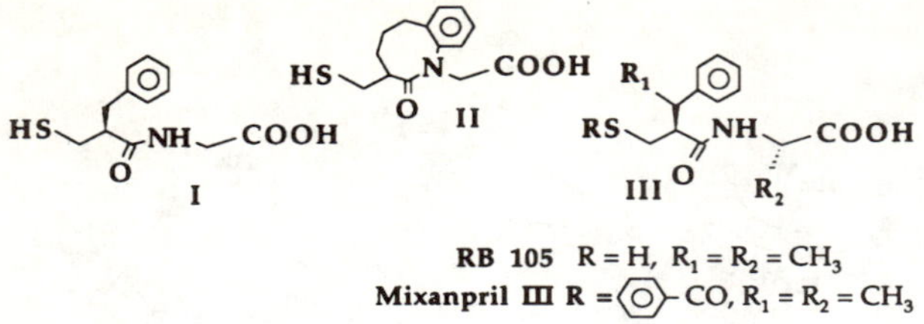

Fig. 2.2 Formulae of the NEP inhibitor, thiorphan (I), the ACE inhibitor (II) [3-(mercaptomethyl)-3,4,5,6-tetrahydro-2-oxo-^{1}H-1-benzazocine-1-acetic acid] and the mixed NEP/ACE inhibitor RB 105 (III).

TLN, however, NEP possesses an Arg102 residue located at the edge of the active site which is probably responsible for the dipeptidylcarboxypeptidase activity of NEP as observed with the enkephalins (Beaumont *et al.*, 1991). The replacement of Arg102 by Glu has allowed the specificity of the enzyme to be changed by charge polarity reversal (Beaumont *et al.*, 1992). The mutated enzyme has also been used to assign the position of an inhibitor into the S_1–S_2' subsites of NEP (Gomez-Monterrey *et al.*, 1993). ACE, aminopeptidase A (APA) and APN, were recently cloned and also shown to contain the consensus sequence VxxHExxH (Turner, 1993).

Several classes of potent and selective inhibitors of NEP, ANP or ACE have been rationally designed by taking into account the similarities and differences in the active site of these peptidases. The residual cross-reactivity with ACE found in the first synthetic NEP inhibitor thiorphan (Fig. 2.2) was eliminated by retroinversion of the amide bond in retrothiorphan. Both inhibitors have been co-crystallized with TLN (Roderick *et al.*, 1989), confirming our hypothesis about the similarities in the spatial disposition of the oxygen and hydrogen atoms in the natural or retroinverted isomers (Benchetrit *et al.*, 1987) and justifying the use of the TLN active site as a model of the NEP active site for docking experiments. It is interesting to observe that, as for NEP with enkephalins, ACE releases the two terminal amino acids of angiotensin I. In fact, ACE behaves also as an efficient endopeptidase. Its dipeptidylcarboxypeptidase activity is probably due to the presence of an arginine residue (corresponding to Arg102 in NEP) located in the enzyme's S_2' subsite in close proximity to the carboxyl group of the substrate (unpublished results from our laboratory). This interaction seems to be more precise in the case of ACE than in the case of NEP (Roques and Fournié-Zaluski, 1986).

Rational Design of Mixanpril, a Dual Inhibitor of NEP and ACE

Blood pressure and fluid volume homeostasis are critically dependent on regulatory peptides, such as angiotensin II which has vasoconstrictive properties, and atrial natriuretic peptide (ANP) which induces diuresis, natriuresis and a slight vasodilation. The metabolism of these peptides is mainly controlled by two enzymatic systems, ACE and NEP (Ondetti and Cushman, 1984; Roques *et al.*, 1993). ACE belongs to the enzymatic cascade of the renin–angiotensin system and releases the vasoconstrictor peptide angiotensin II from the inactive precursor, angiotensin I. NEP inactivates ANP (Kenny and Stephenson, 1988), and bradykinin is metabolized by both ACE and NEP at endothelial and epithelial sites respectively (Ura *et al.*, 1987). The modulation of the circulating levels of these various endogenous peptides may, therefore, be an efficient way of treating various cardiovascular diseases. Selective inhibitors of ACE (Ondetti *et al.*, 1977; Wyvratt and Patchett, 1985) are clinically useful for the treatment of hypertension and congestive heart failure. In order to increase their effectiveness, these inhibitors are generally associated with classical diuretics. This can, however, evoke secondary effects, such as activation of pressor systems and kaliuresis.

Selective inhibitors of NEP have been developed with the aim of delaying ANP degradation (Sybertz, 1991) and their efficiency in protecting endogenous ANP has been demonstrated in various animal models of hypertension (Sybertz, 1991; Pham *et al.*, 1992). In humans they have significant diuretic and natriuretic effects with no potassium loss (Richards *et al.*, 1990; Burnier *et al.*, 1991). However, these renal effects are not accompanied by significant changes in blood pressure or left ventricular haemodynamic load (Richards *et al.*, 1990).

Taken together, these results suggest a need for a simultaneous inhibition of ACE, to avoid angiotensin II formation, and of NEP, to potentiate ANP action (Roques and Beaumont, 1990). Accordingly, the association of selective inhibitors of both enzymes has been tested in various models of hypertension in rats, and a potentiation of their respective effects has been observed (Seymour *et al.*, 1991; Pham *et al.*, 1993). Nevertheless, for reasons of bioavailability, pharmacokinetic parameters and toxicity, it was more interesting to develop mixed inhibitors of NEP and ACE. The first dual inhibitor of NEP and ACE, *N*-[2-mercapto-methyl-3-phenylpropanoyl]-L-leucine was described over ten years ago (Fournié-Zaluski *et al.*, 1981; Gordon *et al.*, 1983). This compound, also designated SQ 28133, has been found to elicit depressor activity in both desoxycorticosterone acetate (DOCA) hypertensive rats and spontaneously hypertensive rats (SHRs) after i.v. administration at high doses (100–300 mg/kg) (Seymour *et al.*, 1991).

The design of mixed NEP–ACE inhibitors was facilitated by the fact that these enzymes belong to the group of zinc ectopeptidases, whose mechanism of action has been determined from both crystallographic data (Matthews, 1988) and molecular biology experiments (Roques *et al.*, 1993). Moreover, a large number of selective inhibitors have allowed the similarities and differences in the active site of both enzymes to be determined (Fournié-Zaluski *et al.*, 1984b).

Inhibitors interacting with the S_1', S_2' subsites of NEP and ACE and bearing a sulphydryl group as a zinc chelator, such as captopril for ACE and thiorphan for NEP, were selected as models for dual NEP/ACE inhibition. Furthermore, highly efficient and selective ACE inhibitors, such as compound II [3-(mercaptomethyl)-3,4,5,6-tetrahydro-2-oxo-^{1}H-benzazocine-1-acetic acid] (IC_{50} = 4 nM) (Watthey *et al.*, 1984) (Fig. 2.2) have been obtained by introducing cyclic constraints into the structure of captopril. In order to increase the affinity for both NEP and ACE, various conformational restrictions, aimed at reducing the degree of freedom of the dual inhibitors, were introduced in a structure able to fit optimally the active site of both enzymes (Fournié-Zaluski *et al.*, 1994).

Taking into account the fact that the active site of NEP is relatively large, but does not accept an imino acid in the P_2' position (Fournié-Zaluski *et al.*, 1984b), acyclic hydrophobic constraints were introduced onto the benzyl moiety of thiorphan. Introduction of a methyl group into the β position of this residue led to the best superimposition of both the putative biologically active conformation of thiorphan in the active site of NEP (Roderick *et al.*, 1989) and the constrained benzolactam II structure obtained from molecular modelling studies (Plate 2.1).

Furthermore, an important step in designing a dual inhibitor of NEP and ACE was to select a molecule able to reach the endothelial and renal epithelial targets at the same time. The chosen compound possesses L-alanine as the C-terminal residue and corresponds to the (2*S*,3*R*) isomer of *N*-[2-(mercaptomethyl)-1-oxo-3-phenylbutyl] (*S*)-alanine (RB 105) (K_i on ACE = 4.2 ± 0.5 nM; K_i on NEP = 1.7 ± 0.3 nM) (Table 2.1). The hydrophobicity of this compound was further improved by introduction of the lipophilic benzoyl moiety as a mercapto protecting group, leading to mixanpril.

Oral administration of the prodrug mixanpril elicits a long duration and

Table 2.1
Inhibitory potencies of the four stereoisomers of RB 105 on NEP and ACE

	K_i(nM)	
	NEP	ACE
(2*R*, 3*R*)	2.3 ± 0.4	80 ± 10
(2*S*, 3*S*)	2.1 ± 0.4	16 ± 4
(2*S*, 3*R*)	1.7 ± 0.3	4.2 ± 0.5
(2*R*, 3*S*)	0.7 ± 0.1	95 ± 10

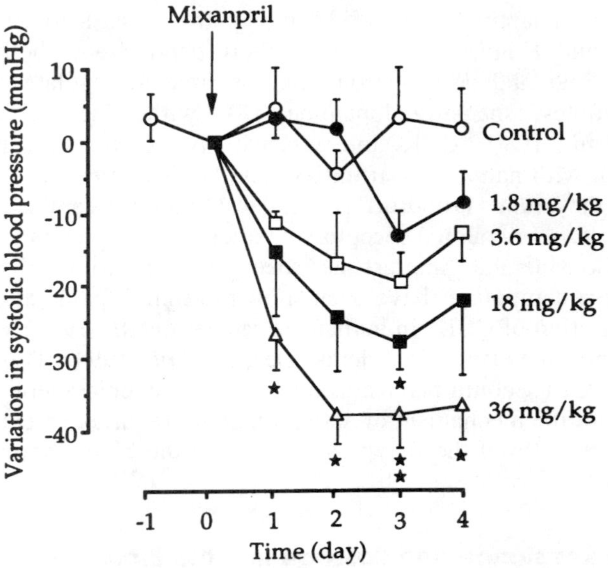

Fig. 2.3 Dose-dependent ($r = 0.6$, $P < 0.01$) effect of orally administered mixanpril on blood pressure in SHR. Mixanpril or its vehicle was administered by gavage twice a day at the indicated doses and systolic blood pressure measured 2 h after oral administration by the tail-cuff method. (★ 0.05; ★★ 0.01).

dose-dependent hypotensive response in the spontaneously hypertensive rat (SHR) (Fig. 2.3) and an inhibition of urinary NEP activity. This shows that a mixed inhibitor can be orally effective on both vascular and renal targets and thus could represent a new therapeutic alternative for the treatment of hypertension. These favourable vasodilator and renal effects could also be beneficial in other cardiovascular diseases such as heart failure (Seymour *et al.*, 1993). Furthermore, angiotensin II has been shown to be a growth factor-like molecule (Berk *et al.*, 1989), and ANP (Itoh *et al.*, 1990) and kinin-induced endothelium nitric oxide (Farby *et al.*, 1992) have been reported to act as antiproliferative agents in smooth muscle cells. Thus, mixed ACE/NEP inhibitors could also have beneficial effects in vascular disease (Mourlon-Legrand *et al.*, 1993) involving hypertrophy or proliferation of smooth muscle cells.

The Design of Cholecystokinin Receptor Ligands: Equality Between Pseudopeptide, Peptidomimetics and Non-peptide Compounds

The sulphated fragment of cholecystokinin, CCK_8 (H–Asp–Tyr(SO_3H)–Met–Gly–Trp–Met–Asp–Phe–NH_2), appears to play a critical role in behavioural, emotional and adaptive processes such as pain, stress, learning and memory (Woodruff and Hughes, 1981). This short peptide acts both as classical neurotransmitter and as a neuromodulator, able to regulate the release of biogenic amines especially dopamine (DA) with which it is co-localized (Hökfelt *et al.*, 1980). CCK_8 interacts with two distinct receptors, CCK-A and CCK-B, with nanomolar affinities. The latter is present in large concentrations in the brain (Woodruff *et al.*, 1991). Both receptors belong to the group of G-protein coupled receptors characterized by seven transmembrane domains. Considerable interest has been devoted to CCK-B antagonists because these compounds have been shown to inhibit panic attacks triggered by administration of CCK_4 in humans (Bradwejn *et al.*, 1991) and to produce antidepressant-like effects in rodents (Derrien *et al.*, 1994). This suggests that endogenous CCK_8 could behave as a natural anxiogenic agent. Nevertheless, exploration of the mechanism of action of CCK_8 requires potent and selective agonists, especially of the B type able to cross the blood–brain barrier.

Peptidase Resistance and Passage into the Brain of a Systemically Active, Highly Potent and Selective Agonist for Central CCK Receptors

When incubated with brain tissue, CCK_8 was shown to be cleaved by aminopeptidase A releasing the N-terminal Asp residue (Deschodt-Lanckman, 1985; Migaud *et al.*, 1995) and by NEP at the Trp–Met and Asp–Phe–NH_2 bonds (Nadjouski *et al.*, 1985; Durieux *et al.*, 1985). In addition, the Nle28–Gly29 bond was shown to be cleaved by a thiol protease (Durieux *et al.*, 1986). A serine protease has also been claimed to be involved in the metabolism of CCK_8 (Rose *et al.*, 1988). These peptide bonds were protected by introduction of a Boc or propionyl group in place of Asp, by retroinversion of the Met–Gly bond, by changing Met residues to the non-oxidizable norleucine (Nle) residues, which occurs without loss of affinity, and by methylation of the Trp–Nle amide bond. This led to a highly enzyme-resistant compound, BC 264, Boc–Tyr(SO_3H)–gNle–mGly–Trp–*N*(Me)Nle–Asp–Phe–NH_2 (Fig. 2.4), endowed with a high affinity and a 500-fold selectivity for central CCK receptors (Charpentier *et al.*, 1988). An analogue of BC 264, made by replacing the Boc group by a propionyl residue (pBC 264) has also been prepared. This could be radiolabelled in the propionyl residue. The resulting [^{3}H]pBC 264 had a specific activity of 98 Ci/mmol and has been used for binding studies with mouse, rat and guinea-pig brain cortex membranes (Durieux *et al.*, 1991). Steady-state conditions were established from association kinetics of 0.2 nM [^{3}H]pBC 264, and in both rat and guinea-pig, equilibrium was reached in 45 min at 25°C. Saturation experiments were carried out using [^{3}H]pBC 264 from 5×10^{-11} M to 6×10^{-9} M at 25°C (incubation time

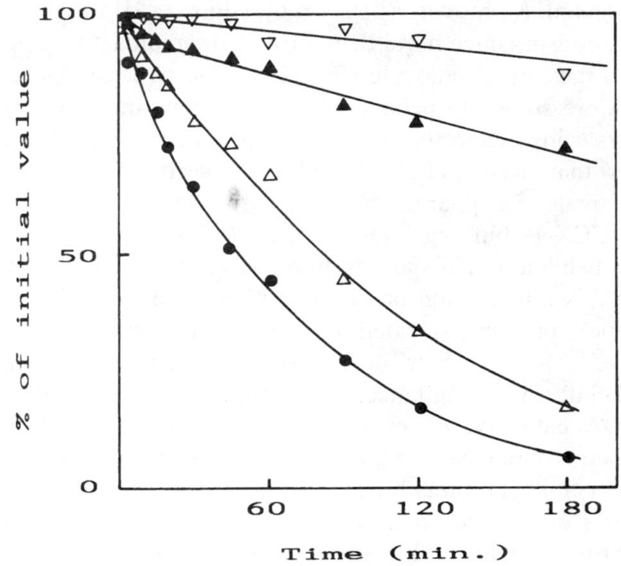

Fig. 2.4 Time course for the hydrolysis of CCK_8 analogues by rat brain homogenate. Substrates (10^{-4} M) were incubated for varying times at 37°C with crude membrane fractions of rat brain (2.7 mg of protein/ml). ●, CCK_8, Δ, Boc–Tyr(SO_3H)–Nle–Gly–Trp–Nle–Asp–Phe–NH_2; ▲, Boc–Tyr(SO_3H)–Nle–Gly–Trp–*N*(Me)Nle–Asp–Phe–NH_2; ∇, BC 264 (Boc–Tyr(SO_3H)–gNle–mGly–Trp–*N*(Me)Nle–Asp–Phe–NH_2, where the standard three-letter notation preceded by the prefix g represents the gem-diaminoalkyl residue derived from the specific amino acid; the prefix m represents the malonic acid residue derived from the amino acid residue specified by the three-letter notation.

60 min): Scatchard analysis of the binding isotherm to membranes of guinea-pig cortex showed that the tritiated probe interacts with high affinity (K_D = 0.15 ± 0.01 nM) to a single class of binding sites (B_{max} = 39.8 ± 2.7 fmol/mg protein). The specific binding was 90% at the K_D concentration and 70% at saturation (2 nM). [^{3}H]pBC 264 also showed a high affinity (K_D ~ 0.2 nM) for rat, cat, monkey and human brain.

The selectivity of pBC 264 was determined by competitive experiments using [^{3}H]pCCK_8 as a non-selective ligand and membranes from cortex (CCK-B sites) or pancreas (CCK-A sites) of guinea-pig and rat. pBC 264 was found to have an affinity approximately 1000 times higher for CCK-B than for CCK-A receptors, with the following K_i values: guinea-pig, 0.06 nM for brain receptors vs. 62.3 nM for pancreas receptors; rat, 0.16 nM for brain receptors vs. 153 nM for pancreas receptors (Durieux *et al.*, 1991). Studies on the bioavailability of [^{3}H]pBC 264 have been carried out in the mouse (Ruiz-Gayo *et al.*, 1990). The radioactivity present in the brain 15 min after i.v. injection of [^{3}H]pBC 264 (50 pmol) represented 1.4/10 000 of the total radioactivity injected. Moreover, as shown by HPLC, [^{3}H]pBC 264 was very resistant to metabolism, since more than 85% of the radioactivity in the brain corresponded to the intact molecule (Fig. 2.5). The two analogues, BC 264 and pBC 264, were shown to behave as highly potent and selective CCK-B receptor agonists using electrophysiological experiments (Daugé *et al.*, 1990). The results show that these modified peptides can be administered by systemic routes to investigate the pharmacological responses induced by selective stimulation of CCK-B binding sites. When administered i.p. to monkeys, BC 264 led to behavioural responses mimicking panic attacks in humans, suggesting that this effect could be due to activation of the CCK-B receptor type (or subtype), probably located in a particular brain area. However, interestingly BC 264 at lower doses led to a set of pharmacological responses, especially hypervigilance, suggesting an activation of the meso-corticolimbic DA pathway. Accordingly, i.p. administration of BC 264 at 3 μg/kg increased DA release in vigilant rats implanted with a microdialysis probe in the N-accumbens (unpublished results from our laboratory). Therefore, BC 264 has drawn the attention of clinicians to its use as a possible psychostimulant for patients with neurodegenerative diseases. Due to the low

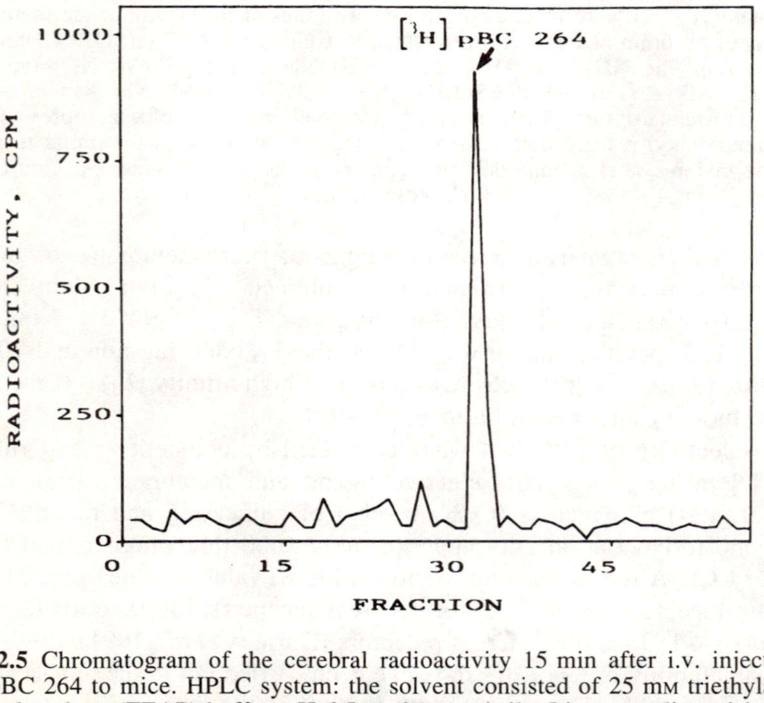

Fig. 2.5 Chromatogram of the cerebral radioactivity 15 min after i.v. injection of [^{3}H]pBC 264 to mice. HPLC system: the solvent consisted of 25 mM triethylammonium phosphate (TEAP) buffer, pH 6.5, and acetonitrile. Linear gradient rising from 28 to 38% of acetonitrile in 30 min at a flow rate of 1.2 ml/min.

doses required, the development of this compound as a possible drug is conceivable.

Criteria for Agonist Versus Antagonist Properties: An Excursion in Receptor Structure-based Design

CCK-B antagonists belonging to the classes of peptidomimetics such as PD-134,308 or non-peptide ligands such as L-365,260, RP-102,682 and LY-288513, have been recently synthesized.

Only the peptoid PD-134,308, has been designed following a rational approach in which the conformational characteristics of CCK_8 and the essential amino acids present in CCK_4 for recognition of the CCK-B receptor (Belleney *et al.*, 1989), have been taken into account (Hughes *et al.*, 1990). Interestingly most of the non-peptide ligands synthesized for interaction with peptide receptors have antagonist properties. One may speculate that the conformational restriction present in these heterocyclic molecules prevents the transfer of information which is believed to follow the binding of an agonist to its receptor. Nevertheless, a relatively rigid molecule could present an agonist property provided that it stabilizes a conformation of the receptor which allows the transduction process to occur.

During the development of CCK_4-derived pseudopeptides, we were quite surprised to observe that bis methylation of the terminal carboxamide group in the selective CCK-B agonist

Boc–Trp–Phg–Asp–(1-Nal)–NH_2 (**1**)

(Phg = phenylglycine; 1-Nal = 1-napthylalanine) results in a CCK-B selective antagonist

Boc–Trp–Phg–Asp–(1-Nal)–*N*$(Me)_2$ (**2**)

(Corringer *et al.*, 1993). The opposing pharmacological activities of these two structurally related peptides suggested that bis methylation alone is responsible for the antagonist properties displayed by **2**. However, whether this opposite pharmacological response is related to conformational changes induced by the presence of the dimethyl group or to the lack of an essential hydrogen bond involving the $CONH_2$ group and appropriate donor and/or acceptor groups in the receptor, still remains to be answered. Therefore, the solution conformation of the two peptides was examined by ^1H NMR in a d_6-DMSO/H_2O (80:20) mixture. ^1H–^1H distance constraints, derived from 2D NOESY and ROESY experiments, were used as inputs for subsequent restrained molecular dynamics simulations (unpublished results from our laboratory). Comparison of the NMR and molecular modelling data indicates

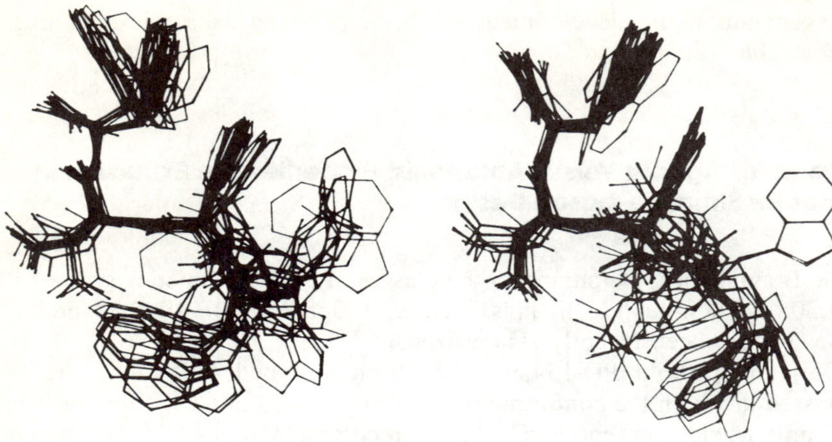

Fig. 2.6 Superposition (backbone atoms only) of the 30 structures generated by the restrained simulated annealing procedure for Boc–Trp–Phg–Asp–(1-Nal)–NH_2 (left) and Boc–Trp–Phg–Asp–(1-Nal)–*N*$(Me)_2$ (right). For clarity, hydrogen atoms are not shown.

distinct conformational preferences for these two peptides with a different spatial orientation of the Trp residues (Fig. 2.6).

The conformations of the cholecystokinins (CCK_4, CCK_5, CCK_6, CCK_7, CCK_8) have been extensively studied by NMR spectroscopy, circular dichroism, X-ray crystallography and theoretical calculations. These studies have shown that these peptides are able to adopt a large range of conformations, going from folded to more extended structures which can allow, in some cases, conformational adaptation to both CCK-A and CCK-B receptors (Fournié-Zaluski *et al*., 1986; Nadzan *et al*., 1992). Interestingly, the conformations that were obtained in the present study for the selective CCK-B agonist Boc–Trp–Phg–Asp–(1-(Nal)–NH_2 (**1**), are related to the conformations that we have previously determined for another selective CCK-B agonist, Boc–Trp–*N*Me–(Nle)–Asp–Phe–NH_2 (Goudreau *et al*., 1994). Indeed, as can be seen in Plate 2.2, both sets of conformations display a similar spatial relationship of their aromatic side chains, specifically those in positions 1 and 4, which are known to play a key role in the interaction with the receptor. Moreover, as pointed out before in the study of Boc–Trp–*N*(Me)–Nle–Asp–Phe–NH_2, these conformations are also in agreement with the 'bioactive' conformation that Nadzan *et al*. (1992), proposed for their A-63387 constrained analogue (Ctp–t–3PP–Asp–Phe–NH_2). Indeed, it can be noted that all three conformations are more or less characterized by an S-shape form with a similar spatial arrangement of the aromatic rings in positions 1 and 4 which point in opposite directions. In contrast, in the set of conformers generated for the selective CCK-B antagonist, Boc–Trp–Phg–

Asp–(1-Nal)–NMe_2 (**2**), the side chains of the biologically relevant Trp and Nal residues do not display the same spatial relationship as observed within the agonists, which could account for their different pharmacological activity (Fig. 2.6). Moreover, the antagonist **2** seems overall less flexible than the agonists, as appears to be the general case among the different families of CCK-B antagonists. Furthermore, an interesting feature of the conformers that we obtained for this antagonist, is that they have some similarities with the low energy conformations proposed for two other CCK-B antagonists, namely L-365,260 and LY-288513 (Howbert *et al.*, 1993). Indeed, Howbert *et al.*, have performed a comparative conformational analysis on these two antagonists. They have shown that although the origins and development of these two compounds are completely independent, their low energy conformations show remarkable three-dimensional homology, most specifically regarding the disposition of the three aromatic domains contained in each compound. In Plate 2.3, we show these two compounds in their reported low energy conformations along with one of our NMR-derived conformers for peptide **2**. Again, we can observe the spatial correspondence of the three aromatic rings of peptide **2** with those of the other two antagonists. However, apart from the three aromatic groups, there seemed to be no other overlaps between the backbone of **2** and the pyrazolidinone ring of LY-288513 or the diazepine ring of L-365,260, suggesting that the pharmacophore for the CCK-B antagonists is mainly defined by the presence of three aromatic and/or cyclic residues. Provided that the difference in the receptor activities of peptide **1** and peptide **2** is primarily based on the molecular conformations of these peptides and not on other factors such as the lack of an essential hydrogen bond with appropriately located donor and/or acceptor groups in the receptor, it is tempting to assume that the conformational mobility of the N-terminal Trp residue plays an important role in discriminating between agonist and/or antagonist activity.

Though there is no a priori reason to believe that the preferred solution conformation is the active conformation at the receptor, the above conformational results can still provide insights into some of these requirements since it is conceivable that the CCK-B receptor selects the biologically active form of these ligands from the ensemble of conformations existing in solution. Therefore, we could hypothesize that both peptides are recognized by their C-terminal ends, which display similar conformations, through an interaction with a common subsite of the receptor, while their opposite pharmacological activities would result from a different interaction of their N-terminal Trp residue with the receptor. In addition, it has already been suggested for some other G-protein coupled receptors, through computer modelling studies, that agonists and antagonists might have distinct binding sites at the receptor (Maloney Huss and Lybrand, 1992; Hibert *et al.*, 1993; Strosberg, 1993).

These possibilities have been investigated by computer modelling and site-directed mutagenesis since the rat CCK-B receptor has been cloned

(Jagerschmidt *et al.*, 1994) and expressed in Cos-7 cells (unpublished results from our laboratory) for binding experiments or in CHO cells for studies of the pharmacological profile of CCK_8 and related compounds using mutants (unpublished results from our laboratory). Thus, CCK-B agonists and antagonists can be easily distinguished by measurement of the release of inositol phosphate in the culture medium. Mutations of the His and Tyr residues located in the seventh transmembrane domain suggested that these amino acids could be involved in the receptor-bound transduction process. The antagonist properties induced by *N,N′*-methylation of the C-terminal amide group could be related to a change in the localization of the Trp residue in a hydrophobic pocket constituted by aromatic side chains of residues belonging to three transmembrane domains. This change would hinder the formation of the hydrogen bond necessary for receptor activation.

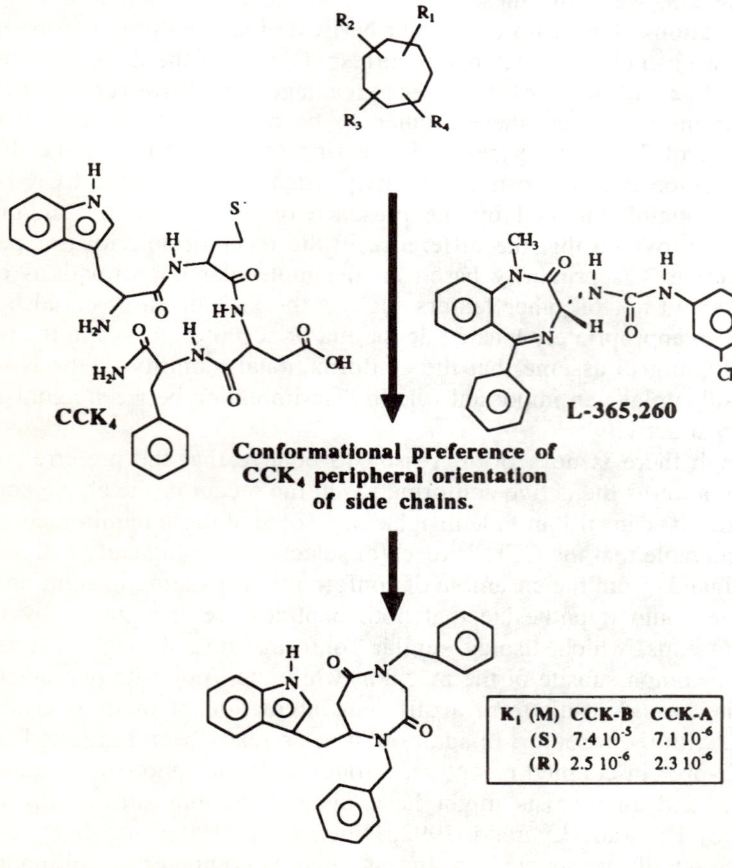

K_i (M)	CCK-B	CCK-A
(S)	$7.4\ 10^{-5}$	$7.1\ 10^{-6}$
(R)	$2.5\ 10^{-6}$	$2.3\ 10^{-6}$

Fig. 2.7 Rational design of non-peptide analogues of CCK_4.

Based in part on these observations, two strategies have been followed to design CCK-B agonists. The first one was to introduce on a rigid scaffold the side chains of CCK_4 expected to be essential for CCK-B receptor recognition. This preliminary approach, still not confirmed by molecular modelling studies, led to compounds such as a diazepinone (Fig. 2.7) which have modest affinities but some selectivity for CCK receptors, since these molecules are able to interact with more than 30 other receptors including amino and peptide binding sites at concentration $\geq 10^{-3}$ M (Corringer, 1990). Unexpectedly, these molecules were endowed with antagonist properties.

Another strategy consisted of deriving constrained compounds based on the results of the conformational analysis of the CCK-B agonist Boc–Trp–(*N*-Me)Nle–Asp–Phe–NH_2 (Goudreau *et al.*, 1994). This led us to synthesize interesting ligands which exhibit favourable selectivity and affinity for the B receptor (unpublished results from our laboratory). These molecules could serve as a lead for designing CCK-B agonists with improved affinity.

Progress in Structure-based Drug Design

Genetic studies have progressed in the definition of the proteins or nucleic acid sequences which need to be targeted to correct deficiencies in physiological pathways. In addition, improvements in solid phase peptide synthesis allow the preparation of large quantities of proteins with a high degree of purity. Several small proteins such as the SH_3 domains of GAP and Grb_2, the 1–93 domain of human synaptobrevin and the nucleocapsid protein NCp7 of HIV-1 have been recently synthesized (de Rocquigny *et al.*, 1992; Cornille *et al.*, 1994; Yang *et al.*, 1994; Goudreau *et al.*, 1994) and their structures analysed (Plate 2.4).

The nucleocapsid protein NCp7 of the human immunodeficiency virus type I (HIV-1) is a 72 amino acid peptide containing two zinc fingers of the type $CX_2CX_4HX_4C$ linked by a short basic sequence ^{29}RAPRKKG^{35}. NCp7 was shown to activate *in vitro* both viral RNA dimerization and replication primer $tRNA^{Lys,3}$ annealing to the initiation site of reverse transcription (Darlix and Roques, 1993). In order to clarify the possible structural role of the zinc fingers in the various functions of NCp7, complete sequence-specific ^1H NMR assignment of the entire protein has been achieved by two-dimensional NMR experiments (Morellet *et al.*, 1994). Moreover, to characterize the role of the peptide linker in NCp7 folding, a synthetic analogue with an inversion of the Pro31 configuration has been studied by NMR and fluorescence techniques. Several long-range NOEs implying proximal amino acid protons from the folded zinc fingers and the spacer (such as Ala25 and Trp37, Phe16 and Trp37, Arg32 and Trp37, Lys33 and Trp37, Cys18 and Lys33, disappeared in the D-Pro31(12–53)NCp7, confirming the spatial proximity of the two CCHC boxes observed in the (13–51)NCp7 (Plate 2.5). This was also confirmed by iodide fluorescence quenching experiments. The N- and C-terminal parts of NCp7 displayed a large flexibility except for two short sequences Tyr56–Gly58 and Tyr64–Gly66 which seemed to oscillate between random-coil and helical conformations. The biological relevance of the structural characteristics of NCp7 was studied *in vitro* and *in vivo*. Substitution of Pro31 by D-Pro31 in the active (13–64)NCp7 peptide led to a severe reduction of dimerization *in vitro*. Moreover, site-directed mutagenesis, substituting Leu for Pro31, resulted in the formation of non-infectious and immature viral particles. These results suggest that the spatial proximity of the zinc fingers induced by the peptide linker plays a critical role in encapsidation of genomic RNA and morphogenesis of HIV-1 infectious particles. On the other hand, the replacement of His23 by Cys in the N-terminal zinc fingers of NCp7 led to a slight change in the structure of this domain but without loss of the zinc atom. Nevertheless, this slight conformational modification was sufficient to increase the distance between the two zinc fingers with subsequent large loss in RNA binding affinities. Transposed in the virus, this mutation yielded a complete loss of virus infectivity, probably related to the inability of the Cys23 NCp7 to protect the genomic RNA from nucleases (Déméné *et al*., 1994). The complex of NCp7 with ACGCC corresponding to a possible site of binding of the protein on the HIV-1 genome has been solved by ^{1}H NMR. It could serve as a model for *de novo* design of drugs able to inhibit the critical functions of NCp7.

References

Bateman, Jr, R.C., Jackson, D., Slaughter, C.A., Unnithan, S., Chai, Y.G., Moomaw, C.A. and Hersh, L.B. (1989). *J. Biol. Chem.* **264**, 6151–6157.

Bateman, Jr, R.C., Young, A.E., Slaughter, C. and Hersh, L.B. (1990) *J. Biol. Chem.* **265**, 8365–8368.

Beaumont, A., Le Moual, H., Boileau, G., Crine, P. and Roques, B.P. (1991). *J. Biol. Chem.* **266**, 214–220.

Beaumont, A., Barbe, B., Le Moual, H., Boileau, G., Crine, P. and Roques, B.P. (1992). *J. Biol. Chem.* **267**, 2138–2441.

Belleney, J., Gacel, G., Fournié-Zaluski, M.C., Maigret, B. and Roques, B.P. (1989). *Biochemistry* **28**, 7392–7400.

Benchetrit, T., Fournié-Zaluski, M.C. and Roques, B.P. (1987). *Biochem. Biophys. Res. Commun.* **147**, 1034–1040.

Benchetrit, T., Bissery, V., Mornon, J.P., Devault, A., Crine, P. and Roques, B.P. (1988). *Biochemistry* **27**, 592–597.

Berk, B.C., Wekshtein, V., Gordon, H.M. and Tsuda, T. (1989). *Hypertension* **13**, 305–314.

Boden, P.R., Higginbottom, M., Hill, D.R., Horwell, D.C., Hughes, J., Rees, D.C., Roberts, E., Singh, L., Suman-Chauhan, N. and Woodruff, G.N. (1993). *J. Med. Chem.* **36**, 552–565.

Bradwejn, J., Koszycki, D. and Shriqui, C. (1991). *Arch. Gen. Psych.* **48**, 603–610.

Burnier, M., Granslmayer, M., Perret, F., Porchet, M., Kosoglou, T., Gould, A., Nussberger, J., Waeber, B. and Brunner, H.R. (1991). *Clin. Pharmacol. Ther.* **50**, 181–191.

Charpentier, B., Durieux, C., Pélaprat, D., Dor, A., Rubaud, M., Blanchard, J.C. and Roques, B.P. (1988). *Peptides* **9**, 835–841.

Cornille, F., Goudreau, N., Ficheux, D., Niémann, H. and Roques, B.P. (1994). *Eur. J. Biochem.* **222**, 173–181.

Corringer, P.J. (1990). PhD thesis, Synthèse et activités biologiques d'analogues peptidiques et peptidomimétiques de la CCK, University of Paris V.

Corringer, P.J., Weng, J.H., Ducos, B., Durieux, C., Boudeau, P., Böhme, A. and Roques, B.P. (1993). *J. Med. Chem.* **36**, 166–172.

Darlix, J.L. and Roques, B.P. (1993). *Médecine Sci.* **9** 952–958.

Daugé, V., Böhme, G.A., Crawley, J.N., Durieux, C., Stutzmann, J.M., Féger, J., Blanchard, J.C. and Roques, B.P. (1990). *Synapse* **61**(1), 73–80.

Déméné, H., Dong, C.Z., Ottmann, M., Rouyez, M.C., Jullian, N., Morellet, N., Mely, Y., Darlix, J.L., Fournié-Zalvski, M.C., Saragosti, S., and Roques, B.P. (1994). *Biochemistry* **33**, 11707–11716.

de Rocquigny, H., Gabus, C., Vincent, A., Fournié-Zaluski, M.C., Roques, B.P. and Darlix, J.L. (1992). *Proc. Natl. Acad. Sci. USA* **89**, 6472–6476.

Derrien, M., Durieux, C. and Roques, B.P. (1994) *Brit. J. Pharmacol.* **111**, 956–960.

Deschodt-Lanckman, M. (1985). *Ann. N.Y. Acad. Sci.* **448**, 87–98.

Devault, A., Lazure, C., Nault, C., Le Moual, H., Seidah, N.G., Chretien, M., Kahn, P., Powell, J., Mallet, J., Beaumont, A., Roques, B.P., Crine, P. and Boileau, C. (1987). *EMBO J.* **6**, 1317–1322.

Devault, A., Sales, N., Nault, C., Beaumont, A., Roques, B.P., Crine, P. and Boileau, G. (1988a). *FEBS Lett.* **231**, 54–58.

Devault, A., Nault, C., Zollinger, M., Fournié-Zaluski, M.C., Roques, B.P., Crine, P. and Boileau, G. (1988b). *J. Biol. Chem.* **263**, 4033–4040.

Durieux, C., Charpentier, B., Fellion, E., Gacel, G., Pélaprat, D. and Roques, B.P. (1985). *Peptides* **6**, 495–501.

Durieux, C., Charpentier, B., Pélaprat, D. and Roques, B.P. (1986). *Neuropeptides* **7**, 1–9.

Durieux, C., Ruiz-Gayo, M. and Roques, B.P. (1991). *Eur. J. Pharmacol.* **209**, 185–193.

Farby, R.D., Hu, K.L., Carretero, O.A. and Scicli, A.G. (1992). *Biochem. Biophys. Res. Commun.* **182**, 283–288.

Fournié-Zaluski, M.C., Llorens, C., Gacel, G., Malfroy, B., Swerts, J.P., Lecomte, J.M., Schwartz, J.C. and Roques, B.P. (1981). *In* 'Peptides' (K. Brunfeld, ed.), pp. 476–481. Scriptor, Copenhagen, Denmark.

Fournié-Zaluski, M.C., Chaillet, P., Bouboutou, R., Coulaud, A., Chérot, P., Waksman, G., Costentin, J. and Roques, B.P. (1984a). *Eur. J. Pharmacol.* **102**, 525–528.

Fournié-Zaluski, M.C., Lucas, E., Waksman, G. and Roques, B.P. (1984b). *Eur. J. Biochem.* **139**, 267–274.

Fournié-Zaluski, M.C., Belleney, J., Lux, B., Durieux, C., Gerard, D., Gacel, G., Maigret, B. and Roques, B.P. (1986) *Biochemistry* **25**(13), 3778–3787.

Fournié-Zaluski, M.C., Coric, P., Turcaud, S., Rousselet, N., Gonzalez, W., Barbe, B., Pham, I., Jullian, N., Michel, J.B. and Roques, B.P. (1994). *J. Med. Chem.* **37**, 1070–1083.

Gomez-Monterrey, I., Turcaud, S., Lucas, E., Bruetschy, L., Roques, B.P. and Fournié-Zaluski, M.C. (1993). *J. Med. Chem.* **36**, 87–94.

Gordon, E.M. Cushman, D.W., Tung, R., Cheung, H.S., Wang, F.L. and Delaney, N.G. (1983). *Life Sci.* **33**, 113–116.

Goudreau, N., Cornille, F., Duchesne, M., Parker, F., Tocqué, B., Roques, B.P. and Garbay, C. (1994). *Nature Struc. Biol.* **1**, 898–907.

Goudreau, N., Weng, J.H. and Roques, B.P. (1994). *Biopolymers* **34**, 155–169.

Hibert, M.F., Hoflack, J., Trumpp-Kallmeyer, S. and Bruinvels, A. (1993). *Med. Sci.* **9**, 31–40.

Hökfelt, T., Rehfeld, J.F., Skviboll, L., Ivenark, B., Goldstein, M. and Markey, K. (1980). *Nature* **285**, 476–478.

Howbert, J.J., Lobb, K.L., Britton, T.C., Mason, N.R. & Bruns, R.F. (1993). *Bioorg. Med. Chem. Lett.* **3**, 875–880.

Hughes, J., Boden, P., Costall, B., Domeney, A., Kelly, E., Horwell, D.C., Hunter, J.C., Pinnock, R.D. and Woodruff, G.N. (1990) *Proc. Natl. Acad. Sci. USA*, **87**, 6728–6732.

Itoh, H., Pratt, R.E. and Dzau, V.J. (1990). *J. Clin. Invest.* **86**, 1690–1697.

Jagerschmidt, A., Popovici, T., O'Donohue, M. and Roques, B.P. (1994). *J. Neurochem.* **63**, 1199–1206.

Jolles, G. and Wooldridge, K.R.H. (eds) (1984) 'Drug Design, Fact or Fantasy?' Academic Press, London.

Kenny, A.J. and Stephenson, S.L. (1988). *FEBS Lett.* **232**, 1–8.

Kerr, M.A. and Kenny, A.J. (1974a). *Biochem. J.* **137**, 489–495.

Kerr, M.A. and Kenny, A.J. (1974b). *Biochem. J.* **137**, 477–488.

Le Moual, H., Devault, A., Roques, B.P., Crine, P. and Boileau, G. (1991). *J. Biol. Chem.* **266**, 15670–15674.

Maloney Huss, K. and Lybrand, T.P. (1992). *J. Mol. Biol.* **225**, 859–871.

Matthews, B.W. (1988). *Acc. Chem. Res.* **21**, 333–340.

Migaud, M., Chauvel, E.N., Viereck, J., Soroca-Lucas, E., Ducos, B., Coric, P., Fournié-Zaluski, M.C., Roques, B.P. and Durieux, C. (1995) *Mol. Pharmacol.* (submitted).

Morellet, N., de Rocquigny, H., Mély, Y., Jullian, N., Déméné, H., Ottmann, M., Gérard, D., Darlix, J.L., Fournié-Zaluski, M.C. and Roques, B.P. (1994). *J. Mol. Biol.* **235**, 287–301.

Mourlon-Legrand, M.C., Poitevin, P., Benessiano, J., Duriez, M., Michel, J.C. and Lévy, B.I. (1993). *Arterioscler. Thromb.* **13**, 640–650.

Nadjouski, T., Collette, N. and Deschodt-Lanckman, M. (1985). *Life Sci.* **37**, 827–834.

Nadzan, A.M., Garvey, D.S., Holladay, M.W., Shiosaki, M.D., Tufano, M.D., Shue, Y.K., Chung, J.Y.I., May, C.S., Lin, C.W., Miller, T.R., Witte, D.G., Bianchi, B.R., Wolfram, C.A.W., Burt, S. and Hutchins, C.W. (1992). *In* 'Peptides: Chemistry, Structure and Biology (Proceedings of the 12th American Peptide Symposium)' (J.E. Rivier and J.A. Smith, eds), pp. 100–102. ESCOM, Leiden.

Ondetti, M.A. and Cushman, D.W. (1984). *Crit. Rev. Biochem.* **16**, 381–411.

Ondetti, M.A., Rubin, B. and Cushman, D.W. (1977). *Science* **196**, 441–444.

Pham, I., El Amrani, A.I.K., Fournié-Zaluski, M.C., Corvol, P., Roques, B.P. and Michel, J.P. (1992). *J. Cardiovasc. Res.* **20**, 847–857.

Pham, I., Gonzalez, W., El Amrani, A.I.K., Fournié-Zaluski, M.C., Philippe, M., Laboulandine, I., Roques, B.P. and Michel, J.B. (1993). *J. Pharmacol. Exp. Ther.* **265**(3), 1339–1347.

Richards, M., Espiner, E., Frampton, C., Ikram, H., Yandle, T., Sopwitch, M. and Cussans, N. (1990). *Hypertension* **16**, 269–276.

Roderick, S.L., Fournié-Zaluski, M.C., Roques, B.P. and Matthews, B.W. (1989). *Biochemistry* **28**, 1493–1497.

Roques, B.P., Fournié-Zaluski, M.C., Soroca, E., Lecomte, J.M., Malfroy, B., Llorens, C. and Schwartz, J.C. (1980). *Nature* **288**, 286–288.
Roques, B.P. and Fournié-Zaluski, M.C. (1986). *Natl. Inst. Drug Abuse Res. Monogr. Ser.* **70**, 128–154.
Roques, B.P. (1988) *In* 'Proceedings of the IVth SCI-Royal Society of Chemistry Medicinal Chemistry Symposium, Topics in Medicinal Chemistry' (P.R. Leeming, ed.), vol. 65, pp. 22–42. Royal Society of Chemistry, Cambridge, UK.
Roques, B.P. and Beaumont, A. (1990) *Trends Pharmacol. Sci.* **11**, 245–249.
Roques, B.P. (1993). *Biochem. Soc. Trans.* **21**, 678–685.
Roques, B.P., Noble, F., Daugé, V., Fournié-Zaluski, M.C. and Beaumont, A. (1993). *Pharmacol. Rev.* **45**(1), 87–147.
Rose, K. (1994). *J. Am. Chem. Soc.* **116**, 30–33.
Rose, C., Camus, A. and Schwartz, J.C. (1988). *Proc. Natl. Acad. Sci. USA.* **85**, 8326–8330.
Ruiz-Gayo, M., Delay-Goyet, P., Durieux, C., Corringer, P.J., Baamonde, A., Gacel, G. and Roques, B.P. (1990). *J. Control. Rel.* **13**, 147–155.
Seymour, A.A., Swerdel, J.N. and Abboa-Offei, B. (1991). *J. Cardiovasc. Pharmacol.* **17**, 456–465.
Seymour, A.A., Asaad, M.M., Lanoce, V.M., Laugen-Bacher, K.M., Fennell, S.A. and Rogers, W.L. (1993). *J. Pharmacol. Exp. Ther.* **266**, 872–883.
Strosberg, A.D. (1993). *Protein Sci.* **2**, 1198–1209.
Sybertz, E.J. (1991). *Clin. Nephrol.* **36**, 187–191.
Turner, A.J. (1993). *Biochem. Soc. Trans.* **21**, 697–701.
Ura, N., Carretero, O.A. and Erdos, E.G. (1987). *Kidney Int.* **32**, 507–513.
Watthey, J.W.H., Gavin, T. and Desai, M. (1984). *J. Med. Chem.* **27**, 816–818.
Woodruff, G.N., Hill, D.R., Roden, P., Pinnock, R., Singh, L. and Hughes, J. (1991). *Neuropeptides* **19**, 45–56.
Woodruff, G.N. and Hughes, J. (1991). *Annu. Rev. Pharmacol. Toxicol.* **31**, 469–501.
Wyvratt, M.J. and Patchett, A.A. (1985). *Med. Res. Rev.* **5**, 483–531.
Yang, Y.S., Garbay, C., Duchesne, M., Cornille, F., Jullian, N., Fromage, N., Tocqué, B. and Roques, B.P. (1994). *EMBO J.* **6**, 1270–1279.

Discussion

M.J. Ashton
I found it surprising in the angiotensin converting enzyme (ACE)–neutral endopeptidase (NEP) series that when there is a change from *R* to *S* in configuration of some of the compounds, it did not appear (unless I misunderstood) that there was large change in the biological activity of those molecules. I would have thought that they would have been much more stereospecific than was apparent.

B.P. Roques
It is well known – and has been demonstrated previously – that in the case of NEP the S_1 subsite of this enzyme has no real stereospecificity. With ACE, there is some stereospecificity but not a great deal; for instance, about a 100-fold difference in the affinity between the two stereoisomers.

M.J. Ashton

When the agonist activity of BC 264 on the CCK-B receptor was compared to the natural ligand, and functional activity was also examined, there were differences in the way the animals responded. You elaborated a little on the rationale behind this, but could you explain in more detail why the natural ligand appeared to give a different profile of response in the monkeys compared to the response to the synthesized agonist BC 264?

B.P. Roques

There are probably several reasons. First, CCK_{-4} probably does not enter the brain at the same concentration as BC 264. The other reason is probably because at very low concentration BC 264 can interact with high affinity with the CCK-B receptor located in the mesolimbic pathway. This is probably not the case with CCK_{-4}, which has only about a 25 nM affinity for the B receptor.

The stranger effect is that of CCK_{-4}, which could possibly be considered as interacting not only in the central nervous system but also at the periphery. For instance, one hypothesis is that CCK_{-4} can interact at the periphery with CCK-B receptors located in the intestine, stomach, etc., and the interaction can be relayed via the vagus nerve to the brain, followed obviously by a neuronal activation in different cortical areas.

I.M. McLay

You described some lovely work docking agonist and antagonist into the CCK receptor. Could you give some details about how those docking studies were done?

B.P. Roques

These are very preliminary results, which have not yet been published – even site-directed mutagenesis experiments have not yet been published. We used a classical strategy, in which the Henderson model of rhodopsin was used in order to provide an orientation of the seven transmembrane helices in the membrane. Then, by classical docking experiments and using the Biosyn package, the compound was introduced into the binding pocket. The pocket is formed by the different aromatic rings which have been proven important by site-directed mutagenesis. Such mutagenesis abolishes part of the affinity, so it seems that these different amino acids constitute a part of the active site. Following that, we minimized the complex by classical strategies. These are clearly preliminary results, and dynamic studies have now to be performed – what we have obtained so far is not yet the result of molecular dynamics studies.

3

Topochemistry and Inhibition of Carbohydrate-Mediated Cell Adhesion

C.-H. WONG

Department of Chemistry, The Scripps Research Institute, 10666 North Torrey Pines Road, La Jolla, CA 92037, USA

Complex carbohydrates and their conjugates in biological systems are either structural or informational molecules. Many cell surface carbohydrates of glycoconjugates are involved in various types of biochemical recognition processes (Varki, 1993). These carbohydrates often exist in minute quantities and are difficult to isolate, characterize and synthesize in quantities large enough for biological study and therapeutic evaluation. Although only 7–8 monosaccharides are commonly found as building blocks in mammalian systems, the multifunctionality of these monomers can lead to the assembly of an immense variety of complex structures. Many million different tetrasaccharide structures, for example, can be constructed from this small number of building blocks, when considering the branching, stereochemistry of glycosylation and other modifications. Oligosaccharides therefore represent an effective class of molecules that can code for vast amounts of information required in various biological recognition processes.

The shape of a complex carbohydrate under the influence of anomeric and exo-anomeric effects (Deslongchamps, 1993) and the topographic orientation of the hydroxyl and charged groups contribute significantly to carbohydrate recognition. The synthesis of natural and analogous complex carbohydrates together with structural studies of these complex molecules and their interaction with receptors are often important steps that will lead to a basic understanding of carbohydrate-mediated recognition processes. The pace of development of carbohydrate-based pharmaceuticals has, however, been

New Perspectives in Drug Design
ISBN 0–12–208070–X

slower than that of other classes of biomolecules. Part of the reason is due to the lack of technologies required for the study of complex carbohydrates. There is no method to amplify oligosaccharides for sequence analysis. There is no machine available for automated synthesis of oligosaccharides. In addition, the possibly poor bioavailability and difficulties in the large-scale synthesis of carbohydrates have undoubtedly contributed to this slow pace. Presented here are several enzymatic and chemoenzymatic methods for the large-scale synthesis of oligosaccharides and analogues, including those involved in E-selectin recognition, and some strategies for inhibiting glycosidases and glycosyltransferases. An ultimate goal of research in this field is to develop simple and easy-to-make carbohydrates or carbohydrate mimetics to control carbohydrate-mediated biological processes in a specific manner.

Sialyl Lewis X and Related Structures as Ligands for E-Selectin

Carbohydrate-mediated cell adhesion is an important event which can be initiated by tissue injury and infection and is involved in metastasis (Lasky, 1992). One such adhesion process which was recently discovered is the interaction between the glycoprotein E-selectin (formerly called endothelial leucocyte adhesion molecule or ELAM-1), which is expressed on the surface of endothelial cells during inflammation, and an oligosaccharide structure displayed on the surface of neutrophils. The ligand recognized by E-selectin has been identified to be the tetrasaccharide sialyl Lewis X, which is present at the terminus of glycolipids displayed on the surface of neutrophils (Phillips *et al.*, 1990). The adhesion process is stimulated by signalling molecules (cytokines) or other inflammatory factors (e.g. toxins, lipopolysaccharides, leucotrienes) which induce the production of E-selectin. After binding to the endothelial cells, the white blood cells roll along the surface of the endothelium. Further adhesion occurs by protein–protein interactions, mediated by integrins on white blood cells and an RGD (Arg–Gly–Asp)-containing protein ligand called intercellular adhesion molecule-1 (ICAM-1) on endothelial cells. The white blood cells are then able to squeeze through gaps between endothelial cells and enter the adjacent tissue to help repair injury (Fig. 3.1). However, if too many white blood cells are recruited to the site of injury, normal cells can also be destroyed. This can occur in the condition of septic shock, in chronic inflammatory diseases such as psoriasis and rheumatoid arthritis, and in the reperfusion tissue injury that occurs following heart attack, stroke and organ transplant. High levels of sialyl Lewis X have also been found on the surfaces of certain tumour and cancer cells (e.g. colon and lung cancer cells), suggesting that cancer cells may exploit this phenomenon of adhesion to metastasize, or spread throughout the body, after entering the bloodstream. In addition to E-selectin, two other carbohydrate-binding

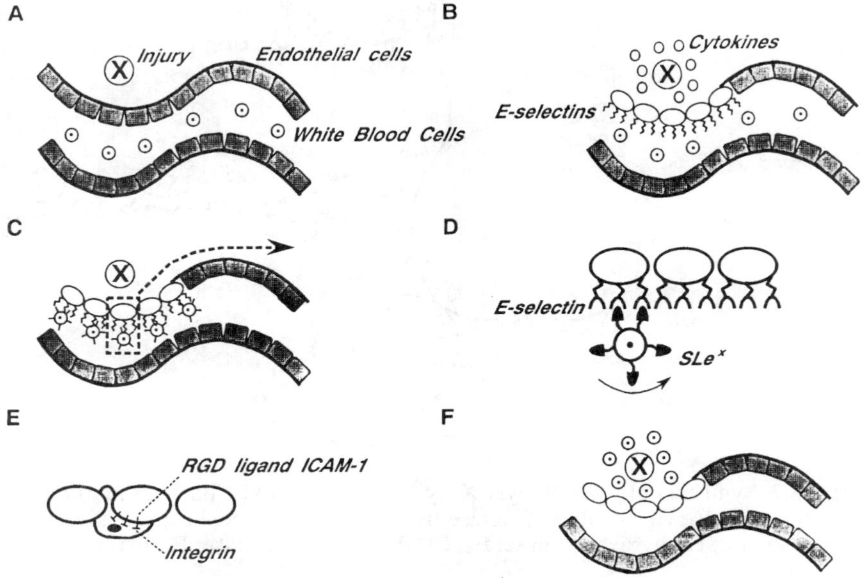

Figure 3.1 Recruitment of white blood cells during inflammation. A, injury occurs; B, cytokines released, E-selectins produced; C, adhesion occurs; D, white blood cell rolling; E, further adhesion mediated by integrins, extravasation; F, white blood cells reach injury site.

proteins, P- and L-selectin, also recognize sialylated ligands in cell-adhesion processes.

The finding that the ligand for E-selectin is sialyl Lewis X provides a new opportunity for the development of therapeutic agents for the treatment of inflammation-related diseases and cancers. Since sialyl Lewis X in solution competes with the white blood cells for binding to E-selectin, thus inhibiting the adhesion process, it may be useful as an anti-inflammatory or anti-cancer agent. On the other hand, understanding the active conformation of sialyl Lewis X recognized by E-selectin may also lead to the development of simple and easy-to-make inhibitors which are analogues or non-carbohydrate mimetics of sialyl Lewis X with better bioavailability. Another approach is to inhibit the enzymes (such as the α-1,3-fucosyltransferase) associated with the biosynthesis of sialyl Lewis X.

Considerable research has been directed toward the chemical synthesis of sialyl Lewis X; however, these syntheses typically require multiple protection and deprotection steps, making large-scale production difficult. Enzymatic syntheses of sialyl Lewis X based on glycosyltransferases proceed regio- and stereoselectively in aqueous solution, without the need for protecting groups.

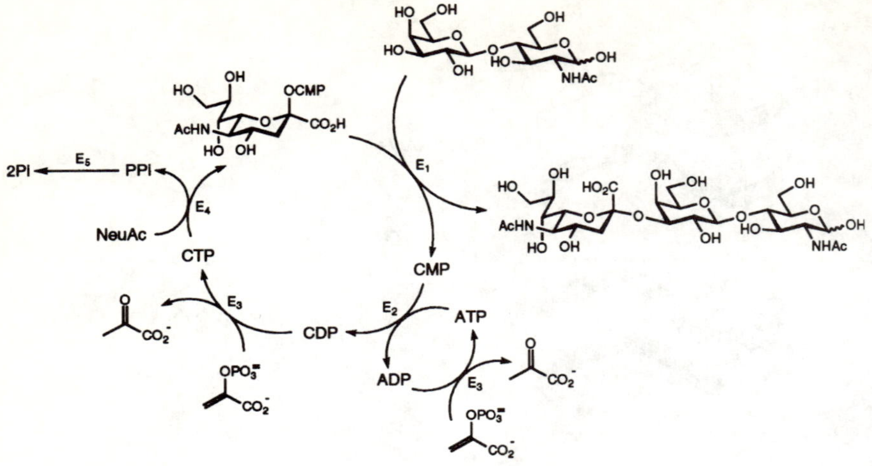

Fig. 3.2 Synthesis of sialyl Lewis X by enzymatic sialylation with *in situ* cofactor regeneration, E_1, α2,3-sialyltransferase; E_2, nucleoside monophosphate kinase or adenylate kinase; E_3, pyruvate kinase; E_4, CMP-NeuAc synthetase; E_5, pyrophosphatase.

The glycosyltransferase reactions coupled with *in situ* regeneration of sugar nucleotides (Ichikawa *et al.*, 1992) have been developed for the synthesis of oligosaccharides on a large scale (Figs. 3.2 and 3.3). With the advances in recombinant DNA technology for the cloning and overproduction of enzymes, sialyl Lewis X can now be produced in large quantities. (Cytel Co. in San Diego is producing SLe^x in kilogram quantities as a drug candidate for treatment of reperfusion tissue injury).

The enzymatic method has also been used for the synthesis of (Gal-1-^{13}C)-

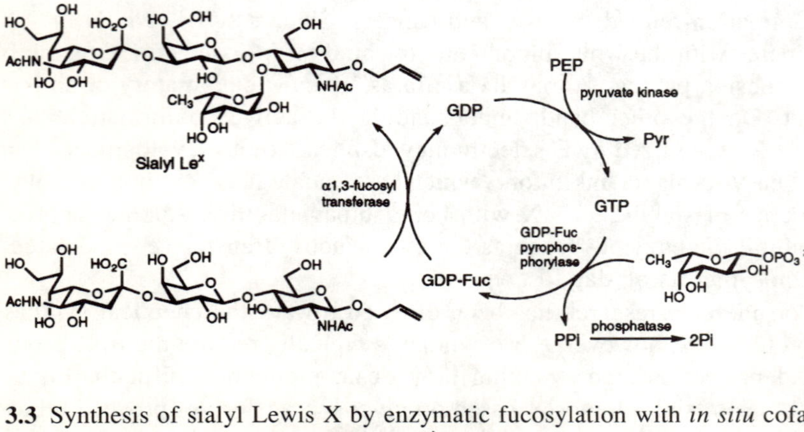

Fig. 3.3 Synthesis of sialyl Lewis X by enzymatic fucosylation with *in situ* cofactor regeneration.

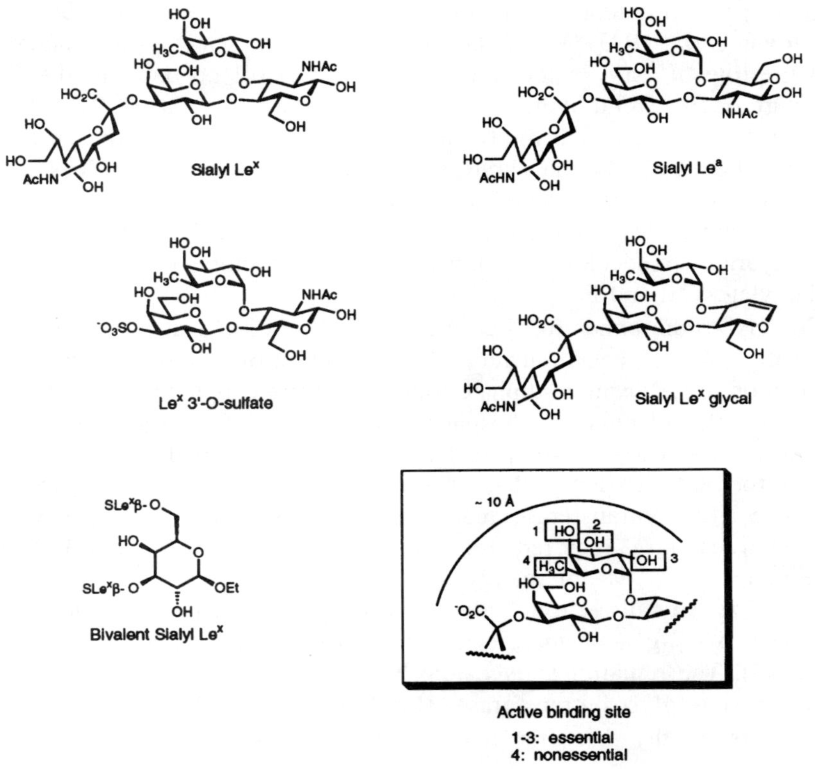

Fig. 3.4 Ligands for E-selectin. Inset shows active binding site. 1–3, essential; 4, non-essential.

labelled sialyl Lewis X which was used for conformational analysis by NMR spectroscopy. In addition, sialyl Lewis a (SLe^a), SLe^x glycal, and Le^x3' sulfate were also found to be conformationally similar to and biologically as active as SLe^x (Fig. 3.4). The results of these studies indicate that the active binding domain of sialyl Lewis X consists primarily of the galactose, fucose and the carboxylate group of the sialic acid. The methyl group of the fucose is not essential, as the fucose residue can be replaced with arabinose. The three hydroxyl groups of the fucose, however, are required (DeFrees *et al.*, 1993).

Further studies of the nature of ligand recognition revealed that a bivalent sialyl Lewis X anchored onto ethyl β-galactoside by β-1,3- and β-1,6-linkages was fivefold better at blocking adhesion (IC_{50} = 0.4 mM) than SLe^x, suggesting the possibility of a multivalent ligand–receptor interaction (DeFrees *et al.*, 1993). All these activities were measured *in vitro* based on an ELISA assay. The level of *in vivo* activity of sialyl Lewis X is, however, not very clear. The

IC_{50} for protecting lung injury in rats appears to be, for example, about 1 μM (Mulligan *et al.*, 1993). While the structure of the E-selectin–ligand complex and the role of Ca^{2+} in the ligand binding are still not known (the X-ray structure of E-selectin alone is now available (Graves *et al.*, 1994)), further experiments with defined multivalent ligands or mimetics with appropriate spacers should clarify the nature of E-selectin-mediated cell adhesion and may suggest new approaches to the discovery and development of anti-adhesion molecules. Of particular interest will be the development of non-carbohydrate molecules to mimic the topostructure composed of the carboxylate, Gal and Fuc of SLe^x.

The glycosidic bonds in SLe^x, SLe^x glycal and Le^x can be formed enzymatically using glycosyltransferases. Introduction of a sulphate group to the 3′ position of Le^x using a sulphate-transfer enzyme coupled with regeneration of 3′-phospho-adenosyl-5′-phosphosulphate (PAPS) for large-scale process, however, has not been developed. The synthesis of the bivalent SLe^x was very straightforward, starting with a chemically prepared trisaccharide followed by three glycosyltransferase reactions (DeFrees *et al.*, 1993). Since the glycosyltransferase required for the synthesis of the Galβ-1,3-GlcNAc core unit of SLe^a is not readily available, this disaccharide was prepared chemo-enzymatically from glucal via subtilisin-catalysed acetylation followed by β-galactosidase-catalysed galactosylation and azidonitration (Fig. 3.5). The remaining glycosidic bonds were then formed with the use of appropriate glycosyltransferases (Look *et al.*, 1993a).

It is noteworthy that though enzymatic synthesis of oligosaccharides is

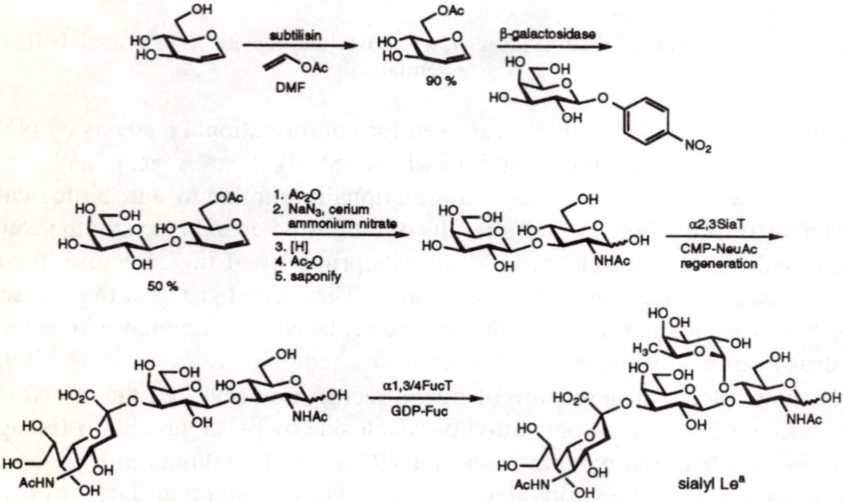

Fig. 3.5 Chemoenzymatic synthesis of sialyl Lewis A.

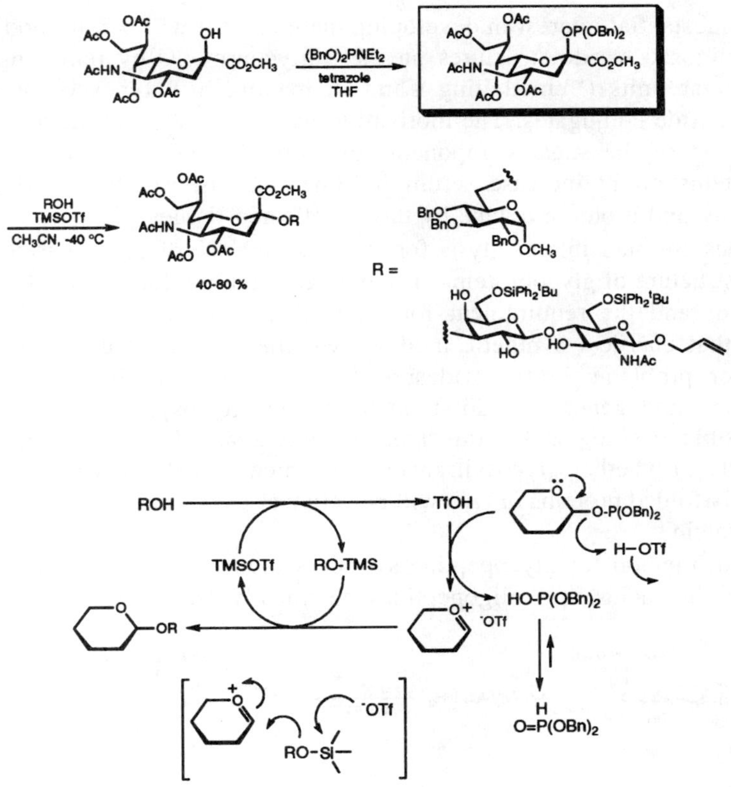

Fig. 3.6 Chemical glycosylation using glycosyl phosphites.

potentially useful for large-scale processes, the method is quite limited, as many oligosaccharide analogues cannot be prepared enzymatically. Synthesis of modified oligosaccharides thus often require the use of chemical glycosylation methods. The use of recently developed glycosyl phosphites in glycosylation has been examined in detail regarding the scope and mechanism (Kondo *et al.*, 1994), and the method appears to be particularly effective for sialylation. Mechanistic study of the glycosylation reactions indicates that triflic acid is involved in the activation when TMSOTf is used in catalytic amounts (Fig. 3.6).

Glycopeptide Synthesis

A number of the proteins of interest as human pharmaceuticals (tissue plasminogen activator, juvenile human growth hormone, CD4) are glycoproteins.

There is substantial interest in developing methods that will permit modification of oligosaccharide structures on these glycoproteins by removing and adding sugar units ('remodelling') and in making new types of protein–oligosaccharide conjugates. The motivation for these efforts is the hope that modification of the sugar components of naturally occurring or unnatural glycoproteins might increase serum lifetime, increase solubility, decrease antigenicity and promote uptake by target cells and tissues.

Enzymes are plausible catalysts for manipulating the oligosaccharide content and structure of glycoproteins. The delicacy and polyfunctional character of proteins and the requirement for high selectivity in their modification indicate that classical synthetic methods will be of limited use. There are two major problems in the widespread use of enzymes in glycoprotein remodelling and generation. First, many of the glycosyl transferases that are plausible candidates for this area are not available. Second, there is uncertainty in whether glycosyltransferases which probably act on unfolded or partially folded proteins *in vivo* will be active at the surface of a completely folded protein.

A useful method for glycopeptide synthesis involves the incorporation of glycosylamino acids into oligopeptides chemically (Bielfeldt *et al.*, 1992;

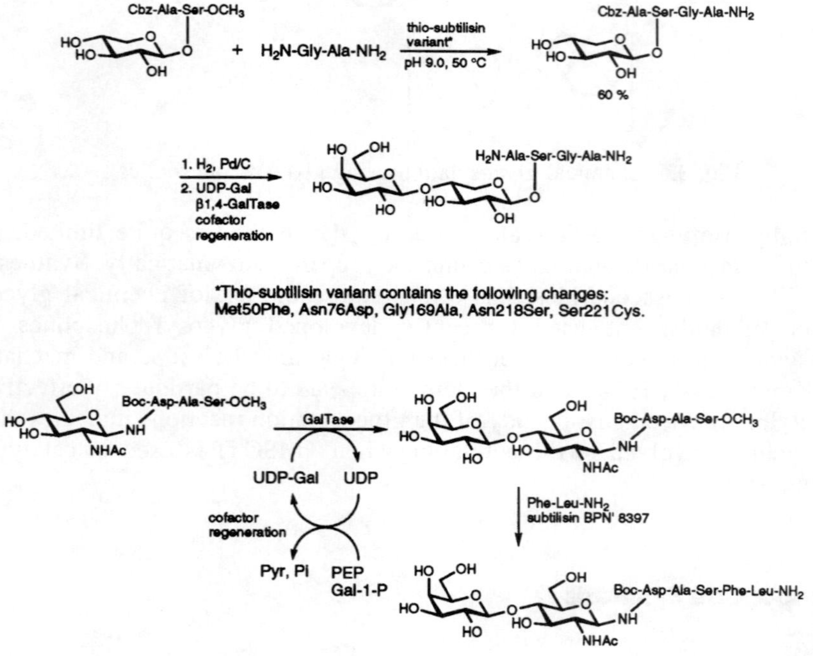

Fig. 3.7 Synthesis of glycopeptides using subtilisin and galactosyltransferase.

Kunz, 1993) or enzymatically (Wong *et al.*, 1993), followed by introduction of additional sugars by glycosyltransferases. Enzymatic formation of peptide and glycoside bonds in certain cases is quite effective as both procedures can be carried out in aqueous solution, thus minimizing protection/deprotection steps in peptide synthesis. Glycosyl amino acids can be used as the P_2, P_3, P_2' or P_3' residue in subtilisin-catalysed glycopeptide segment condensation. Using a thermostable variant developed by site-directed mutagenesis, with the active-site Ser converted to Cys, the enzymatic coupling of glycopeptide segments can be carried out effectively at 60°C in aqueous solution (Fig. 3.7) (Wong *et al.*, 1993). The enzyme prefers aminolysis over hydrolysis by a factor ~10 000, and kinetic studies indicate that the selectivity comes from the acyl-enzyme intermediate which reacts more selectively with the amine nucleophile than does the wild-type enzyme. The strategy of chemical synthesis of glycopeptides followed by enzymatic glycosylation also works very well on aminopropyl-silica support (Schuster *et al.*, 1994). A key element is to attach a proper acceptor-spacer group with a selectively cleavable bond. This strategy allows a rapid iterative formation of peptide and glycosidic bonds in organic and aqueous solvents, respectively, and enables the release of glycopeptides from the support enzymatically (Fig. 3.8).

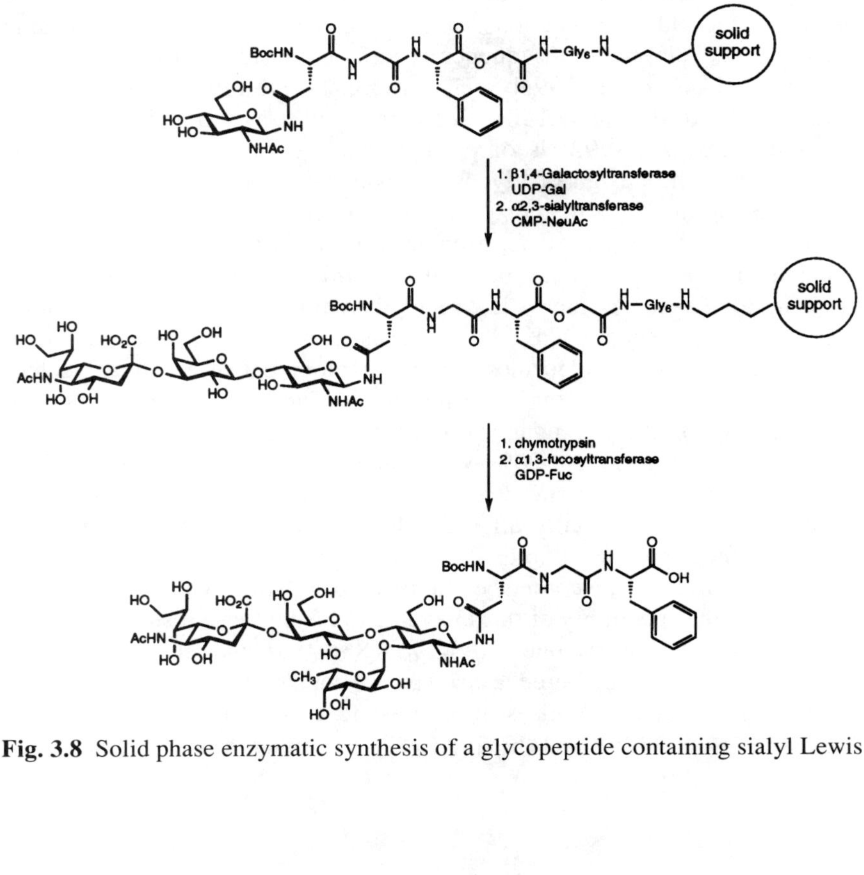

Fig. 3.8 Solid phase enzymatic synthesis of a glycopeptide containing sialyl Lewis X.

Inhibition of Glycosidases and Glycosyltransferases, Especially α-1,3-Fucosyltransferase

Glycosidases and glycosyltransferases are important enzymes for the processing of various oligosaccharide-containing glycoproteins and glycolipids. The profound impact of these enzymes on life processes has made them desirable targets for inhibition. Glycoprocessing inhibitors have been used to treat diabetes and other metabolic disorders, and have been implicated in the blocking of infection, inflammation and metastasis. The mechanisms for glycosidases and to some extent for glycosyltransferases have been studied (Sinnott, 1990). It is generally believed that the reactions proceed through a half-chair (or twist-boat) transition state with substantial sp^2 character at the anomeric carbon. This positively charged, transition-state structure is generated via general acid and general base catalysis, presumably from carboxylic acid and carboxylate residues in the active site of the enzyme. Compounds which resemble the transition-state structure of the glycosidic cleavage or glycosyltransfer reactions are therefore potent inhibitors of the enzyme. Azasugars seem to be transition-state like inhibitors as they show potent inhibition activities. Both five- and six-membered azasugars can easily be prepared via the aldolase reactions, and they can be considered as building blocks for the development of sequence-specific glycosidase or glycosyltransfer inhibitors (Look *et al.*, 1993b). The synergistic inhibition of α-1,3-fucosyltransferase with the fucosyl-like five-membered azasugars and GDP (Fig. 3.9) (Ichikawa *et al.*, 1992) is of particular interest, as it provides a new direction toward the design of glycosyltransferase inhibitors. Another interesting observation is that most naturally occurring glycosyltransferase inhibitors do not have the pyrophosphate moiety. Perhaps sugars (e.g. that in tunicamycin) or peptides can be used to mimic the pyrophosphate-Mn^{2++} component of the sugar nucleotide in glycosyltransferase reactions. Other mimics of pyrophosphate-Mn^{2++} complexes may be useful as a linker between azasugars and nucleosides for the development of azasugar nucleosides as synthetic glycosyltransferase inhibitors. Though the non-covalent or covalent adduct of the azasugar (or its mimetics) is a strong inhibitor of fucosyltransferase (more than 90% of the enzyme activity is inhibited in the presence of 50 μM of GDP and 8 mM of the azasugar), the inhibition is not sequence-specific and virtually all fucosyltransferases will be inhibited. To develop sequence-specific inhibitors of α-1,3-fucosyltransferase, it is necessary to understand the acceptor specificity of α-1,3-fucosyltransferase. Fig. 3.10 illustrates the specificity of this enzyme, and from these results it appears that the azadisaccharide (the one with IC_{50} = 8 mM) or analogues perhaps can be linked to the five-membered azasugars to construct a sequence-specific inhibitor of this enzyme. Work is in progress to accomplish this goal.

The issue of stability and bioavailability associated with sugar-based

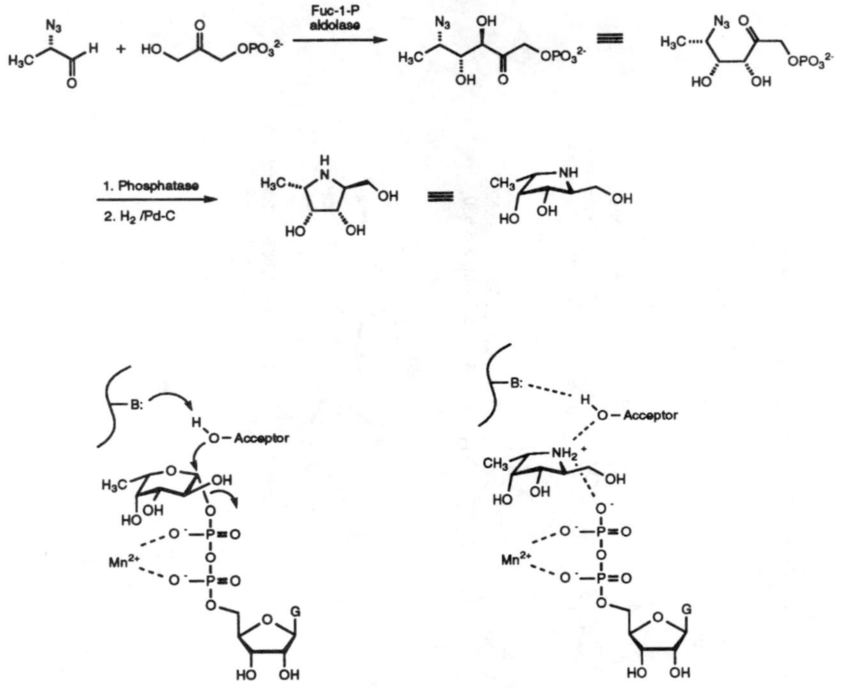

Fig. 3.9 Chemoenzymatic synthesis of an azasugar and the synergistic inhibition of fucosyltransferase by the azasugar and GDP.

inhibitors will have to be further examined if carbohydrates are to be considered as drug candidates. The discovery that *C*-linked glycosides possess the same conformation as the parent *O*-linked glycosides (Wu *et al.*, 1987) is important, as *C*-linked glycosides may be metabolically stable. Similarly, *C*-linked aza glycosides, guanidosugar-containing glycosides and *O*-linked carbocycles may have desirable conformations and may be useful as sequence-specific endoglycosidase and glycosyltransferase inhibitors (Fig. 3.11). With regard to the preparation of inhibitors to block the multivalent interaction of receptors or enzymes with their ligands or inhibitors, the phospholipase D-catalysed transphosphatidylation (Wang *et al.*, 1993) may offer a new method for the preparation of multivalent inhibitors, as phospholipids tend to form a liposome *via* self-assembly.

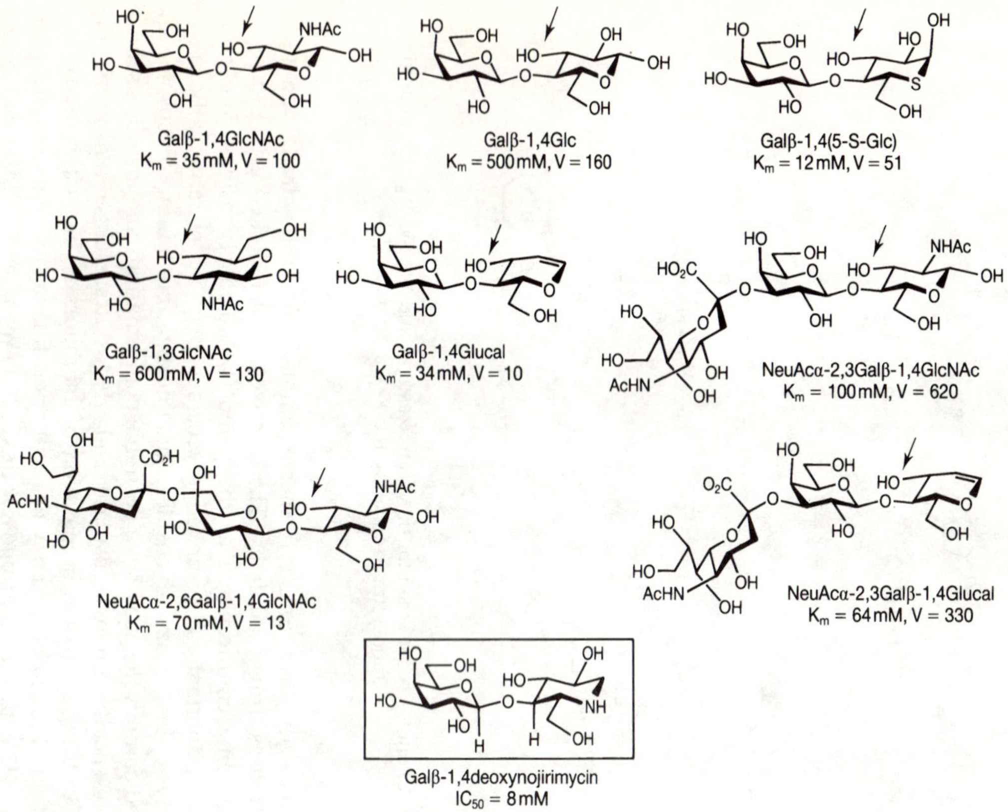

Fig. 3.10 Acceptor specificity for α-1,3-fucosyltransferase.

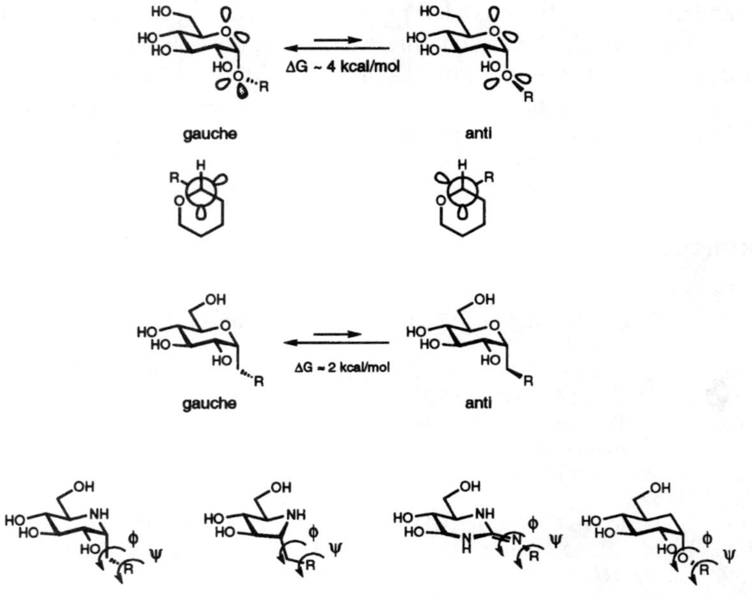

Fig. 3.11 Conformational equilibria of glycosides and their analogues.

Conclusion

The pace of development of carbohydrate-derived pharmaceutical agents has, in general, been slower than that of more convenient classes of materials. The difficulties in the synthesis and analysis of carbohydrates have undoubtedly contributed to this slow pace, but at least three areas of biology and medicinal chemistry have redirected attention to carbohydrates. First, interfering with the assembly of bacterial cell walls remains one of the most successful strategies for the development of antimicrobials. As bacterial resistance to penams and cephams becomes more widespread, there is increasing interest in interfering with the biosynthesis of the characteristic carbohydrate components of the cell wall, especially 3-deoxy-D-manno-2-octulosonate (KDO), heptulose, lipid A and related materials. Interest in cell wall constituents is also heightened by their relevance to vaccines and leads toward non-protein immunomodulating compounds. Second, cell surface carbohydrates are central to cell–cell communication, cell adhesion, infection, differentiation and development, and may be relevant to abnormal states of differentiation, such as those characterizing some malignancies. Syntheses of these cell surface ligands on large scales by enzymatic or chemoenzymatic methods for therapeutic evaluation are beginning to be realized. The enzymes involved in the biosynthesis of these ligands also represent interesting targets for therapeutic development. Third, the broad interest in diagnostics has finally begun to generate interest in carbohydrates as markers of human health. Enzymatic and chemo-enzymatic methods of synthesis, by rendering carbohydrates more accessible, will contribute to further research in all of these areas.

References

Bielfeldt, T., Peters, S., Meldal, M., Bock, K. and Paulsen, H. (1992). *Angew Chem. Int. Ed. Engl.* **31**, 857–859.

DeFrees, S.A., Gaeta, F.C.A., Lin, Y.-C., Ichikawa, Y. and Wong, C.-H. (1993). *J. Am. Chem. Soc.* **115**, 7549–7550.

Deslongchamps, P. (1993). *Pure Appl. Chem.* **65**, 1161–1178.

Graves, B.J., Crowther, R.L., Chandran, C., Rumberger, J.M., Li, S., Huang, K.-S., Presky, D.M., Familletti, P.C., Wolitzky, B.A. and Burns, D.K. (1994). *Nature* **367**, 532–538.

Ichikawa, Y., Lin, Y.-C., Dumas, D.P., Shen, G.-J., Garcia-Junceda, E., Williams, M.A., Bayer, R., Ketcham, C., Walker, L.E., Paulson, J.C. and Wong, C.-H. (1992). *J. Am. Chem. Soc.* **114**, 9283–9298.

Kondo, H., Aoki, S., Ichikawa, Y., Halcomb, R.L., Ritzen, H. and Wong, C.-H. (1994). *J. Org. Chem.* **59**, 864–877.

Kunz, H. (1993). *Pure Appl. Chem.* **65**, 1223–1226.

Lasky, L.A. (1992). *Science* **258**, 964–969.

Look, G.C., Ichikawa, Y., Shen, G.-J. and Wong, C.-H. (1993a). *J. Org. Chem.* **58**, 4326–4330.

Look, G.C., Fotsch, C.H. and Wong, C.-H. (1993b). *Acc. Chem. Res.* **26**, 182–190.

Mulligan, M.S., Paulson, J.C., DeFrees, S.A., Zheng, Z.-L., Lowe, J.B. and Ward, P.A. (1993). *Nature* **364**, 149–151.

Phillips, M.L., Nudelman, E., Gaeta, F.C.A., Perez, M., Singhal, A.K., Hakomori, S. and Paulson, J.C. (1990). *Science* **250**, 1130–1132.

Schuster, M., Wang, P., Paulson, J.C. and Wong, C.-H. (1994). *J. Am. Chem. Soc.* **116**, 1135–1136.

Sinnott, M.L. (1990). *Chem. Rev.* **90**, 1171–1202.

Varki, A. (1993). *Glycobiology* **3**, 97.

Wang, P., Schuster, M., Wang, Y.-F. and Wong, C.-H. (1993). *J. Am. Chem. Soc.* **115**, 10487–10491.

Wong, C.-H., Schuster, M., Wang, P. and Sears, P. (1993). *J. Am. Chem. Soc.* **115**, 5893–5901.

Wu, T.-C., Goekjian, P.G. and Kishi, Y. (1987). *J. Org. Chem.* **52**, 4819–4823.

Discussion

S. Perez

It is possible, of course, to disagree with the statement about the conformational rigidity of carbohydrates. I would say that, in general, carbohydrates are very flexible molecules, except in the case of the blood group antigens which you have also studied. These are fairly rigid, and essentially display one, two or perhaps three stable conformations.

With regard to the role and location of calcium in the binding of E-selectin to a ligand like sialyl Lewis X, did you say that calcium stabilizes a particular intramolecular conformation?

C.-H. Wong

No, I did not say that. I was trying to locate the calcium. Calcium does not affect the conformation of sialyl Lewis X. Based on nuclear magnetic resonance studies, when 10-molar equivalents of calcium ions are added the conformation is unchanged. We also did transfer NOE studies, and the bound conformation of the ligand sialyl Lewis X is essentially the same as in solution. Oligosaccharide conformations are somewhat confined due to the *exo*-anomeric effects.

S. Perez

There has been some speculation about the occurrence of several sialyl Lewis Xs that would together form a patch. The patch could be held together by mediation of calcium ions. Have you any comments on this particular model?

C.-H. Wong

I have no evidence for that – but it is possible. We know that there is a multivalent interaction. We do not know how many ligands on the surface of the cells are involved together in binding. We know that bivalent sialyl Lewis X is better than monovalent sialyl Lewis X. There is in fact a lot of controversy about the inhibition constant; it depends on how the assay is done. If a sugar is linked via a lipid attached to a microtitreplate, and an ELISA performed, there is very good inhibition. The best example I know, so far, is a pentasaccharide sulphate made by Dr Nicolaou's group. If a lipid is attached to the surface of the well, it mimics a multivalent type of interaction and there is very good inhibition. Sialyl Lewis X has an *in vivo* IC_{50} of 1 μM, but *in vitro* it is 1–2 mM – there is something occurring *in vivo* which I do not understand.

E. Westhof

Can the manganese be replaced in the α-glycosidase reaction by any other ion, for example, magnesium or cobalt?

C.-H. Wong

No, it cannot be replaced; it is manganese-specific. Some glycosyl transferases are magnesium-specific. Sialyl Lewis X is calcium-specific; the calcium cannot be replaced with magnesium or manganese. The specificity problem is interesting and an area that needs to be further investigated.

M.J. Ashton

I was intrigued to see that it was possible to get an enzyme which was stable at 50°C by changing some of the amino acids in the sequence. Was there a logic to this, or was it a haphazard process just by experimentation?

C.-H. Wong

The crystal structure of that particular enzyme, subtilisin, is known. It was modified logically. Molecular modelling suggested that if an asparagine was changed to aspartic acid there would be an improvement in the calcium binding interaction. The hydrophobic interaction was also improved by replacing methionine with phenylalanine. Doing things like that, step by step, we see a cumulative effect of individual mutations.

4

The Interplay between Intuition and Computer Assistance in the Design of Enzyme Inhibitors: Macrocyclic Phosphonamidates as Inhibitors of Thermolysin

P.A. BARTLETT, H.-J. PYUN, G. LAURI and B.P. MORGAN

Department of Chemistry, University of California, Berkeley, CA 94720, USA

Introduction

Phosphorus-containing peptide analogues have been studied as peptidase inhibitors for some time. Their ability to mimic some of the geometric and electronic characteristics of the tetrahedral intermediate involved in peptide hydrolysis, and the transition state leading to this intermediate, has been demonstrated in a number of systems and invoked as an explanation for their potent inhibition (Bartlett and Marlowe, 1983; Hanson *et al.*, 1989; Bartlett *et al.*, 1990; Kaplan and Bartlett, 1991; Morgan *et al.*, 1991; Sampson and Bartlett, 1991; Phillips *et al.*, 1992). This exploration has extended to the zinc, aspartic and serine peptidases, and has been supported by structural investigations in many cases (Holden *et al.*, 1987; Tronrud *et al.*, 1987; Matthews, 1988; Kim and Lipscomb, 1990; Bone *et al.*, 1991; Fraser *et al.*, 1992). The structures of the complexes between these peptidases and their respective inhibitors provide information not only on the specific interactions between protein and ligand, but also on the bound conformation of an acyclic

New Perspectives in Drug Design
ISBN 0–12–208070–X

peptide. There is considerable interest in the development of strategies for elaboration of peptide leads for a variety of receptors into higher affinity, or non-peptidic ligands. The complexes between thermolysin and the phosphorus-containing inhibitors represented a good test system in this regard, since high-quality structural information was available at the outset (Matthews, 1988), along with a quantitative assay for binding affinity.

Two straightforward strategies for enhancing binding affinity involve reducing conformational flexibility and incorporating substituents that bring additional binding interaction. Extending a bridging unit from one end of an acyclic inhibitor to the other, thus converting it into a macrocyclic structure, can accomplish the first of these goals, and may also provide an opportunity for the second as well. In this report, we describe two macrocyclic analogues of the thermolysin inhibitor Cbz–Gly–(PO_2^--NH)–Leu–Leu (Morgan *et al.*, 1994), and discuss the roles that intuition and computer assistance played in their design.

Our first efforts in this area were initiated several years ago and were based almost entirely on intuition. Computational assistance came in the form of a computer graphics facility and programs that allowed us to visualize the thermolysin binding site and gauge visually whether the designed inhibitors would fit. In the course of pursuing this and related projects, we recognized a common element to many of the steps that we were taking, and the potential advantage that could be gained from automating them. The program CAVEAT was developed as a result; it provides assistance in structure-based design by allowing a chemist to identify structural templates or other fragments that satisfy a specified relationship between bonds (Bartlett *et al.*, 1989; Lauri and Bartlett, 1994). Although CAVEAT was not available for our initial design of constrained thermolysin inhibitors, it served to bolster our confidence in this design, and to suggest an alternative structure from which we have gained considerable additional insight.

Design of a Rigid Linker

Our design was based on the structures of thermolysin complexes with Cbz–Gly–(PO_2^--NH)–Leu–Leu and Cbz–Phe–(PO_2^--NH)–Leu–Ala (Holden *et al.*, 1987; Matthews, 1988). In both complexes, the inhibitor backbone follows a similar path through the active site from the C-α atom at P_1 to the C-terminal carboxylate at P_2', with a β-like turn at the P_1'–P_2' linkage (Fig. 4.1). The terminal carboxylate and the side chain at P_1 are close to the surface of the protein, by the entrance to the active site, hence spanning the α-carbons at P_1 and P_2' presented a logical approach to a macrocyclic structure. The constraints that we perceived were several-fold. First, the phosphonamidate oxygens of the parent inhibitors are coordinated to the zinc atom, and the

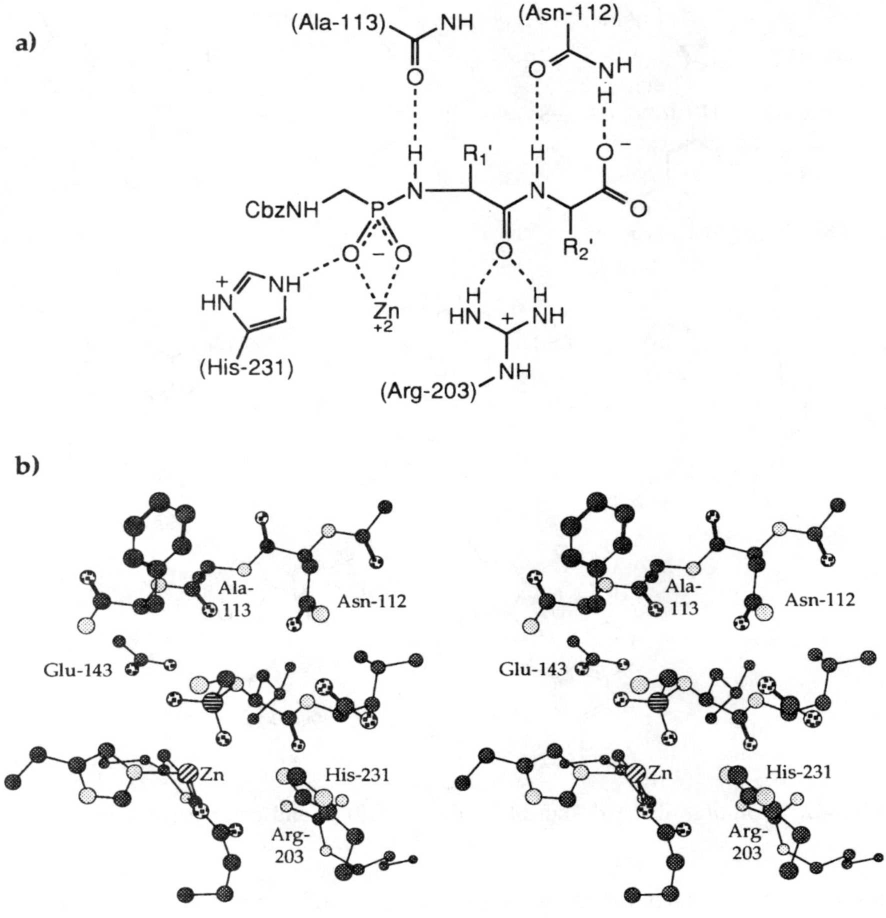

Fig. 4.1 Binding orientation of Cbz–Gly–(PO_2^--NH)–Leu–Leu in the active site of thermolysin. (a) Schematic of hydrogen bonding and other polar interactions. (b) Stereoview of active site; the Cbz moiety of the inhibitor has been removed in this image.

other O and NH moieties are involved in hydrogen bonds with the active site; we did not want to disrupt these interactions. Second, the entrance to the active site is very narrow, with the side chains of Asn112 and His231 representing the upper and lower jaws. Since both of these side chains are involved in specific interactions with the parent inhibitors, we did not want to perturb the positions of these groups either.

Simple model constructions with Dreiding models convinced us that a four-atom linkage would span the distance between the Cα carbons (Fig. 4.2). An

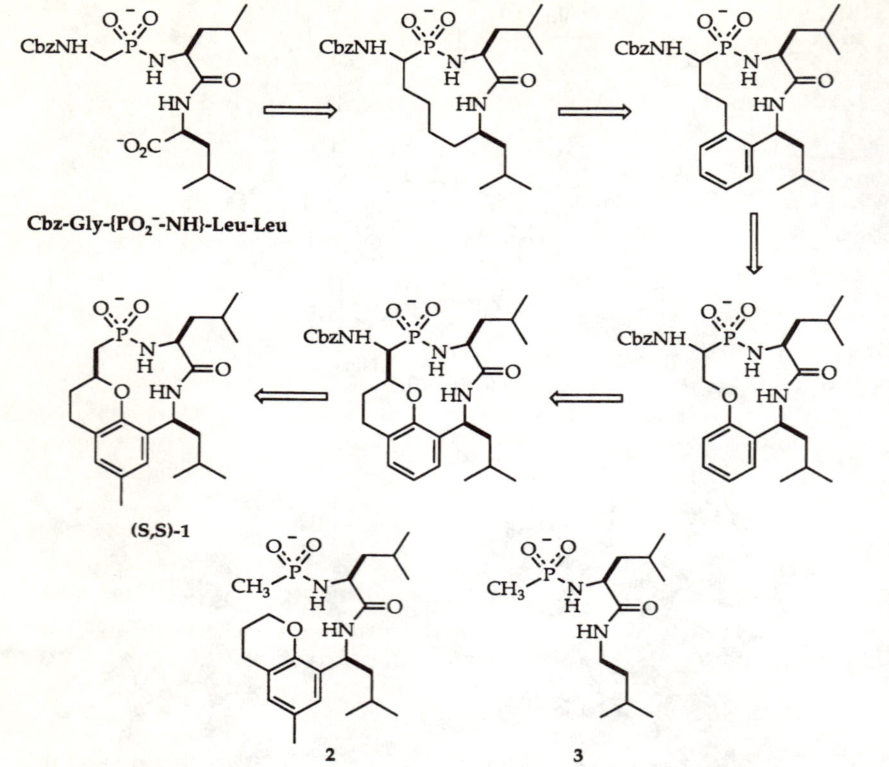

Fig. 4.2 Evolution of the design of inhibitor ***(S,S)*-1**, and comparison compounds **2** and **3**.

aromatic ring was fused at one end, both to confer rigidity and because we needed a very slim unit to fit between the jaws of Asn112 and His231. To avoid transannular interactions arising from hydrogen substituents, an ether oxygen was designated as the central atom of the linker. Although the oxygen was incorporated into the design purely on steric grounds, it turned out that this atom can serve as a favourable hydrogen-bonding site as well. An additional ring was incorporated in the bridging unit for extra rigidity. The structure was simplified by removal of the Cbz-amino moiety, because this group can adopt a variety of conformations in the P_2–P_3 binding sites (Holden *et al.*, 1987; Matthews, 1988), and it would not be affected by the macrocyclization strategy anyway. Finally, a methyl group was added at the para position of the aromatic ring to facilitate the synthesis; this position projects into solvent, so a substituent was not anticipated to have any significant affect on binding. ***(S,S)*-1** was thus the target inhibitor.

Two comparison compounds were selected to help us gauge the success of this design. In structure **2**, a bond is broken between the rigid bridging unit and the carbon α to the phosphonamidate moiety; in another, $MePO_2^-$–Leu–isoamylamide (**3**), the bridging moiety is simply removed from the structure. These structures were intended to measure the impact of the entire bridging process, and to distinguish the contributions from rigidification and specific interactions between the protein and the bridging moiety itself.

Synthesis

The macrocyclic inhibitor **1** was assembled according to the scheme summarized in Fig. 4.3. The desired ortho,ortho′ substitution of *p*-cresol was ensured by the presence of the methyl group, and the desired functionality on the bicyclic chroman unit was introduced at appropriate stages by reduction of carbonyl precursors. In the case of the phosphonomethyl group, the equilibrium mixture of hydroxyketone and hemiketal precursors was subjected to BF_3-catalysed reduction with triethylsilane, which trapped the cyclic ether. At the other position, the amino group was introduced by reduction of the methoxime derivative; attempts to carry out this reduction asymmetrically did not prove to be practical. After coupling to leucine and deprotection, the amino acid was closed to the macrocyclic lactam, the methyl esters were cleaved, and the anionic inhibitors were purified by ion exchange chromatography.

This synthetic route led to all four steroisomers of **1**. By separating various

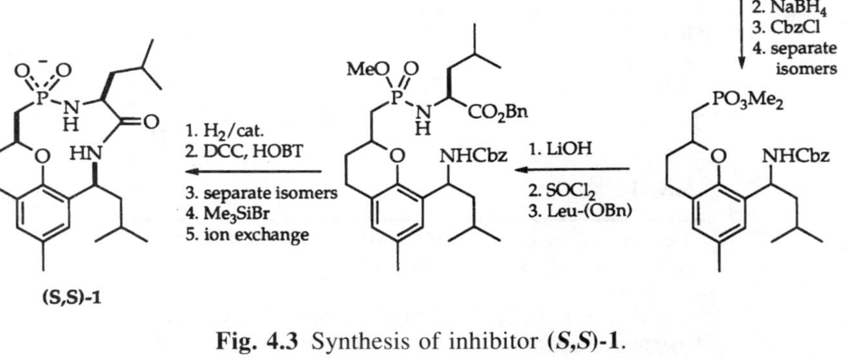

(S,S)-1

Fig. 4.3 Synthesis of inhibitor **(*S,S*)-1**.

diastereomers at key points in the synthesis and carrying out the subsequent reactions in parallel, we were able to obtain each of the stereoisomers in pure form. Although aspects of their relative configurations were known from the synthetic sequence, final assignment of the *R,R*- and *S,S*-diastereomers was ultimately based on crystallographic determination. The assignment of the *R,S*- and *S,R*- isomers was only inferred from their relative binding affinities and remains tentative.

Binding Affinity

The four diastereomers, along with the comparison compounds, were evaluated as reversible, competitive inhibitors of thermolysin, and the inhibition constants listed in Table 4.1 were determined. The stereoisomer that turned out to have the *S,S*-configuration as designed proved to be the most potent inhibitor, with a K_i value significantly lower than those of the other isomers, as well as the comparison compounds. The *ca.* 50-fold enhancement in binding affinity of this isomer over the bare-bones phosphonamidate **3** indicates that the overall strategy was effective, and the 20-fold enhancement over the intact but acyclic analogue **2** suggested that most of this improvement came from conformational constraint, rather than specific interactions of the chroman unit with the protein.

Protein crystallography provided critical insight into both of these conclusions (Morgan *et al.*, 1994). The co-crystal structure of the most potent of the macrocyclic analogues with thermolysin confirmed that the inhibitor had the (*S,S*)-stereochemistry and the binding orientation as designed (Fig. 4.4a).

Table 4.1
Inhibition of thermolysin by macrocyclic phosphonamidates

Inhibitor	K_i(nM)[a]
(*R,R*)-1	> 10 000
(*R,S*)-1[b]	> 10 000
(*S,R*)-1[b]	500
4	500
3	190
2	80
(*S,S*)-1	4

[a] Determined in 0.1 M MOPS buffer, 2.5 M NaBr, 10 mM $CaCl_2$, and 2.5% v/v DMF at pH 7.0 at 25°C (Morgan *et al.*, 1994).
[b] Assignments of **(*R,S*)-1** and **(*S,R*)-1** are tentative ((**(*R,S*)-1** is epimeric with **(*S,S*)-1** at the chroman ring position).)

a)

b)

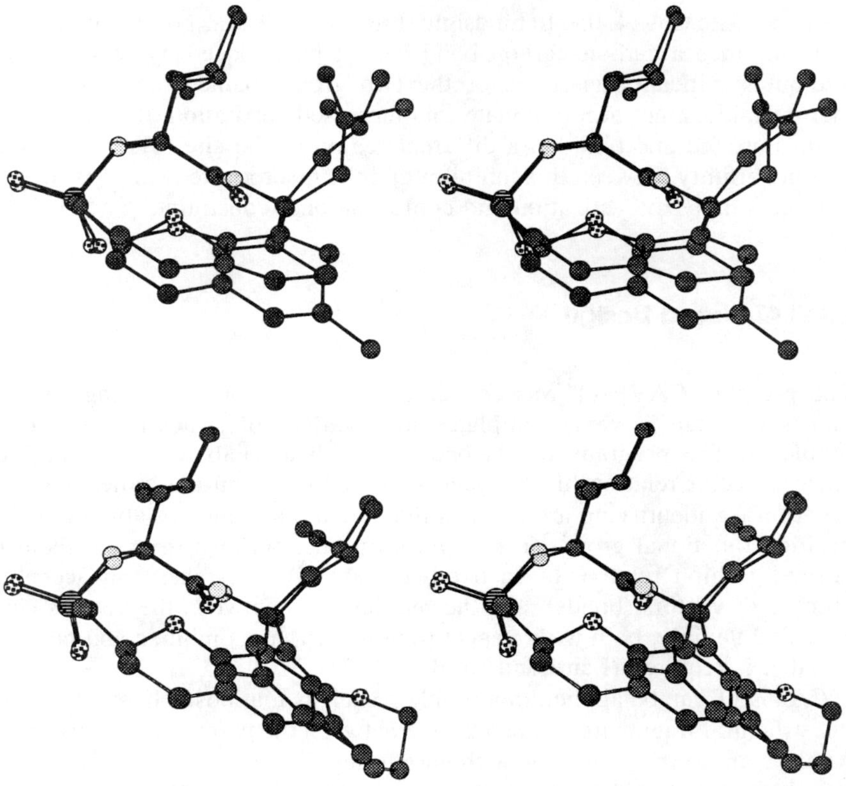

Fig. 4.4 (a) Comparison of the modelled and experimentally determined conformations of the chroman-linked inhibitor **(S,S)-1** bound to thermolysin (the modelled inhibitor lacks the methyl substituent on the aromatic ring). (b) Comparison between the bound conformations of the cyclic inhibitor **(*S*,*S*)-1** and acyclic analogue **3**.

Deviations from the 'modelled' structure are found in two respects. First, the aromatic ring of the inhibitor is pushed away from the Asn112 side chain; this displacement is accommodated by the His231 side chain on the other side by a *c*. 0.4 Å movement of the latter. This orientation of the bicyclic moiety may improve the hydrogen bonding interaction between the ether oxygen and the amide NH of the Asn112 side chain, which in turn is accommodated by a slight rotation of this group about the Cβ–Cγ bond. Because of the displaced orientation of the bicyclic unit relative to the modelled orientation, the isobutyl side chain corresponding to the P_2' residue must adopt a different conformation than that found for the acyclic inhibitor Cbz–Gly–(PO_2^--NH)–Leu–Leu in order to avoid steric interaction with the Asn112 side chain.

The crystal structure of the intact but acyclic comparison compound **2** revealed a completely different orientation of the bicyclic chroman unit in the active site (Fig. 4.4b). In hindsight, this molecule was poorly designed as a control, since a carbon–carbon bond cannot be replaced by two hydrogens without significant separation of the two groups. Since the active site of thermolysin cannot accommodate this increased separation, the bicyclic unit swings around and binds in a different region of the site. The difference in binding affinity between this inhibitor and the macrocycle **(*S*,*S*)-1** is therefore not due simply to cyclization and conformational constraint.

CAVEAT-based Design

The program CAVEAT was conceived as a tool for identifying structural motifs that can serve as templates in a variety of structure-based design problems. The program allows one to search a database of 3D structures using a vector relationship between specified bonds in the molecules as the criterion for identifying a hit. Thus, the structures found are able not only to position functional groups in specific locations, but also to orient them in a desired fashion relative to each other. CAVEAT searches can accept any number of vectors (bonds), and the relationships between the vectors can be specified flexibly, both with respect to how they are combined and how close a match is required (Lauri and Bartlett, 1994).

CAVEAT can be applied to a problem such as that posed here, by identifying structural fragments that can bridge between the two Cα positions and that would bond to these carbons without altering the orientation of the intervening chain. CAVEAT databases (e.g. the 'intra' database (Lauri and Bartlett, 1994)) have been constructed with this specific application in mind, using as vectors bonds that are contained within macrocyclic ring structures. The program is thus able to identify chains of atoms that already adopt the desired conformation in some other macrocyclic structure.

In addition to the search algorithm, CAVEAT also has a post-search filtering and clustering module called CLASS. This utility screens out hits that contain undesirable structural motifs or that would encounter steric or conformational problems, and groups the remaining molecules on the basis of their structural similarity. By assisting in the evaluation of hit structures, CLASS accelerates the design process significantly, and allows one to open up the search tolerances and net a greater diversity of structural motifs.

In applying CAVEAT to the design of a conformationally constrained thermolysin inhibitor, we selected as vectors the Cα-to-P bond of the Gly^P residue and the C-to-Cα bond of the terminal leucine from the crystal structure of the complex with Cbz–Gly–(PO_2^--NH)–Leu–Leu (5TMN in the Protein Databank (Bernstein *et al.*, 1977)). CAVEAT searches involving two bonds (i.e. a single vector-pair, as in this case) typically yield many hits, hence tight tolerances in both the base-to-base distance *d* and in the solid

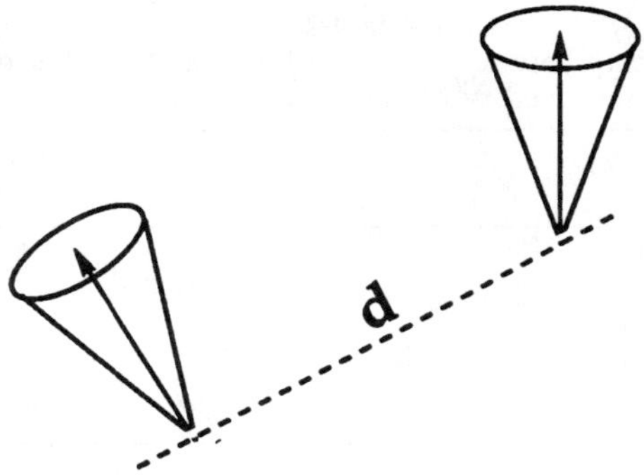

Fig. 4.5 Representation of the tolerance permitted in definition of a vector-pair relationship.

angles (tolerance cones) of each vector (Fig. 4.5) are needed to produce a manageable number. Using an 'intra' database constructed from some 5000 macrocyclic molecules from the Cambridge Structural Database (CSD) (Allen *et al.*, 1983), the number of hits obtained as a function of the tolerances is indicated in Table 4.2.

The hits were screened according to a number of criteria. First, no structure was accepted if the biconnected component of the linking unit was closer than 1.0 Å to the enzyme (the biconnected component represents those atoms which require two bond-disconnections to be detached from the linking unit). This screen effectively removed from consideration linking units that would experience severe steric interactions with the enzyme active site. Second, the potential for eclipsing interactions across the bonds to be formed between the linking unit and the inhibitor chain was evaluated for each hit, and only those which would result in a staggered conformation were accepted. In addition, a subset of structures was selected which contain cyclic moieties as part of the linking unit, on the assumption that these linkers are inherently more rigid. A number of the hits that passed these three selection criteria are shown in Fig. 4.6a. While there was no single hit that incorporated a bicyclic structure, the superposition of these various hits clearly suggests the bicyclic structure of **(*S*,*S*)-1**, which we had designed earlier by a considerably more laborious process.

Without selecting for ring-containing linkers, and clustering the hits based on backbone motif, CLASS identifies some eleven crown ethers as one group of hits. The superposition of these molecules shows the usefulness of the clustering approach (Fig. 4.6b). All these molecules represent the same structural motif, and it would be a waste of time to have to look at each one individually in the course of evaluating the hits. Attractive features of this motif are the ether oxygen, which is located at the same position as the earlier bicyclic design **1**, where it can hydrogen-bond to the Asn112 side chain, and

Table 4.2
Relationship between tolerance limits and number of molecules retrieved from the CAVEAT intra database[a,b]

Tolerance[c]	Number of hits
(0.03 0.03 0.03)	17
(0.05 0.03 0.03)	21
(0.03 0.05 0.05)	175
(0.05 0.05 0.05)	221
(0.05 0.07 0.07)	748

[a] The 'intra' database is a CAVEAT vector database derived from *c.* 5000 macrocyclic structures from the Cambridge Structural Database.
[b] The Cα–P (P_1 residue) and C–Cα (P_2' residue) bonds in the bound form of Cbz–Gly–(PO_2^--NH)–Leu–Leu defined the vector pair to be matched.
[c] The three numbers indicate permitted variation in distance between the base atoms of the vector pair (in Å) and in the angular deviations of vector 1 and vector 2, respectively (in radians).

the fact that it is more accessible synthetically. On the other hand, this linking unit is considerably more flexible than the bicyclic chroman moiety of **(*S,S*)-1**, and there was a question as to whether incorporating it into a macrocycle would decrease or increase the available conformations.

The monocyclic, macrocyclic phosphonamidate **4** was synthesized as shown in Fig. 4.7. Chain elongation of L-leucine via the Arndt–Eistert synthesis, followed by reduction, provided the basic 1,3-aminoalcohol building block. The ether linkage was formed by rhodium-catalysed carbene insertion, and the phosphonate was introduced by an Arbusov reaction on the bromoethyl derivative. Coupling to L-leucine and formation of the macrocyclic lactam proceeded as described above for the more rigid analogue.

Inhibition of thermolysin by the macrocyclic ether **4** was determined as described before, and the results are also recorded in Table 4.1. It is apparent that the flexible linker does not offer any enhancement in binding affinity over the simple acyclic phosphonamidate **2**; indeed, as an inhibitor, compound **4** is a factor of 2 or 3 worse. While we do not have a co-crystal structure of this material in the active site of thermolysin, and thus lack confirmation of our assumptions and the details of the interaction, it is reasonable to presume that the peptidyl-phosphonamidate chain adopts its usual orientation in the active site. If this is indeed the case, it appears that the anticipated orientation for the linking unit is the only one available. At this point, additional information that would help us to assess why this compound is not bound with higher affinity than the acyclic control is unfortunately not available. For example, it would be desirable to know the low-energy conformation of the inhibitor in solution, a)

b)

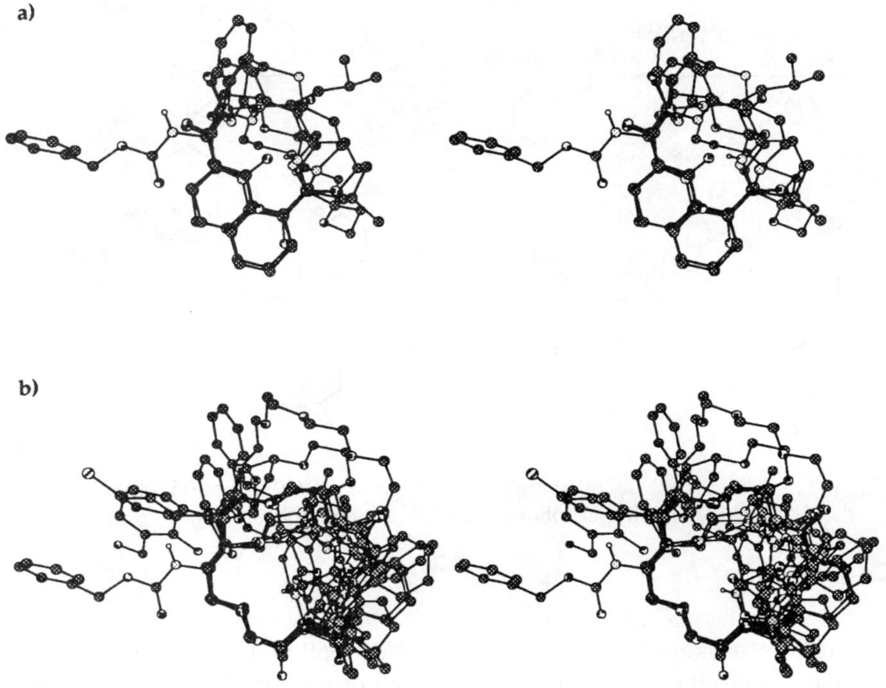

Fig. 4.6 (a) Superposition of macrocyclic structures retrieved from the Cambridge Structural Database illustrating potential ring-containing linking units. (b) Superposition of a number of crown ethers from the CSD illustrating the linear ether linking group.

in the unbound state, and (more importantly) to understand its conformational flexibility.

There is inherently a penalty to be paid for incorporating *more* rotatable bonds in an inhibitor structure, since there will be an unfavourable entropy associated with freezing out the additional conformational motion on binding. Only if the incorporation of this group leads to a greater reduction in the conformational freedom of the rest of the molecule is an advantage to be expected. Such does not appear to be the case with the simple macrocyclic inhibitor: the entropic advantage of cyclizing the simple inhibitor is offset by the additional entropy required to fix the conformation of the large ring. Further exploration of this phenomenon, and a more quantitative assessment of the factors involved, may be obtained from intermediate designs incorporating one of the two annelated rings of inhibitor **(*S*,*S*)-1**.

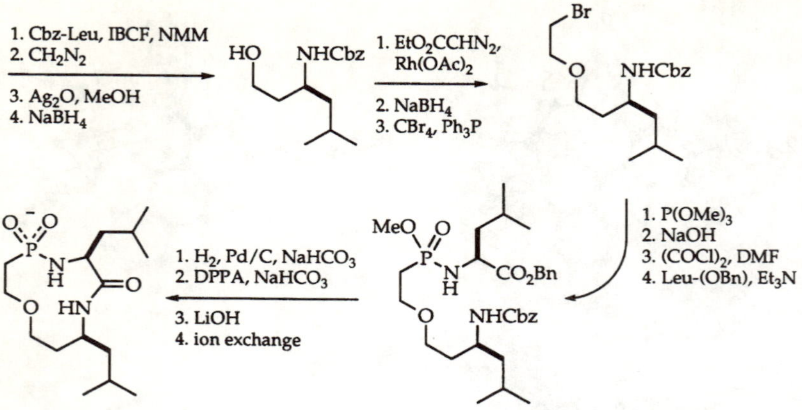

4

Fig. 4.7 Synthesis of the ether-linked inhibitor **4**. IBCF, isobutyl chloroformate; NMM, *N*-methylmorpholine; DPPA, diphenylphosphoryl azide.

Conclusions

The results described here demonstrate that both intuition and computer assistance can play important roles in inhibitor design. Our original design, invented in a laborious process and synthesized by a route that proved to be even more laborious, was successful in enhancing the affinity of the phosphonamidate inhibitor. The same design could now be anticipated much more readily, and with more conviction, due to the availability of CAVEAT and CLASS. In addition, this approach can suggest new designs. However, it seems unlikely that the design process will become wholly automated. We have often stressed that programs such as CAVEAT are tools, designed to assist chemists in coming up with ideas, rather than answers. While these tools may sharpen our intuition, they will never supplant it, and it will always remain a necessary ingredient in the design process.

References

Allen, F.H., Kennard, O. and Taylor, R. (1983). *Acc. Chem. Res.* **16**, 146–153.

Bartlett, P.A. and Marlowe, C.K. (1983). *Biochemistry* **22**, 4618–4624.

Bartlett, P.A., Shea, G.T., Telfer, S.J. and Waterman, S. (1989). *In* 'Molecular Recognition: Chemical and Biological Problems' (S.M. Roberts, ed.), pp. 182–196. Royal Society of Chemistry, London.

Bartlett, P.A., Hanson, J.E. and Giannousis, P.P. (1990). *J. Org. Chem.* **55**, 6268–6274.

Bernstein, F.L., Koetzle, T.F., Williams, G.J.B., Meyer, E.F., Jr., Brice, M.D., Rodgers, J.R., Kennard, O., Shimanouchi, T. and Tasumi, M. (1977). *J. Mol. Biol.* **185**, 535–542.
Bone, R., Sampson, N.S., Bartlett, P.A. and Agard, D.A. (1991). *Biochemistry* **30**, 2263–2272.
Fraser, M.E., Strynadka, N.C.J., Bartlett, P.A., Hanson, J.E. and James, M.N.G. (1992). *Biochemistry* **31**, 5201–5214.
Hanson, J.E., Kaplan, A.P. and Bartlett, P.A. (1989). *Biochemistry* **28**, 6294–6305.
Holden, H.M., Tronrud, D.E., Monzingo, A.F., Weaver, L.H. and Matthews, B.W. (1987). *Biochemistry* **26**, 8542–8553.
Kaplan, A.P. and Bartlett, P.A. (1991). *Biochemistry* **30**, 8165–8170.
Kim, H. and Lipscomb, W.N. (1990). *Biochemistry* **29**, 5546–5555.
Lauri, G. and Bartlett, P.A. (1994). *J. Comput.-Aided Mol. Design,* **8**, 51–66.
Matthews, B.W. (1988). *Acc. Chem. Res.* **21**, 333–340.
Morgan, B.P., Scholtz, J.M., Ballinger, M., Zipkin, I. and Bartlett, P.A. (1991). *J. Am. Chem. Soc.* **113**, 297–307.
Morgan, B.P., Bartlett, P.A., Holland, D.R. and Matthews, B.W. (1994). *J. Am. Chem. Soc.* **116**, 3251–3260.
Phillips, M.A., Kaplan, A.P., Rutter, W.J. and Bartlett, P.A. (1992). *Biochemistry* **31**, 959–962.
Sampson, N.S. and Bartlett, P.A. (1991). *Biochemistry* **30**, 2255–2263.
Tronrud, R.E., Holden, H.N. and Matthews, B.W. (1987). *Science* **235**, 571–574.

Discussion

C. McCarthy

Referring to the earlier part of the presentation, was there any marked difference between the kinetics of binding of the restricted conformation compounds and the prototype?

P.A. Bartlett

That is an interesting question because something that we have looked at and worried about over the years, particularly with our phosphorus inhibitors of thermolysin, has been the slow binding behaviour which is observed. Interestingly, the constrained compounds were no slower in their association rate with the enzyme than the typical phosphorus inhibitors. All the phosphorus inhibitors for thermolysin are, on an absolute scale, slow binding inhibitors, with on-rates between 10^3 and 10^5/mol/s. α-Substituted inhibitors – that is, with P_1 residues, which are substituted phosphonic acids – tend to be at the lower end, around 10^3/mol/s. The macrocyclic structure does not seem to be even that slow; it is no more slow binding than the flexible acyclic molecules.

B.P. Roques

You have rightly underlined the role of the hydrogen bond between the NH of histidine 231 and the oxygen of the phosphonate group. We have recently mutated this residue in thermolysin and replaced it by phenylalanine. Curiously, this change modulated very strongly the recognition of bidentate and phosphonate ligands, but did not change the recognition of thiorphan and retrothiorphan, for instance. When the affinity of phosphoramidon and your best inhibitor is compared, is one of the possible causes of this change the distance between the NH in both compounds and the oxygen of the phosphonate group?

P.A. Bartlett
The effect on the binding of replacing the histidine with a neutral phenylalanine is an interesting result. *[B.P. Roques*: It is very strong – about ten to the power four]. With thermolysin, with the various inhibitors for which Brian Matthews has determined the structure, all kinds of orientations are seen between the tetrahedral phosphorus and the zinc. As I recall, phosphoramidon has a relatively symmetrical orientation: the two oxygens are relatively similarly disposed to the zinc. With our glycine-containing inhibitor, it is quite asymmetric, with one of the oxygens closer to the zinc than the other. With our α-substituted inhibitors, like phenylalanine at P_1, it is much more symmetrical.

Our feeling is that there is not much energy difference between these orientations. I am not sure how much of this is influenced by the peripheral substituents and how much comes from the specific energy of the interaction with the zinc.

B.P. Roques
You do not remember exactly the distance here? [*P.A. Bartlett*: No.] When we looked at this kind of change, replacement of histidine by phenylalanine, and the fact that we found no change in the binding of monodentate ligands . . .

P.A. Bartlett
[*interrupting*] That makes sense, I think: the fact that the thio compounds do not have a significant affinity change, whereas the bidentate compounds do, means that the thio compounds are not dependent upon the interaction with histidine. Rather, they are dependent on the interaction directly with the zinc.

In collaborative work with Professor William Rutter's group (University of California, San Francisco), using the rat carboxypeptidase (which is structurally very similar to the human carboxypeptidase), they did the mutations and we made a series of inhibitors for that zinc peptidase. They replaced the arginine (which takes the position of the histidine in carboxypeptidase) with lysine, methionine and alanine, and determined the influence of these mutations on the catalytic activity of the enzyme, and we looked at the influence of these mutations on the binding affinity of a series of phosphorus inhibitors. These mutations had a relatively small effect (about an order of magnitude) on the ground-state binding – on the K_m values – but a fantastic effect on the catalytic ability, and exactly the same effect on binding the inhibitors.

B.P. Roques
And that is very different in the case of thermolysin?

P.A. Bartlett
It would be interesting to see what is the direct relationship, but if we compare the $K_{m/}K_{cat}$ values for the substrates with the K_i values of the inhibitors, over five orders of magnitude there is an exact correlation of inhibitor binding with transition state binding, and no correlation with the ground-state binding. There clearly is an important interaction between the phosphorus and the cationic group that is present.

P.M. Dean
How thoroughly have you tested the search for these vectors? Have the algorithms been given a well spaced, but essentially randomly distributed, set of vectors simply to test how often it gets it right as opposed to how often it cannot actually find any? Are there any vectors that it could never find?

P.A. Bartlett
There certainly are not any vectors that it cannot find. Let me answer the question from a different direction to see if it gets to the answer for which you are looking. In the early days of developing CAVEAT we developed some histograms which indicated how frequently the different possible values for the vector parameters are encountered – that is, the distribution of values across the parameter ranges. As would be expected, there are many more vector combinations with low values for the distance parameter, for example, than high values, because all molecules have bonds that are close together but only a few have bonds that are far apart. For the dihedral angle parameter, there is a fairly even distribution across the range of possibilities. In contrast, the external angles are heavily biased toward values less than $\pi/2$ – less than 90°. There are relatively few molecules in which the vectors (of substituent groups) point inward because there are relatively few macrocyclic structures in most databases.

Nevertheless, there is representation across all the vector parameter ranges. I am not sure how we would test what you are asking, whether there is some combination of vectors that could not be found. I am sure there is some combination of vectors, say, three or more vectors, where we will not find any molecules in which they are represented. Is that the question?

P.M. Dean
In part. Secondly, have you tried scoring the hits in terms of some sort of

energy of interaction of the site? [*P.A. Bartlett assented.*] Does that give good values?

P.A. Bartlett
When we do the clustering, the filtering and the screening we are not looking at the entire molecule. There is an algorithm within CLASS which senses what are the biconnected components of a structure, that is, the core that does not include side chains and unnecessary parts of the ring system. It counts only the core in all the scoring, filtering and clustering algorithms. For example, all the steroids will cluster together, but if the vectors are on the A and B rings a host of other tetracyclic and tricyclic structures will also cluster with them if their core consists of the same decalin-type system.

All the scoring, whether against the surface or some other criterion which we have, is done only on the core, so in effect it is a superstructure that is being scored. The scores are used completely subjectively: we may take a structure and say that it scores better than another, but we are still going to modify the structure and go on with the design.

My sense is that the intuitive scoring which the chemist brings in front of the graphics screen in these sorts of problems is ultimately better than any sort of quantitative score that we would use. We are still trying to figure out this ease-of-synthesis scoring possibility.

A.P. Johnson
Clearly, the tolerances that are used will greatly influence the number of answers obtained. How are they chosen?

P.A. Bartlett
Before we had CLASS, the tolerances were used to get a manageable number of hits. They would be set to net perhaps 100 hits – which was about our attention span for putting one structure after another up on the screen. We were uneasy about this because the tolerances were being defined in physically unrealistic terms. We were narrowing down the tolerances to limit the number of hits, even reducing them beyond the accuracy of the crystal structure with which we were working. It made no physical sense.

With the advent of CLASS, we can now handle hundreds and thousands of hits. In a typical search we will usually open up the tolerances to get between 1000 and 3000 hits. We know that the useless molecules can be filtered out and the remainder can be clustered so that, for example, all the crown ethers are put in one group and only a representative example has to be looked at. We can get rid of siloxanes, cut out molecules with three-membered rings and so on – we can be much more realistic about how the tolerances are set and net a much greater diversity of structures this way.

In addition, it was frustrating to have to reduce the tolerances to get a manageable number of hits – and then discover that 50 of these molecules represented the same information, crown ethers, for example. It is much more realistic now because of that.

A.P. Johnson

Secondly, in working with *de novo* ligand design, we and others in this field have found that the very large number of answers is a problem. One way in which these can be filtered is by ease-of-synthesis – or estimated ease-of-synthesis. We have tried to develop a computer program that does precisely that. It would be interesting to match it against some synthetic chemists' ease of synthesis criteria.

P.A. Bartlett

One of the applications of CAVEAT that I passed over is to try to use it for *de novo* design, turning into a vector problem what is, in many respects, a volumetric match that we are looking for with DOCK or with many of the genetic algorithms for growing molecules in active sites. This is done by picking hydrogen bonding sites and asking what we can find that will match that. CLASS, in its ability to sense volume and structure, or three-dimensionality of interaction, is then used to accept only those molecules which will fit as well. This, again, gives supermolecules that fill active sites but have vectors pointing in certain directions. It will be important and extremely useful to incorporate some sense of ease-of-synthesis.

5

Total Synthesis of Taxol and Designed Taxoids

K.C. NICOLAOU*† and R.K. GUY*

*Department of Chemistry, The Scripps Research Institute, 10666 North Torrey Pines Road, La Jolla, CA 92037, USA
†Department of Chemistry, University of California, San Diego, CA 92037, USA

Introduction

Taxol (Fig. 5.1, **1a**) (Kingston, 1993; Nicolaou *et al.*, 1994a) is an antineoplastic agent originally isolated from *Taxus brevifolia*, the Pacific yew. Wani and Wall first reported taxol's activity and structure in 1971 (Wani *et al.*, 1971). Taxol has proven itself effective in the treatment of many cancers including breast, ovarian, skin, lung, and head and neck types (Rowinsky *et al.*, 1992, 1993). Due to its rapidly expanding medical purview, taxol has seen intensive development as an anti-cancer agent (Borman, 1991).

Taxol exerts its cytotoxicity through binding to β-tubulin (Manfredi and

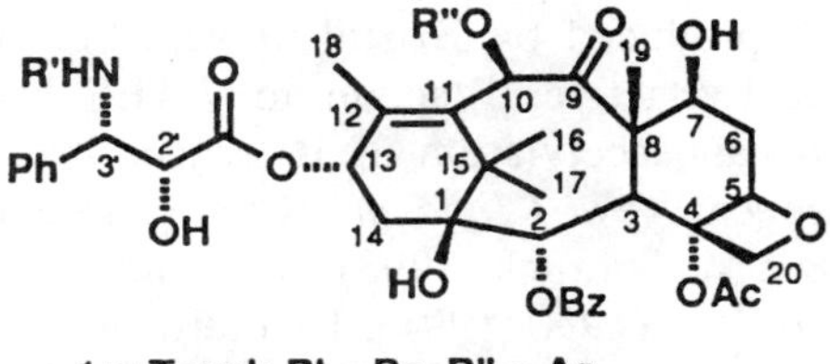

1a: Taxol; R' = Bz, R" = Ac
1b: Taxotere; R' = tBOC, R" = OH

Fig. 5.1 The structure of taxol.

New Perspectives in Drug Design
ISBN 0–12–208070–X

Horwitz, 1984), one of the principal substituents of microtubules. Once bound to this receptor, taxol encourages the polymerization of tubulin into microtubules and stabilizes the resulting structures to breakdown (Schiff *et al.*, 1979). Horwitz's group reinforced their theory of this unique mechanism by observing the formation of stable, discrete and non-functional bundles of microtubules in HeLa cells (Schiff and Horwitz, 1980). Since that time, workers in the field have observed a strong correlation between the freezing out of microtubules *in vitro* and cytotoxicity *in vivo*.

Taxol entered into clinical trials in the early 1980s. Rowinsky and his colleagues first noticed its dramatic effects during phase I trials with drug-resistant ovarian carcinoma (McGuire *et al.*, 1989). A high incidence of acute hypersensitivity reactions among the patients almost caused the termination of these early studies (Weiss *et al.*, 1990). After successful control of these side-effects through pretreatment with steroids and antihistamines and extended infusion times, the trials resumed on a limited basis (Brown *et al.*, 1991). In the studies that followed, taxol has shown meaningful effect on ovarian (Einzig *et al.*, 1990; Rowinsky *et al.*, 1991; Pazdur *et al.*, 1992; Caldos and McGuire, 1993), breast (Holmes *et al.*, 1991), lung (Chang *et al.*, 1993; Murphey *et al.*, 1993; Ettinger, 1993), skin (Legha *et al.*, 1990; Einzig *et al.*, 1991), and head and neck cancers (Forastiere, 1993). Clinical trials are still ongoing with this promising new drug. The FDA approved taxol for use in ovarian cancer late in 1993.

Since its discovery, taxol has been the subject of extensive study with regard to its structure–activity relationships (Kingston, 1993; Nicolaou *et al.*, 1994a). Early in these studies, Potier's group discovered (Chauvière *et al.*, 1981; Guéritte-Voegelein *et al.*, 1986) what, so far, has proven the only analogue more effective than taxol, taxotere (Fig. 5.1, **1b**) (Boven *et al.*, 1993). Taxotere has shown clinical characteristics similar to taxol (Lavelle, 1993) and is currently in phase II trials in Europe and the USA. Other studies have succeeded in giving a wealth of information about those areas important to taxol's activity but have not yet yielded a commercially viable drug.

The chemical industry now produces both taxol and taxotere through semisynthesis. Taxol, produced by Bristol-Meyers Squibb, arises from the coupling of an optically active β-lactam to 7-TES baccatin III (TBIII), available by silylation and acetylation of 10-deacetylbaccatin III (10-DAB) derived from the European yew, *T. baccata* (Chauvière *et al.*, 1981; Guéritte-Voegelein *et al.*, 1986; McCormick, 1993) following the method of Ojima *et al.* (1991, 1992) and Holton (1990, 1991). Taxotere, however, comes from the reaction of a protected chiral acid with TBIII, made from 10-DAB also from the European yew (Chauvière *et al.*, 1981; Guéritte-Voegelein *et al.*, 1986). The development of these two efficient coupling methodologies has settled a large amount of concern about the environmental impact of producing taxol by isolation from *T. brevifolia* (Borman, 1991; Hartzell, 1991).

The Total Synthesis of Taxol

As the continued exploration of taxol's structure–activity relationships is clearly important, we undertook the design of a synthetic methodology that would afford not only taxol but also, with minimal manipulation, a host of analogues. With this overriding goal in mind, our examination of taxol's structure yielded several interesting observations. First, several methods already existed for attachment of the side chain (Holton, 1990, 1991; Ojima *et al.*, 1991, 1992) and formation of the oxetane (Ettouati *et al.*, 1991; Magee *et al.*, 1992; Nicolaou *et al.*, 1992b), so these events could be safely left to the endgame. Applying this stratagem retrosynthetically led to taxol's ABC ring system. The presence of vicinal oxygenation at C9–C10 suggested the use of a McMurry pinacol coupling (McMurry, 1989; Lenoir, 1989) as a potential transform. Further examination of this route brought us to the conclusion that the C1–C2 bond could be formed via a Shapiro coupling (Chamberlin and Bloom, 1990) with oxygenation at C1 following later. Finally, the formation of both the A and C rings through Diels–Alder chemistry was particularly attractive due to its flexibility and normally exquisite stereocontrol.

Before embarking on this course, we stopped to consider the potential problems. Taxol is a densely substituted molecule, containing 11 stereocentres, three of them tertiary, four esters, a ketone, an amide, three free alcohols, and the acid-sensitive oxetane ring. One problem caused by this enforced proximity is the epimerization at C7 through a retro-aldol/aldol mechanism (Kingston, 1991, 1993). Another is the opening of the oxetane ring by the C2 alcohol under basic conditions (Wahl *et al.*, 1992; Klein, 1993; Chen *et al.*, 1993; Samaranayake *et al.*, 1993). Both of these problems had to be kept in mind while designing a protection scheme.

The carbon skeleton itself contains a highly strained eight-membered ring with two pseudo-axial methyl groups as well as a fused connection to an anti-Bredt alkene. Indeed the groups of Kende (Kende *et al.*, 1986) and Pattenden (Begley *et al.*, 1990) had already established the difficulty of directly forming this highly strained ring through McMurry coupling. We hoped that newly developed technologies (McMurry and Rico, 1989; McMurry *et al.*, 1989a,b) would provide the results promised by our model studies (Nicolaou *et al.*, 1993).

Finally, we had worries about the differentiation of the electronically less reactive C10 alcohol from its sterically less reactive counterpart at C9. Leaving all of these worries aside, we decided to press on, as shown in Fig. 5.2. Thus our retrosynthetic analysis led us to starting materials that were either commercially available or known in the literature.

As shown in Fig. 5.3, the combination of chloroacrylonitrile **5** and diene **6** (Alkonyi and Szabó, 1967) gave the cyclic adduct **9** in good yield. This material converted to ketone **10** after exposure to basic conditions that also

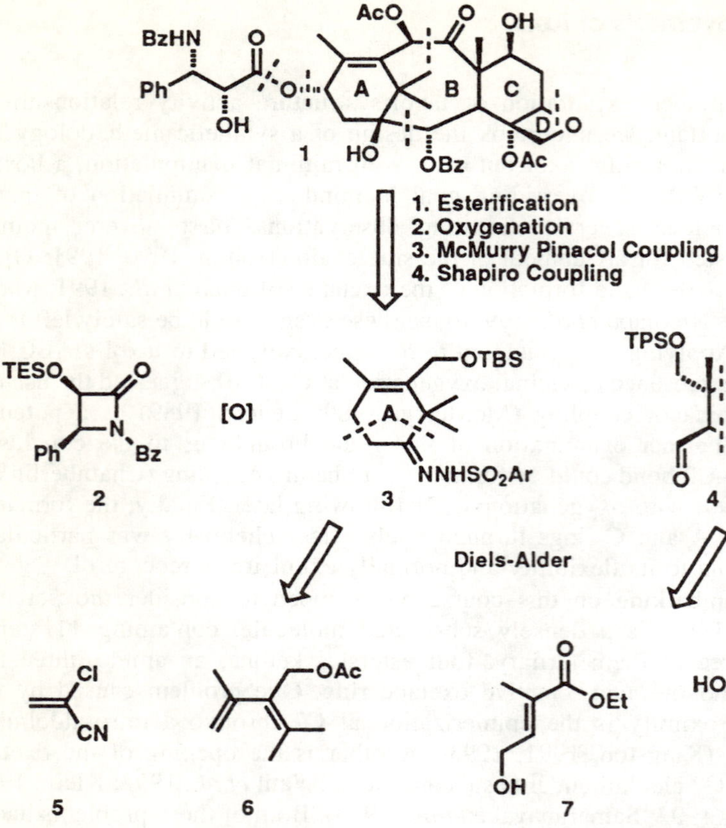

Fig. 5.2 Retrosynthetic analysis of taxol.

removed the acetate group (Madge and Holmes, 1980). Protection of the primary alcohol as the *t*-butyldimethylsilyl ether proceeded cleanly to give **11**. Treatment of this ketone with 2,4,6-triisopropylbenzene-sulphonyl hydrazine generated the hydrazone **3** (Cusack *et al*., 1976).

Problems with regiochemistry and kinetics plagued initial attempts to form the C ring. Concomitant with our efforts, a report by Narasaka *et al*. (1991) of a template-controlled cycloaddition in a system very similar to ours appeared. As shown in Fig. 5.4, the creation of the temporarily unimolecular system **12** by the reaction of **7** (Nicolaou *et al*., 1992b) and **8** (Wiley and Jarboe, 1956) with phenylboronic acid under dehydrating conditions encouraged the intramolecular Diels–Alder reaction between the two. This reaction came about with good yield and excellent stereo- and regiocontrol to give the bridged ring system **13**. This highly strained system rearranged by translactonization *in situ* to give the fused system **14**. Diprotection of the hydroxyl moieties of this molecule proceeded nicely to afford **15**. Selective reduction of the ester

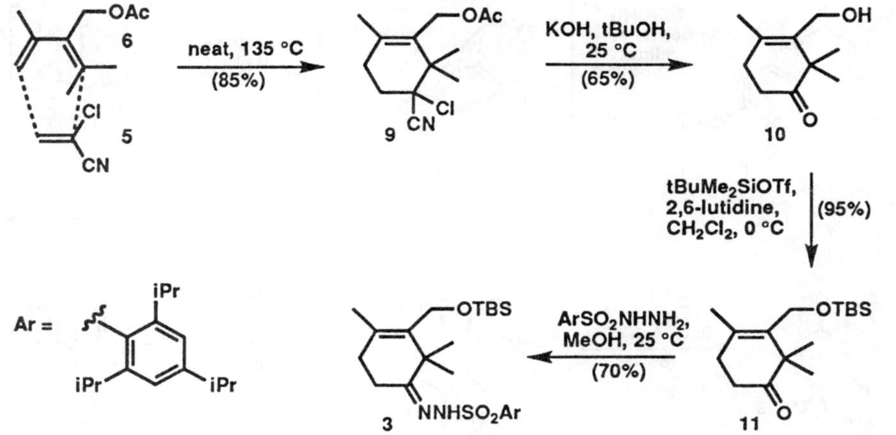

Fig. 5.3 Synthesis of taxol's A ring. The following, less common abbreviations, may be found in Fig. 5.3 and successive figures. TPAP-NMO, tetrapropyl ammonium perruthenate–4-methyl morpholine-*N*-oxide; PCC, pyridinium chlorochromate; TPS, *t*-butyldiphenylsilyl; TBS, *t*-butyldimethylsilyl; TES, triethylsilyl; TBAF, tetrabutyl ammonium fluoride; DMAP, 4-dimethylaminopyridine.

followed by selective cleavage of the less hindered silyl ether formed **16**. Sequential reaction of this material with *t*-butyldiphenylsilyl chloride and benzyl bromide gave **17**. Exhaustive reduction of **17** with lithium aluminium hydride produced triol **18**. Transketalization of **18** with 2,2-dimethoxypropane, followed by oxidation with Ley's TPAP-NMO system (Griffith and Ley, 1990) led to **4**.

As presented in Fig. 5.5, coupling of the vinyl anion of **5**, generated by the method of Martin (Martin *et al.*, 1992), with aldehyde **4** produced allylic alcohol **19** in good yield as a single diastereomer. X-Ray crystallographic analysis of **19** confirmed the relative stereochemistry as that shown. One can explain this high degree of stereoselectivity by chelation control of the conformation of the aldehyde through a lithium cation. Epoxidation of this allylic alcohol by the method of Sharpless (Sharpless and Verhoeven, 1979) gave epoxide **20** as one diastereomer. Reductive opening of the epoxide with lithium aluminium hydride afforded exclusively the 1,2-diol **21**.

Molecular modelling studies had shown that cyclic protection at C1–C2 should enforce the geometry desired for the McMurry reaction. Thus, reaction of **21** with phosgene gave **22**. Deprotection and oxidation of the two hydroxyl groups in **22** produced dialdehyde **23** in good yield. Addition of **23** to the low valency titanium reagent produced by the reduction of titanium trichloride with zinc–copper couple gave the desired diol **24** in modest yield. During attempts to optimize this transformation, we elucidated the structures of the major side products as alkene **25**, 1,4-addition product **26**, and oxidation product **27**.

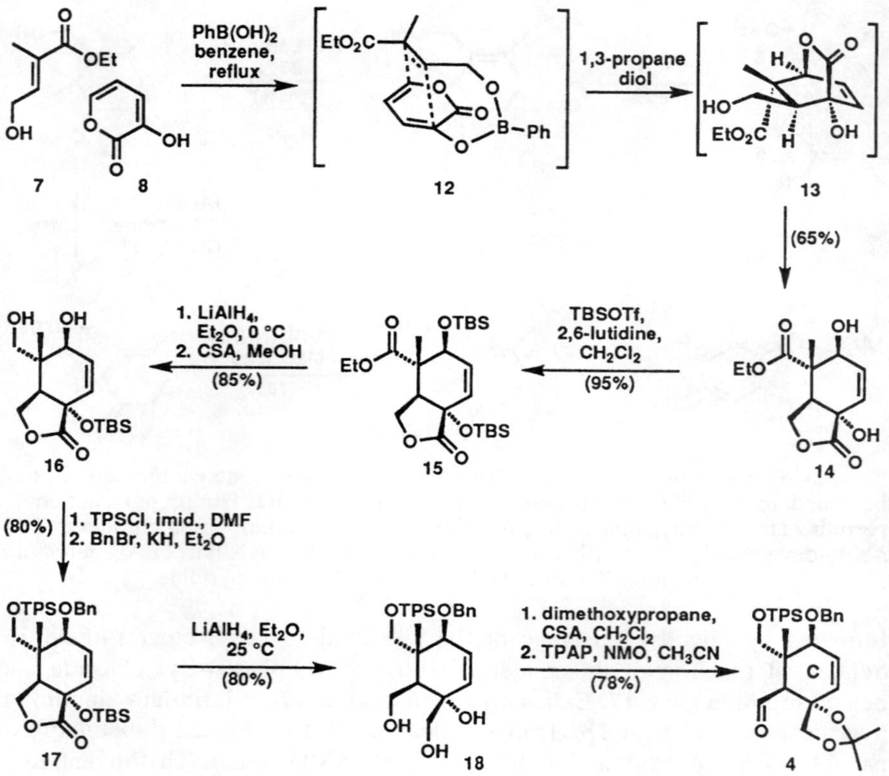

Fig. 5.4 Synthesis of taxol's C ring.

As shown in Fig. 5.6, formation of the diastereomeric esters **28** followed by chromatographic separation allowed the resolution of diol **24**. X-Ray crystallographic analysis of one of these isomers allowed us to choose the correct one for synthetic elaboration. Basic hydrolysis of this ester gave **24** as one enantiomer. Acetylation of **24** produced **29**, which converted, upon treatment with TPAP-NMO, to **30**. Crystallographic analysis of the crystalline benzoate **31**, obtained by PCC oxidation of **30**, confirmed the regiochemistry of this keto-acetate. Next, hydroboration of **30** followed by oxidative workup gave alcohol **32** with fair regiochemistry and excellent stereoselectivity.

As shown in Fig. 5.7, treatment of alcohol **32** with acid, followed by acetylation, produced diol-acetate **33**. Then, exchange of the benzyl ether for a triethylsilyl ether provided **34**, a manoeuvre undertaken so that protection at C7 would match that from our degradative studies (Nicolaou *et al.*, 1994b). Removal of the acetate, selective formation of the primary trimethylsilyl ether, and triflation at the secondary alcohol gave **35**. Treatment of **35**

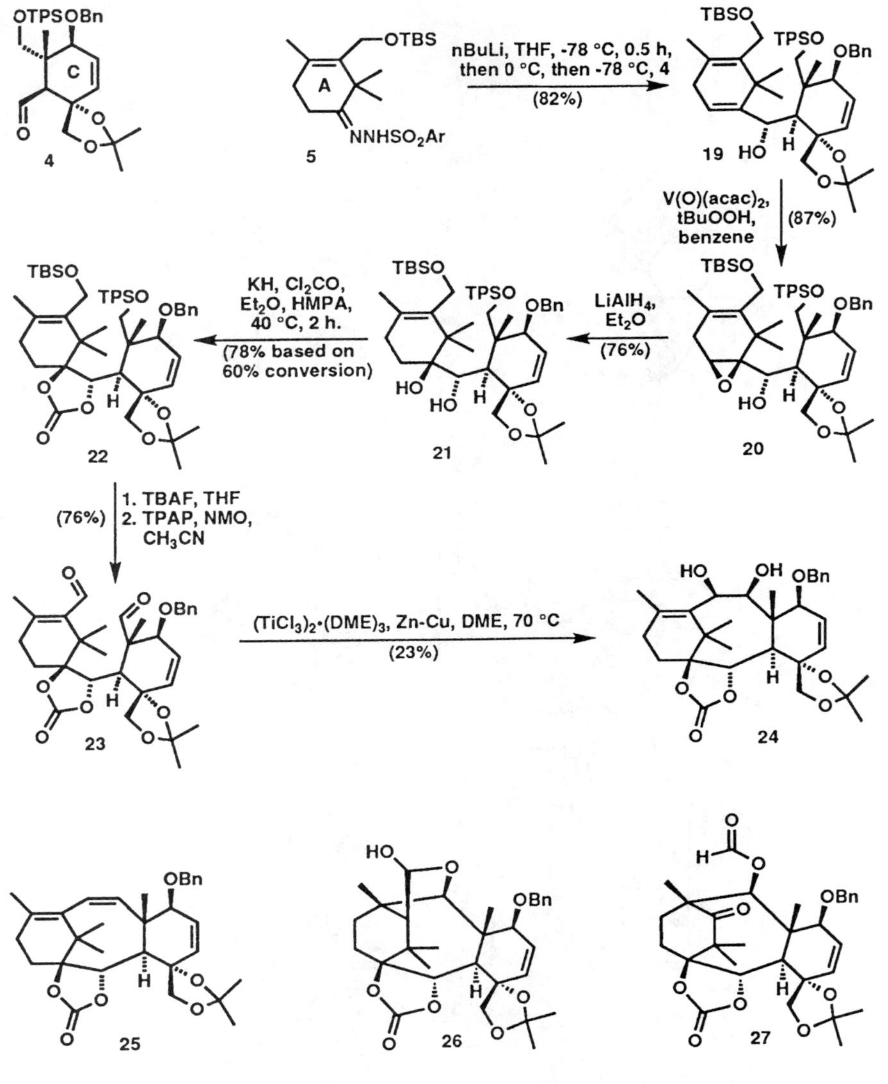

Fig. 5.5 Synthesis of taxol's ABC ring system.

with acid provided, in a manner similar to that of Potier (Mangatel *et al.*, 1989; Ettouati *et al.*, 1991) and Danishefsky (Magee *et al.*, 1992), the ABCD ring system of taxol as **36**. Finally, acetylation of this substrate gave **37**.

As portrayed in Fig. 5.8, **37** was readily transformed into taxol. Thus, treatment of **37** with phenyllithium gave, as a single regioisomer, the benzoate **38**. Reaction of **38** with pyridinium chlorochromate produced the allylic

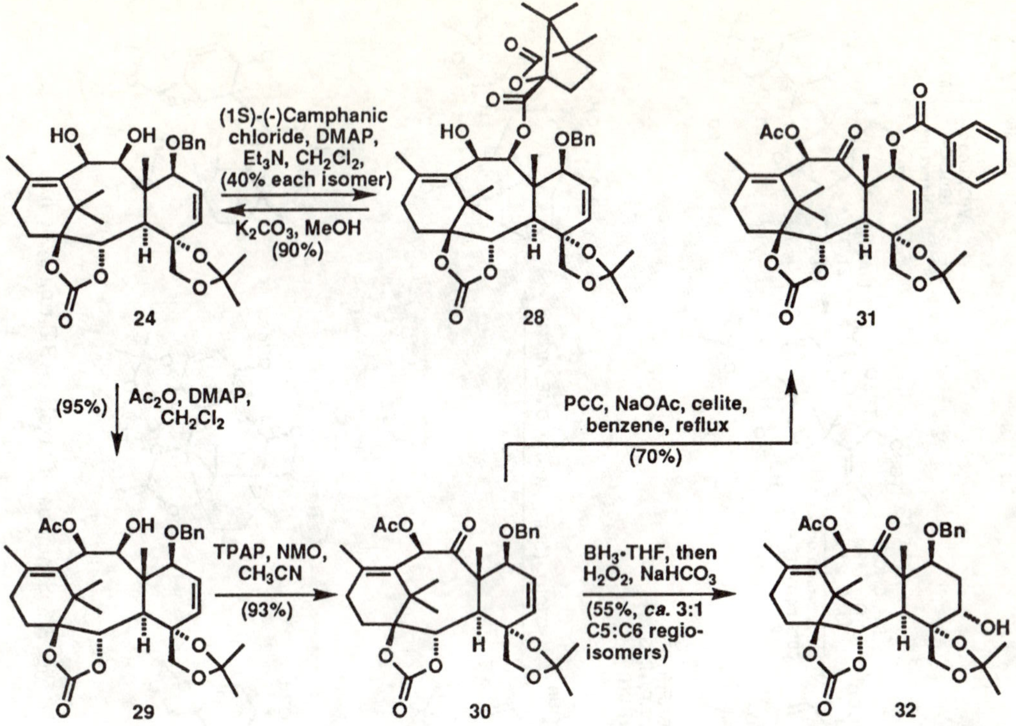

Fig. 5.6 Functionalization of taxol's ABC ring system.

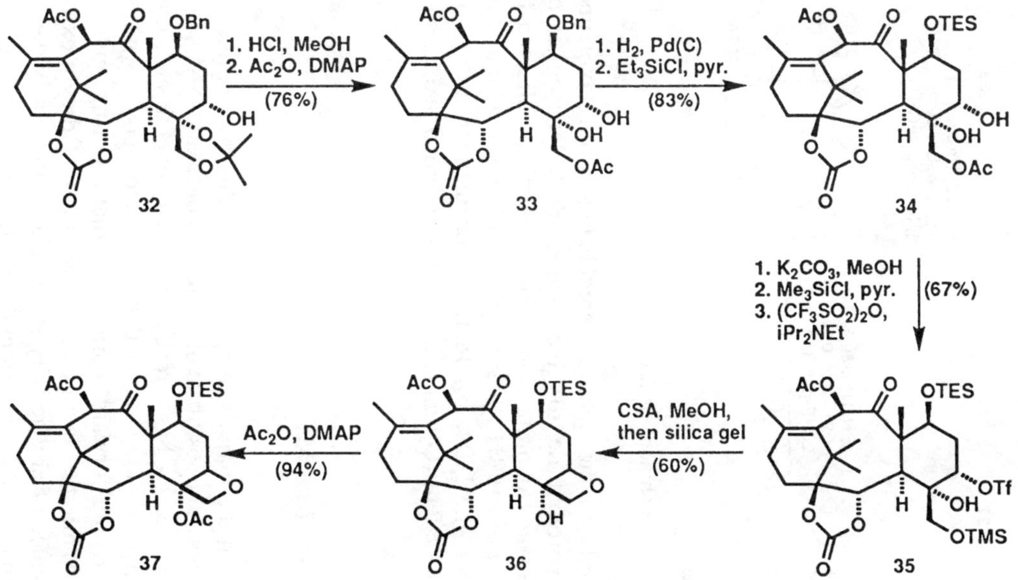

Fig. 5.7 Synthesis of taxol's D ring.

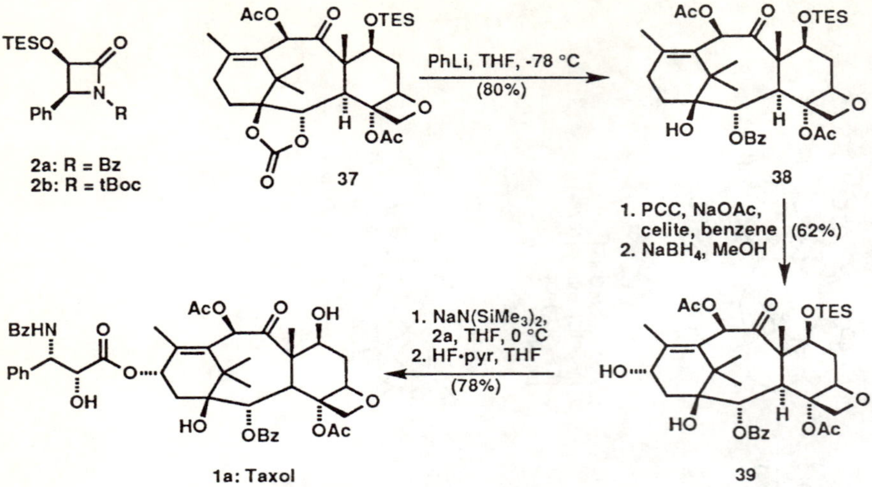

Fig. 5.8 Attachment of taxol's side chain.

ketone that reduced cleanly to the natural stereochemistry for taxol upon treatment with sodium borohydride to give alcohol **39** (Harrison *et al.*, 1966). Finally, attachment and deprotection of the side chain followed the method of Ojima (Ojima *et al.*, 1991, 1992) to give taxol **1a** (Nicolaou *et al.*, 1994c; see also Holton *et al.*, 1994a,b). In the same manner, use of the appropriate side chain equivalent (Ojima *et al.*, 1993) provided taxotere **1b**.

The Synthesis of Designed Taxoids

As mentioned before, one of the major strategic goals of this programme was finding efficient routes to new classes of taxol analogues or taxoids. As shown in Fig. 5.9, our synthetic strategy has already produced several such compounds. Following chemistry analogous to that described above, with the gross simplification of carrying forward a simple aromatic C ring, gives **40** (Nicolaou *et al.*, 1994d). While this compound shows attenuated cytotoxicity relative to taxol, the presence of any activity is singular, particularly in light of its complete lack of tubulin polymerization ability. Other aromatic taxoids are currently under study in these laboratories.

Another area of our studies that revealed competence in the production of derivatives was the nucleophilic opening of carbonate **34**. In our hands, most nucleophiles, including alkyl and aryl lithiates and amines, opened this ring to give the corresponding C2 derivatives (Nicolaou *et al.*, 1994e). Since this material was available in bulk from 10-deacetylbaccatin III (Nicolaou *et al.*,

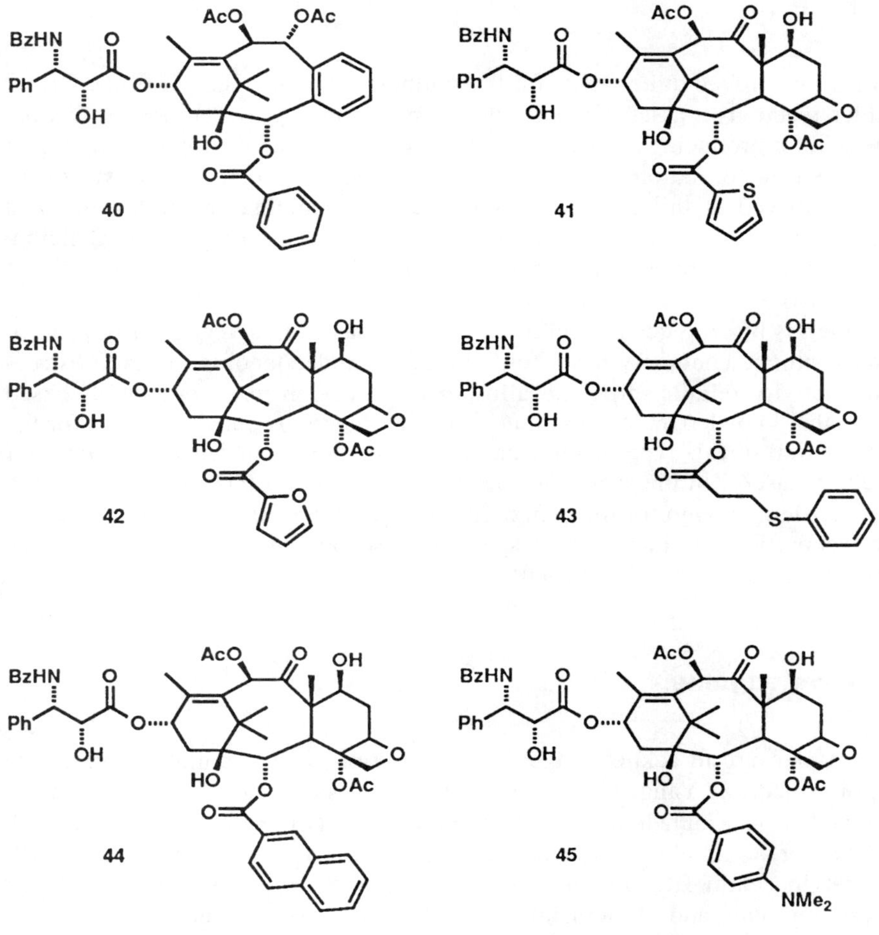

Fig. 5.9 Synthetic taxoids.

1994b), this proved a ready method for the production of these derivatives. Aromatic esters such as **41** and **42** produced through this route exhibited biological characteristics comparable to those of taxol. Aromatic compounds more bulky than these, particularly in the para position, such as **44** and **45** had greatly attenuated cytotoxicities. Compounds such as **43**, available through Michael addition to the condensation product of vinyl lithium and **37**, were also readily available. They, however, exhibited almost no cytotoxicity, suggesting the importance of a cyclic substituent immediate to the ester.

Conclusion

This route proved quite viable for the synthesis of taxol. The use of the Diels–Alder reaction to assemble both the A and C rings provided a very flexible method for producing a variety of synthons that allowed the rapid screening of various ring formation strategies for the B ring. The method that was eventually arrived at utilized the extremely direct combination of Shapiro and McMurry reactions to yield a highly convergent route to the taxane skeleton. Taken together these elements make a useful first generation synthesis of taxol (**1a**) and taxotere (**1b**).

In terms of drug design and discovery this has been a very fruitful project. Our synthetic chemistry has afforded a better understanding of taxol's structure–activity relationships and allowed us to design new compounds based upon that knowledge. We continue to use our general route to taxoids for the elucidation of this type of information and we hope that others will find our methods useful in the search for better taxoids. While this route is presently not efficient enough for the commercial production of taxol, if a novel taxoid proves particularly interesting a specialized second generation synthesis may arise from this body of knowledge.

Acknowledgement

It is a pleasure to acknowledge the contributions of our collaborators in the taxol project: Z. Yang, J.J. Liu, H. Ueno, P.G. Nantermet, C.F. Claiborne, J. Renaud, E.A. Couladouros, K. Paulvannan and E.J. Sorensen. We thank I. Ojima for a sample of β-lactam **2a** and E. Bombardelli for a gift of 10-deacetylbaccatin III. Our deepest gratitude goes to Raj Chadha for X-ray crystallography and W. Wrasidlo for biological assays. We also wish to thank Drs John Taylor, Michel Barreau, Alain Commerçon, of Rhône-Poulenc Rorer and Professor Pierre Potier for stimulating discussions and encouragement during this project. This work was supported by the NIH, the Scripps Research Institute, and fellowships from Mitsubishi Kasei Corporation (H.U.), Rhône-Poulenc Rorer (P.G.N.), the Office of Naval Research USA (R.K.G.), Glaxo, Inc. (C.F.C.), Mr Richard Staley (C.F.C.), NSERC (J.R.), the Agricultural University of Athens (E.A.C.), R.W. Johnson–ACS Division of Organic Chemistry (E.J.S.) and grants from Merck Sharp and Dohme, Pfizer Inc. and Schering Plough.

References

Alkonyi, I. and Szabó, D. (1967). *Chem. Ber.* **100**, 2773–2775.
Begley, M.J., Jackson, C.B. and Pattenden, G. (1990). *Tetrahedron* **46**, 4907–4924.
Borman, S. (1991). *Chem. Eng. News*, 2 September, 11–18.
Boven, E., Venema-Gaberscek, E., Erkelens, C.A., Bissery, M.C. and Pinedo, H.M. (1993). *Ann. Oncol.* **4**, 321–324.
Brown, T., Havlin, K., Weiss, G., Cagnola, J., Koeller, J., Kuhn, J., Rizzo, J., Craig, J., Phillips, J. and Von Hoff, D. (1991). *J. Clin. Oncol.* **9**, 1261–1267.
Caldos, C. and McGuire, W.P. (1993) *Semin. Oncol.* **20**(4 Suppl. 3), 50–55.
Chang, Y., Kim, K., Glick, J., Anderson, T., Karp, D. and Johnson, D. (1993). *J. Natl Cancer Inst. USA.* **85**, 388–394.
Chamberlin, A.R. and Bloom, S.H. (1990). *Org. React.* **39**, 1–83.
Chauvière, G., Guénard, D., Picot, F., Sénilh, V. and Potier, P. (1981). *C.R. Séances Acad. Sci.* (2), **293**, 501–509.
Chen, S.H., Wei, J.M. and Farina, V. (1993). *Tetrahedron Lett.* **34**, 3205–3206.
Cusack, N.J., Reese, C.B., Risius, A.C. and Roozpeikar, B. (1976). *Tetrahedron* **32**, 2157–2162.
Einzig, A.I., Wiernik, P.H., Sasloff, J., Garl, S., Runowicz, C., O'Hanlan, K.A. and Goldberg, G. (1990). *Proc. Am. Assoc. Cancer Res.* **31**, 187 (Abstract 1114).
Einzig, A.I., Hochster, H., Wiernik, P.H., Trump, D.L., Dutcher, J.P., Garowski, E., Sasloff, J. and Smith, T.J. (1991). *Invest. New Drugs.* **9**, 59–64.
Ettinger, D.S. (1993). *Semin. Oncol.* **20**(4 Suppl. 3), 46–49.
Ettouati, L., Ahond, A., Poupat, C. and Potier, P. (1991). *Tetrahedron* **47**, 9823–9838.
Forastiere, A.A. (1993). *Semin. Oncol.* **20**(4 Suppl. 3), 56–60.
Griffith, W.P. and Ley, S.V. (1990). *Aldrichimica Acta* **23**, 13–18.
Guéritte-Voegelein, F., Sénilh, V., David, B., Guénard, D. and Potier, P. (1986). *Tetrahedron* **42**, 4451–4462.
Harrison, J.W., Scrowston, R.M. and Lythgoe, B. (1966). *J. Chem. Soc. C.* 1933–1945.
Hartzell, H. (1991). *In* 'The Yew Tree, A Thousand Whispers'. Hulogosi, Eugene, OR, USA.
Holmes, F.A., Walters, R.S., Theriault, R.L., Forman, A.D., Newton, L.K., Raber, M.N., Buzdar, A.U., Frye, D.K. and Hortobagyi, G.N. (1991). *J. Natl Cancer Inst. USA* **83**, 1797–1805.
Holton, R.A. (1990). European Patent EP400 971; *Chem. Abstr.* (1990) **114**, 164 568q.
Holton, R.A. (1991). US Patent 5 015 744.
Holton, R.A., Somoza, C., Kim, H.B., Liang, F., Biediger, R.J., Boatman, P.D., Shindo, M., Smith, C.C., Kim, S., Nadizadeh, H., Suzuki, Y., Tao, C., Vu, P., Tang, S., Zhang, P., Murthi, K.K., Gentile, L.N. and Liu, J.H. (1994a). *J. Am. Chem. Soc.* **116**, 1597–1598.
Holton, R.A., Kim, H.B., Somoza, C., Liang, F., Biediger, R.J., Boatman, P.D., Shindo, M., Smith, C.C., Kim, S., Nadizadeh, H., Suzuki, Y., Tao, C., Vu, P., Tang, S., Zhang, P., Murthi, K.K., Gentile, L.N. and Liu, J.H. (1994b). *J. Am. Chem. Soc.* **116**, 1599–1600.
Kende, A.S., Johnson, S., Sanfilippo, P., Hodges, J.C. and Jungheim, L.N. (1986). *J. Am. Chem. Soc.* **108**, 3513–3515.
Kingston, D.G.I. (1991). *Pharmac. Ther.* **52**, 1–34.
Kingston, D.G.I. (1993). *Fortschritte Chem. Org. Natur.* **61**, 1–206.
Klein, L. (1993). *Tetrahedron Lett.* **34**, 2047–2050.
Lavelle, F. (1993). *Curr. Op. Invest. Drugs* **2**, 627–635.

Legha, S.S., Ring, S., Papadopoulos, N., Raber, M.N. and Benjamin, R. (1990). *Cancer* **65**, 2478–2481.

Lenoir, D. (1989). *Synthesis* 883–897.

Madge, N.C. and Holmes, A.B. (1980). *J. Chem. Soc. Chem. Commun.* 956–957.

Magee, T.V., Bornmann, W.G., Isaccs, R.C.A. and Danishefsky, S.J. (1992). *J. Org. Chem.* **57**, 3274–3276.

Manfredi, J.J. and Horwitz, S.B. (1984). *Pharmac. Ther.* **25**, 83–125.

Mangatel, L., Adeline, M.T., Guénard, D., Guéritte-Voegelein, F. and Potier, P. (1989). *Tetrahedron.* **45**, 4177–4190.

Martin, S.F., Daniel, D., Cherney, R.J. and Liras, S. (1992). *J. Org. Chem.* **57**, 2523–2528.

McCormick, D. (1993). *Bio/Technology* **11**, 26.

McGuire, W.P., Rowinsky, E.K., Rosenshein, N.B., Grumbine, F.C., Ettinger, D.S., Armstrong, D.K. and Donehower, R.C. (1989). *Ann. Intern. Med.* **111**, 273–279.

McMurry, J.E. (1989). *Chem. Rev.* **89**, 1513–1524.

McMurry, J.E. and Rico, J.G. (1989). *Tetrahedron Lett.* **30**, 1169–1172.

McMurry, J.E., Rico, J.G. and Lectka, T.C. (1989a). *J. Org. Chem.* **54**, 3748–3750.

McMurry, J.E., Rico, J.G. and Shin, Y.N. (1989b). *Tetrahedron Lett.* **30**, 1173–1176.

Murphey, W.K., Winn, R.J., Fossella, F.V., Shin, D.M., Hynes, H.E., Gross, H.M., Davila, E., Leimert, J.T., Dhinga, H.M., Raber, M.N., Krakoff, I.H. and Hong, W.K. (1993). *Proc. Am. Soc. Clin. Oncol.* **85**, 384–388.

Narasaka, K., Shimada, S., Osada, K. and Iwasawa, N. (1991). *Synthesis* 1171–1173.

Nicolaou, K.C., Hwang, C.K., Sorensen, E.J. and Claiborne, C.F. (1992a). *J. Chem. Soc. Chem. Commun.* 1117–1118.

Nicolaou, K.C., Liu, J.J., Hwang, C.K., Dai, W.M. and Guy, R.K. (1992b). *J. Chem. Soc. Chem. Commun.* 1118–1120.

Nicolaou, K.C., Yang, Z., Sorensen, E.J. and Nakada, M. (1993). *J. Chem. Soc. Chem. Commun.* 1024–1026.

Nicolaou, K.C., Dai, W.M. and Guy, R.K. (1994a). *Angew. Chem. Int. Ed. Engl.* **33**, 15–44.

Nicolaou, K.C., Nantermet, P.G., Ueno, H. and Guy, R.K. (1994b). *J. Chem. Soc., Chem. Commun.* 295–296.

Nicolaou, K.C., Yang, Z., Liu, J.J., Ueno, H., Nantermet, P.G., Guy, R.K., Claiborne, C.F., Renaud, J., Couladouros, E.A., Paulvannan, K. and Sorensen, E.J. (1994c). *Nature* **367**, 630–634.

Nicolaou, K.C., Claiborne, C.F., Couladouros, E.A., Nantermet, P.G. and Sorensen, E.J. (1994d). *J. Am. Chem. Soc.* **116**, 1591–1592.

Nicolaou, K.C., Nantermet, P.G., Couladouros, E.A., Renaud, J., Guy, R.K. and Wrasidlo, W. (1994e). *Agnew. Chem. Int. Ed. Engl.* 1581–1583.

Ojima, I., Habus, I., Zhao, M., Georg. G.I. and Jayasinghe, L.R. (1991). *J. Org. Chem.* **56**, 1681–1683.

Ojima, I., Habus, I., Zhao, M., Zucco, M., Park, Y.H., Son, C.M. and Brigaud, T. (1992). *Tetrahedron* **48**, 6985–7012.

Ojima, I., Sun, C.M., Zucco, M., Park, Y.M., Duclos, O. and Kuduk, S. (1993). *Tetrahedron Lett.* **34**, 4149–4152.

Pazdur, R., Ho, D.H., Lassere, Y., Bready, B., Kvakoff, I.H. and Raber, M.N. (1992). *Proc. Am. Soc. Clin. Oncol.* **11**, 111 (Abstract 265).

Rowinsky, E.K., Gilbert, M., McGuire, W.P., Noe, D.A., Grochow, L.B., Forastiere, A., Ettinger, D.S., Lubejko, B.G., Clark, B., Sartorius, S.E., Cornblath, D.R., Hendricks, C.B. and Donehower, R.C. (1991). *J. Clin. Oncol.* **9**, 1692–1703.

Rowinsky, E.K., Onetto, N., Canetta, R.M. and Arbuck, S.G. (1992). *Semin. Oncol.* **19**, 646–662.

Rowinsky, E.K., Eisenhauer, E.A., Chaudhry, V., Arbuck, S.G. and Donehower, R.C. (1993). *Semin. Oncol.* **20**(4 Suppl. 3), 1–15.

Samaranayake, G., Magri, N.F., Jitrangsri, C. and Kingston, D.G.I. (1991). *J. Org. Chem.* **56**, 5114–5119.

Schiff, P.B., Fant, J. and Horwitz, S.B. (1979). *Nature* **277**, 665–667.

Schiff, P.B. and Horwitz, S.B. (1980). *Proc. Natl Acad. Sci. USA* **77**, 1561–1565.

Sharpless, K.B. and Verhoeven, T.R. (1979). *Aldrichimica Acta.* **12**, 63–77.

Wahl, A., Guéritte-Voegelein, F., Guénard, D., Le Goff, M.T. and Potier, P. (1992). *Tetrahedron* **48**, 6965–6974.

Wani, M.C., Taylor, H.L., Wall, M.E., Coggen, P. and McPhail, A.T. (1971). *J. Am. Chem. Soc.* **93**, 2325–2327.

Weiss, R.B., Donehower, R.C., Wiernik, P.H., Ohnuma, T., Gralla, R.J., Trump, D.L., Baker, J.R., Van Echo, D.A., Von Hoff, D.D. and Leyland-Jones, B. (1990). *J. Clin. Oncol.* **8**, 1263–1268.

Wiley, R.H. and Jarboe, C.H. (1956). *J. Am. Chem. Soc.* **78**, 2398–2401.

Discussion

M.N. Palfreyman
How do you explain the regioselectivity at the 2-position when the benzoate was made? Is regioselective opening of the carbonate with phenyl lithium a steric effect or is there a coordination with lithium as in the Shapiro reaction?

K.C. Nicolaou
The only explanation I can offer is the steric explanation that I pointed out earlier, that if the other regio-isomer were made, it would be much more hindered than the one corresponding to taxol. Therefore, I expect the reaction to go in this direction. If there are any electronic reasons, I cannot put my finger on them – perhaps a physical or organic chemist could do better than I.

Incidentally, after we did this chemistry a precedent was found in the literature by Paul Wender who used *t*-butyl lithium to open a carbonate in a different molecule that he made – phorbol ester. Again, there was the same situation: it opened up with *t*-butyl lithium to give the secondary ester as opposed to the tertiary ester. I expect that the steric hindrance of the ester there, would be the driving force, but I am slightly reluctant to swear to this explanation.

M.N. Palfreyman
Is there the same regiospecificity with smaller alkyl lithium regents?

K.C. Nicolaou
It works with a furyl lithium and also with methyl lithium in which case the secondary acetate is formed.

J.N. Barton
Is the carbonate ring-opening performed under metal solvated conditions? Do you not have to worry about the size of the metal alkoxide product as well as the size of the ester group in your steric explanation?

K.C. Nicolaou
I do not know the answer to that question. We used commercially available phenyl lithium. I do not know how it is made and what it contains. In some of the variations I showed with the naphthalene and thiophene we made our own reagent by exchange with *t*-butyl lithium. In these cases, the reactions are done in pure tetrahydrofuran (THF) solution. I do not know what solvent the one (phenyl lithium) we buy comes in, but the reagents we made were all in THF. Since the right product was obtained, I guess we did not bother to investigate it much further or need to do much improvement.

C. McCarthy
At the start of the synthesis, did you always intend to use the McMurry coupling? Samarium chemistry would immediately come to mind to effect that transformation as well.

K.C. Nicolaou
We tried samarium chemistry as well, but unfortunately got no trace of the cyclization product with samarium chemistry. Samarium chemistry gives reduction of the aldehydes to alcohols. There are perhaps bimolecular reactions giving dimers and things like that, but never cyclization – which is interesting – although we tried very hard.

C. McCarthy
Did you also consider the use of radicals generated from acyl selenides?

K.C. Nicolaou
I had a student who was very dedicated to doing that, but she had no success with it.

C.G. Newton
At the beginning of your presentation you talked about the mode of action of these compounds inhibiting the assembly of the normal mitotic spindle. What you have said is more of an observation as opposed to a mechanism in molecular terms. What is known about the molecular basis of the action of these compounds, whether at the enzyme or the receptor they are interfering with. What will be the impact of knowing the exact protein interaction on drug design in this field?

K.C. Nicolaou

I think Susan Horwitz is doing the most advanced work in this field. She gave a lecture in San Diego, which unfortunately I did not attend, but from what I heard she now knows that taxol binds to tubulin, which is the monomer of polymerized tubulins, but there are, so far, only some photo-affinity labelling studies. There is no crystallization of this protein, no X-ray structure and no nuclear magnetic resonance studies. Nobody really knows how the ligand–receptor interactions operate in this system.

This is one of the things that needs to be done much more carefully in order to be able to design drugs based on rational snapshots of this ligand–receptor interaction. We are doing some work on this ourselves in fact – synthesizing small sequences of tubulin and trying to see whether taxol or taxotere will bind or adhere to any of these sequences.

G.A. Petsko

Some tumour cells are resistant to taxol. Is anything known about the mechanism of resistance? Is it multidrug resistance, protein-mediated, for example, and what about some of the analogues that have been made?

K.C. Nicolaou

I do not know the answer to that good question either. I am sure people from Rhône-Poulenc Rorer would be able to answer better. It is true that taxol shows some resistance after a few months, but I do not know the exact mechanism.

E.J. Thomas

Do you have an explanation for the stereochemistry of the McMurry coupling across the 9.10-positions, – how the particular relative configurations are obtained?

K.C. Nicolaou

That is an interesting question, for which I do not really have any explanation. As you notice, we get a *cis* compound – both the hydroxy groups are facing towards us. In this system we get only one compound. In this case, we were lucky to get a single stereochemistry, which made things simple and which was consistent all the time. In other systems – I showed a benzene ring where we made an analogue – we found that the stereochemistry varies depending upon how the McMurry reagent is prepared, the age of the reagent, and so forth. Neither the stereochemistry of these reactions nor the nature of the reagent is very well understood.

A. Laoui

Do you think that it may be possible to replace the baccatin skeleton by a new scaffold, using a 3D searching strategy?

K.C. Nicolaou

In this particular case, I guess we have to be realistic: the answer is no. Baccatin III cannot be replaced with a novel scaffold at present. The essence of our exercise was basically to develop new strategies in general for total synthesis. We knew that it was difficult to replace baccatin III and retain activity, thanks to the work of Potier. The synthesis reveals the weakness of the synthetic chemist, which is much more important a lesson to pay attention to. Compared to the miracles of enzymes, what our bodies can do, and what trees can do, we are still far away from mimicking this kind of chemistry. We should not give up now, but push along this direction, trying to become more efficient in making molecules such as taxol. Even though we cannot compete, we should be striving for more efficient reactions and shorter routes to make these kinds of complex molecules.

A.P. Ijzerman

With high throughput testing and screening following the advances in molecular biology, the time-frame has become so small that organic chemistry seems somehow to lag behind in a way that we have seen from both Dr Nicolaou's and Dr Hirschmann's presentations: that is, many compounds can be made, but at the expense of a considerable amount of time. Do you see ways of speeding up things in organic chemistry to compete with molecular biology findings and with the screening and testing?

K.C. Nicolaou

One approach to speeding up synthetic chemistry to catch up with molecular biology perhaps lies in the chemical libraries which many companies, both small and large, are now setting up programs to generate. The objective is to generate a large number of compounds so that we can screen these molecules simultaneously. It will be a kind of systematic approach, like that of isolating compounds from broths and natural sources like plants. This may be a major new dimension to drug discovery. It has not yet proven itself, but there are companies like Pharmacopea and several others in the USA setting this up, also major companies including Rhône-Poulenc Rorer.

The other approach, of course, will be to keep pushing synthetic chemistry for its own sake. If we really want to make a comparison, as I mentioned, with the miracles of enzymes and living systems, we are still in the Stone Age. This is the science that must still be considered top priority and be pushed, especially in academic institutions.

R.F. Hirschmann

I would like to echo the second sentiment especially. I think we have misled ourselves, and certainly the biologists and the research directors, by making such statements as 'we can synthesize anything' – although this is true in a way, in that we can synthesize taxol, vitamin B_{12} and all kinds of complicated structures.

As K.C. Nicolaou and Gilbert Stork have pointed out repeatedly, we are really not very good organic chemists. I believe that whenever a professor tells a student to do a particular reaction, the chances are statistically high that it will not go the way it was intended. As long as this is true, we will not be good at predicting the outcome of a synthetic scheme.

My worry is that when a reaction yields a major product which NMR or mass spectrometry quickly indicates is not the desired product, such a reaction product often gets thrown away. We have to get on, we are in a big hurry, so people do what is called 'screening reagents'. There are 50 ways of going from A to B. If the first five do not work, we try reagent 6.

That is all right, I guess, but I would prefer to see people find out what *did* happen because I think it is likely to be useful to somebody later on. For example, our pyrrolinone synthesis was provided from a reaction discovered in Japan. The Japanese did not want a pyrrolinone, but we did. If this product had not been characterized, we would have moved much slower in finding a way of making these compounds.

In this age of tremendous competition, the desire to 'get on with it' is huge, but I feel sad when people do not try to find out what has happened because, to me, this is what organic chemistry is all about: find out what happened, then see if organic chemistry can be used to control the reaction and make it work the way you want it to. Many people agree with that, but not everybody.

6

The Age of Structure: The Role of Protein Crystallography in Drug Design

D. RINGE and G.A. PETSKO

Departments of Biochemistry and Chemistry and Rosenstiel Basic Medical Sciences Research Center, Brandeis University, Waltham, MA 02254-9110, USA

The atomic structures of large and small molecules can be determined by X-ray crystallography provided the molecule in question can be crystallized. Most of the three-dimensional structures of proteins, nucleic acids and viruses that are known at present have been determined by X-ray crystallography. In favourable cases, the resolution of such a structure determination is such that the relative positions of all non-hydrogen atoms are known to a precision of a few tenths of an angstrom unit.

Structural information has become so central to drug design, especially second generation design, that an understanding of the process and limitations, as well as the power, of this technique is essential to the modern medicinal chemist. In this article, we attempt to impart this basic information. We begin with a discussion of the most important quantity in any structure determination, the resolution.

Resolution

There are two end-products of a crystallographic structure determination. The objective end-product is an electron density map, which is a contour plot indicating those regions in the crystal where the electrons in the molecule are

New Perspectives in Drug Design
ISBN 0–12–208070–X

to be found. Subjective human beings must interpret this electron density map in terms of an atomic model. The model allows the measurement of the atomic coordinates – the *x*, *y* and *z* values relative to some defined origin – of the non-hydrogen atoms in the structure. The medicinal chemist who wishes to use a protein structure in drug design rarely sees the electron density map. He or she is usually given the atomic coordinate set and must infer from its characteristics and from information in the published papers how reliable the structure is. It is essential to realize that atomic coordinates are only as good as the electron density map from which they were derived.

It is also essential to appreciate the distinction between the *accuracy* of an experimentally determined structure and its *precision*. The latter is much easier to assess than the former. We define the precision of a structure determination in terms of the reproducibility of its atomic coordinates. If the crystallographic data allow the equilibrium position of each atom to be determined precisely, then the same structure done independently elsewhere should yield atomic coordinates that agree very closely with the first set. Precise coordinates are usually reproducible to within a few tenths of an angstrom: this is the sort of root-mean-square deviation that one finds between the equivalent coordinates in two independent, high-quality determinations of the same protein structure.

Accuracy refers to whether or not the structure is correct, but there are two ways to define correctness. A structure may be right but irrelevant: the protein may have been crystallized under conditions of high salt or unusual pH where it is not biologically active. Such cases are very rare, but they have occurred. Those structures are 'right' in that they represent accurate interpretation of the crystallographic data, but they do not represent the form of the molecule that functions in its biological context. In such cases, no human error has been made. However, it is also possible for a structure to be inaccurate due to human error: the crystallographer may interpret the data incorrectly. Various levels of inaccuracy are possible. The complete structure may be wrong (very rare but it has happened), some errors in chain connectivity or in sequence registration may be made (less rare but usually corrected soon after they occur), or certain side chains may be positioned incorrectly (quite common, especially in the early stages of a structure determination; usually corrected in the final stages of an analysis, but not always detectable). For the medicinal chemist, the most important thing to understand is that precision and accuracy are somewhat related, in the sense that the more precise a structure determination is, the less likely it is to have gross errors. What links precision with accuracy is the concept of resolution.

Crystallographers express the resolution of a structure in terms of a distance: if a structure has been determined at 2 Å resolution then any atoms separated by more than this distance will appear as separate maxima in the electron density contour plot, and their positions can be obtained directly to high precision. Atoms closer together than the resolution limit will appear as a fused electron density feature, and their exact positions must be inferred from the shape of the electron density and knowledge of the stereochemistry of amino acids or nucleotides. Since the average C–C single bond distance is 1.54 Å, the precision with which the individual atoms of, say, an inhibitor bound to an enzyme can be located will be much greater at 1.5 Å resolution than in a structure determined at, say, 2.5 Å resolution. Operationally, crystallographers categorize structures as being of

1) low resolution (i.e. about 5–6 Å resolution) if all that can be determined is the overall shape of the molecule;
2) medium resolution (around 3 Å resolution) if the folding of the polypeptide chain and the relative positions of the side chains can be determined to about 0.5 Å precision; and
3) high resolution (2 Å resolution or better) if most of the atoms in the molecule can be located with a precision better than 0.3 Å (Fig. 6.1).

Most structure determinations today, even of rather large structures like viruses, are carried out at medium or high resolution, but sometimes very important biological information can be obtained from even a low-resolution picture (for example, the tunnel in the ribosome revealed by low-resolution structural analysis).

There is no substitute for high resolution. It makes the structure determination easier and more reliable. The closer one gets to true atomic resolution (better than 1.5 Å), the less ambiguity one has in positioning every atom. Atomic resolution allows one to detect mistakes in the amino acid sequence, to correct preliminary incorrect chain connectivity, and to identify unexpected chemical features in the molecule (see the story of aldose reductase, below, for a striking example). Incorrect structures have been obtained at high resolution, but only very rarely. Most of the mistakes that have been made in protein crystallography have been made because a medium-resolution structure has been misinterpreted or overinterpreted. The medicinal chemist should assume that the higher the resolution, the more accurate and precise the information is likely to be.

The steps in solving a protein crystal structure at high resolution are shown in Fig. 6.2. First, the protein must be crystallized. Then, the X-ray diffraction pattern from the crystal must be recorded. Phase values must then be assigned to all of the recorded data; this can be done experimentally or, in some cases, computationally. The phased data are then used to generate an image of the electron density distribution of the molecule. Fitting of an atomic model to the electron density map provides the first picture of the structure of the protein, which is improved by an iterative process called refinement until the model is free from gross errors and the precision theoretically attainable at the resolution of the data is achieved. This flow-chart serves as an outline of our discussion.

A

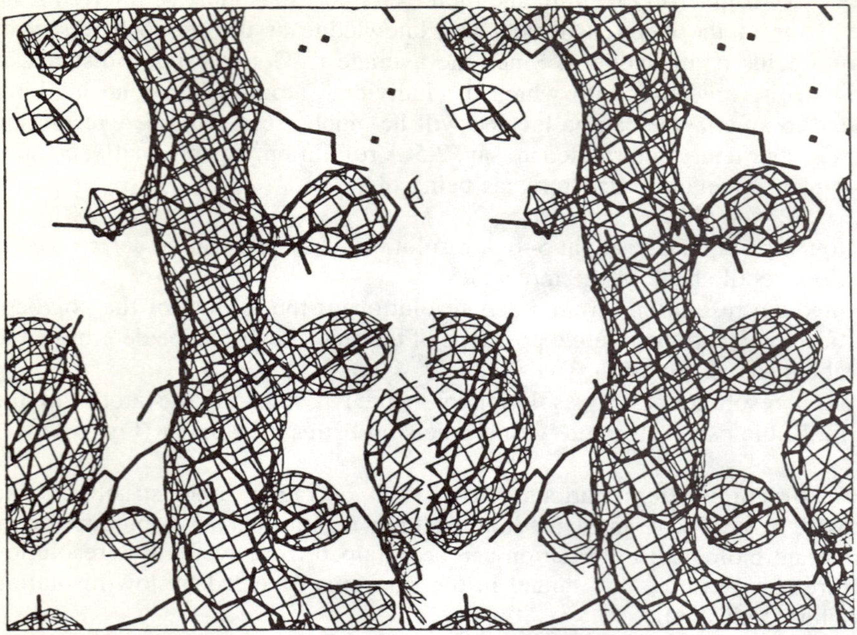

B

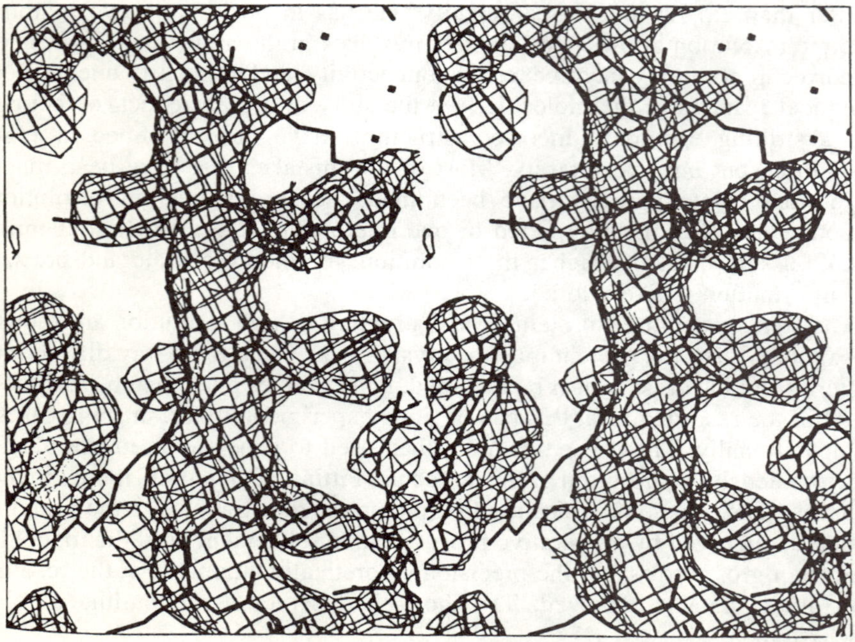

C

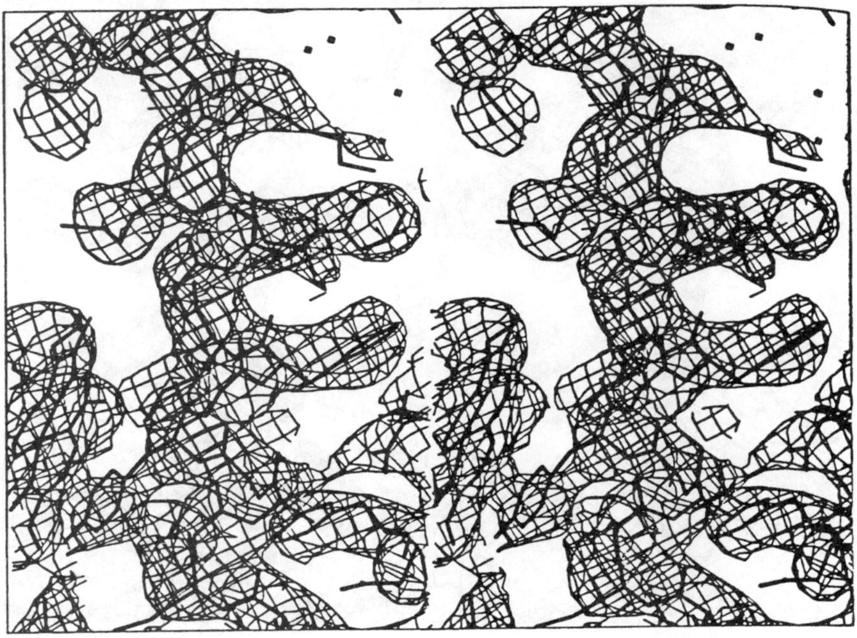

D

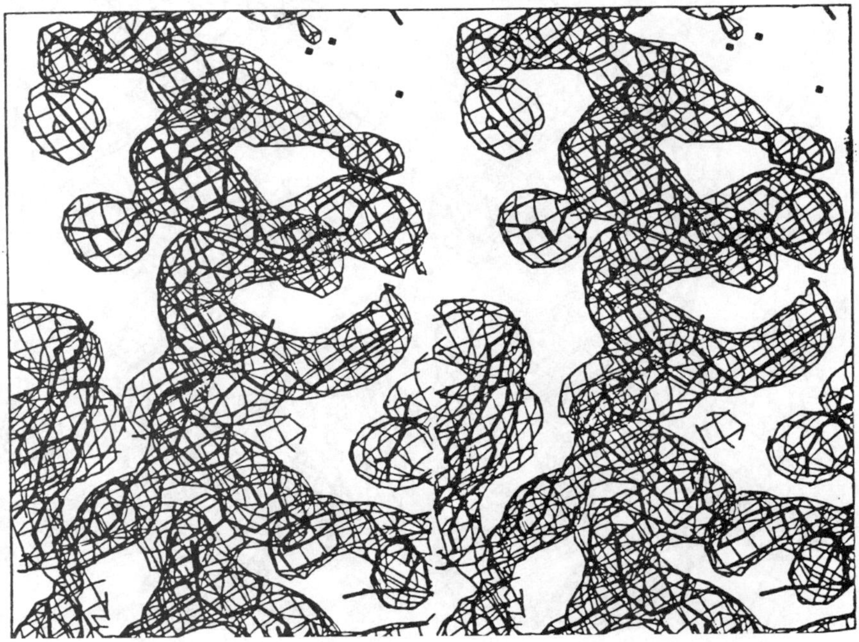

E

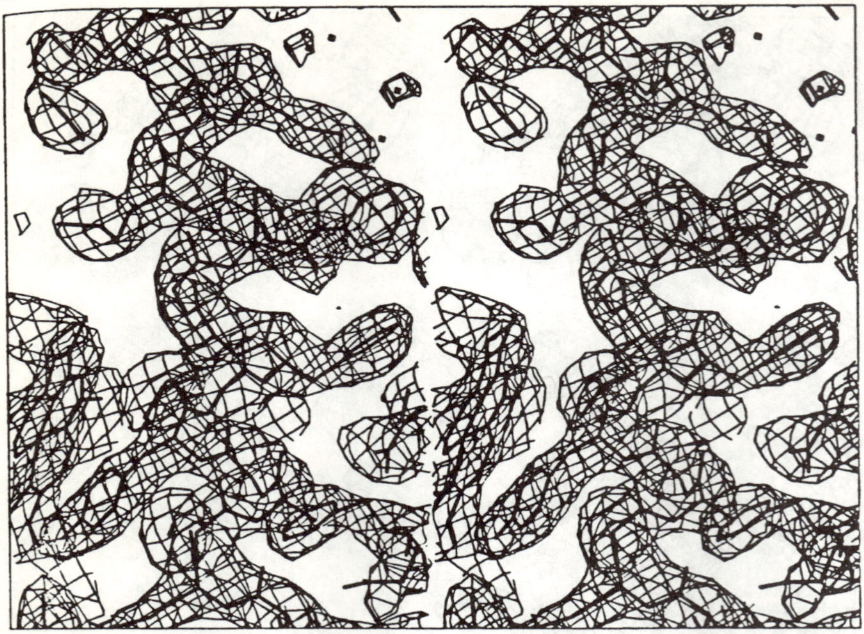

F

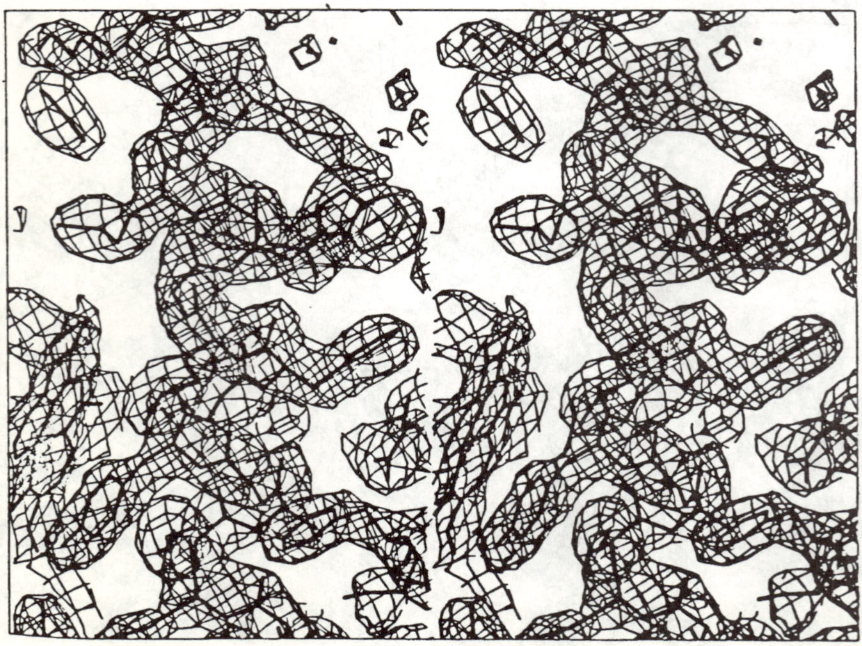

G

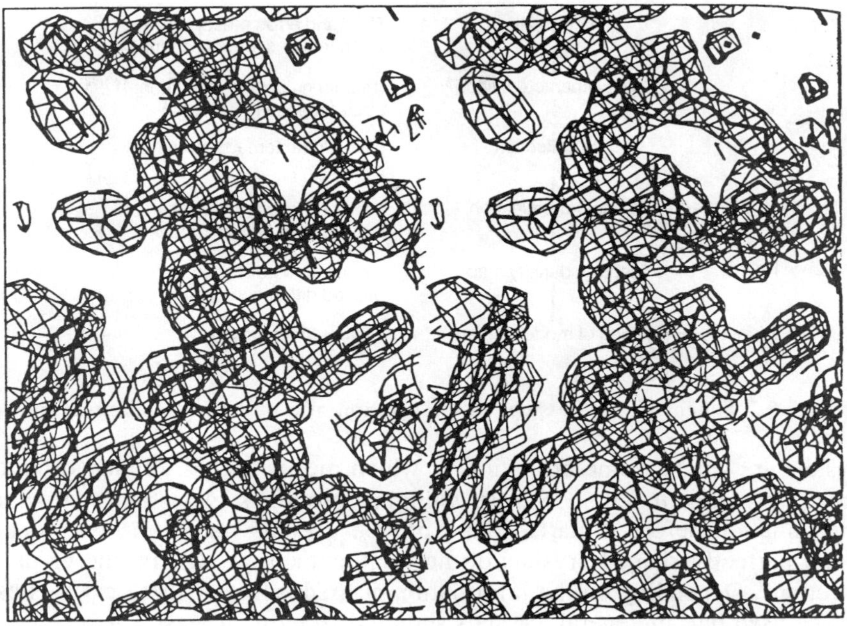

Fig. 6.1 Electron density of an α-helix, in stereo, at different resolutions. (A) 5 Å resolution. A helix at this resolution looks like a cylinder with bumps where the larger side chains protrude. (B) 4.5 Å resolution. The helix now begins to have grooves. (C) 4 Å resolution. There is density for most side chains now. (D) 3.7Å resolution. The turns of the helix are now apparent. (E) 3.3 Å resolution. The chain could be traced unambiguously at 3.5–3.3 Å resolution. (F) 3 Å resolution. The carbonyl bulges are apparent. (G) 2 Å resolution. There is good density for every atom. (Data from D.E. McRee, 'Practical Protein Crystallography', Academic Press, Inc., San Diego, 1993.)

Crystallization

It is remarkable that objects as irregular in shape as proteins or tRNAs crystallize. Yet many of them do so readily. However, forming crystals is one thing, and forming what we call diffraction-quality crystals is quite another. In order to be suitable for a structure determination, protein crystals must be both large and well-ordered. Large means at least a few tenths of a millimetre on an edge (although if two dimensions are at least this big the third can sometimes be smaller). All edge dimensions 0.5–1.0 mm would be ideal. Well-ordered really means two things: the crystal must be a single crystal, and it must scatter X-rays to high resolution in all directions. Not all

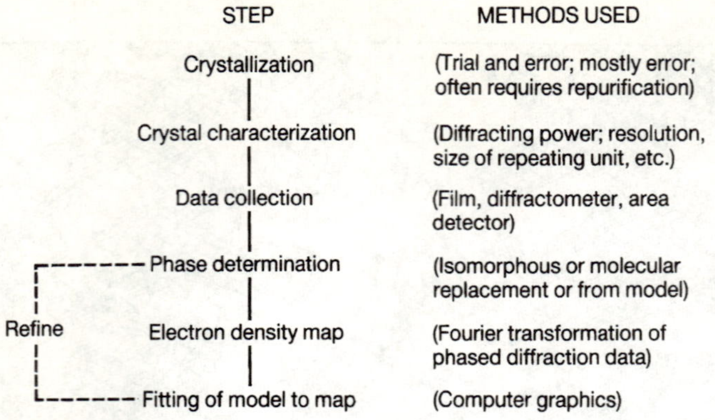

Fig. 6.2 Schematic of the steps in the solution of a protein crystal structure.

crystals are single; some are twinned, which means two differently-oriented lattices growing together. Severe twinning problems can stop a structure determination before it starts. Many protein crystals scatter X-rays weakly (some perfectly shaped crystals do not scatter them at all!) in one or more directions. Depending on the information desired, some of these crystals can still be used but, in general, crystals should diffract to at least 3 Å resolution to be considered suitable.

Protein crystals are not like crystals of sodium chloride or tartaric acid. When proteins crystallize, the large irregular shapes of these macromolecules cause them to make contact with one another at only a few points on their molecular surfaces. Large empty spaces are left in the crystal, and these spaces are filled with the solvent from which the crystals were grown. A typical protein or nucleic acid crystal will be at least 50% solvent by volume. Protein crystals are more like a highly ordered gel than like a crystal of, say, quartz. Sometimes the solvent-filled regions of a protein crystal can be 30 Å in diameter, comparable to the size of the macromolecule itself. Protein and nucleic acid crystals are quite fragile as a result of this and must be maintained in sealed capillary tubes under high humidity so they do not dry out and lose their ordered arrangements.

The high solvent content of protein crystals has three very important consequences: first, the structures of biopolymers determined in the 'crystalline' state will be very similar, if not identical, to the structures these molecules have in aqueous solution. Second, small molecules such as active drugs can be diffused into the crystal lattice, where they will bind to, say, the active site unless it is obstructed by a protein–protein contact. Most crystalline enzymes are active in the 'solid' state, although sometimes the constraints of the neighboring molecules will slow down or inhibit altogether a necessary protein conformational change. Third, the high solvent content of protein crystals usually suggests that they are intrinsically less well-ordered than crystals of smaller molecules. In severe cases, this may mean that the regularity of the crystal is only preserved for the overall shape of the molecule, so that no diffraction data at all can be observed beyond, say, 6 Å resolution. Fortunately, such cases are uncommon, but many protein crystals do not scatter X-rays strongly beyond about 3 Å resolution and in such cases information about their structures is limited in both precision and accuracy.

The rate-limiting step in the determination of the structure of a biomolecule is usually the production of suitable single crystals. The operative word is 'suitable'. As discussed above, to be useful for diffraction, protein crystals must be at least 0.2 mm on an edge, and must be well-ordered. Another aspect of suitability that we have not yet discussed is the protein content of the basic repeating unit of the crystal, because that is what one must actually solve. For ease of structure determination it is desirable that this unit contains the smallest possible number of molecules. For example, if the protein is tetrameric, it is ideal if the repeating unit in the crystal contains only a single monomer.

When one reads a protein crystallography paper, the first thing to look for is the quality of the crystals that have been used. If they were large and diffracted strongly to high resolution, and if the repeating unit was not too big, then the structure is more likely to be of high precision and accuracy.

Although many different techniques have been developed to crystallize proteins, nucleic acids and viruses, all of them are variations on the same general principle that is used to crystallize any molecule: a solution of the desired substance in some buffer conditions in which it is stable is slowly brought to supersaturation, in the hope that crystals rather than amorphous precipitate will form. A variety of methods have been developed to carry out this operation, from microdialysis to vapour diffusion. Most of these methods are designed to use as little of the precious protein sample per experiment as possible, typically, 1–2 μl of protein solution. Unfortunately, protein crystals usually only grow from concentrated solutions. Typical values are 5–40 mg/ml, with 10 mg/ml being the most common. Two microlitres of solution will then have about 20 μg of protein, so at least 1 mg of protein will be used up for every 50 sets of conditions that are tried.

Many hundreds of trials may be needed before the right conditions of protein concentration, pH, temperature and precipitant are found. Sometimes they are never found. It is our belief that, given enough time and effort, most highly purified proteins will crystallize. Unfortunately, this can be like the Eddington monkey problem, and most biochemists do not want to wait an infinite amount of time. If a protein has not crystallized after a year or so of honest effort, the outlook is not promising. But one must be patient: many protein crystals take weeks or months to grow, although some grow overnight; it depends on the protein. And one must supply enough material: if several hundreds of experiments are going to be carried out and different protein concentrations are to be explored, the crystallographer will need tens of milligrams of pure protein. Uncrystallized, precipitated protein frequently cannot be recovered, which places further demands on the supply of pure material. We will start an investigation with 10 mg or so, but we expect to need at least 50 mg for a complete study, and often much more.

A word about purity: although crystallization is a purification step for small organic and inorganic molecules, it is usually not one for proteins. The protein must be pure to begin with. Protein preparations less than 90% pure have crystallized, but not often. Usually at least 95% purity is required and better than 98% is highly desirable. It is worth almost any amount of effort to attain this level of purity, because nothing else has so big an effect on whether or not a protein crystallizes.

Even highly pure protein samples may not be as pure as they appear. Purity is usually assessed by SDS polyacrylamide gel electrophoresis. If the protein runs as a single band on an overloaded, Coomassie-stained gel it is believed to be at least 98% pure. But significant microheterogeneity can still exist even then, and often that will prevent crystallization. Two techniques are particularly good at detecting microheterogeneity: chromatofocusing and isoelectric focusing. Especially if the protein gives only very small or twinned crystals, it is important to use one of these methods to look at the sample. Sometimes three or more closely separated bands can be seen. A striking example of the power of this method is provided by the work of Kuriyan and associates on trypanothione reductase (Kuriyan *et al.*, 1991). The apparently pure sample, which only gave very poor crystals, was found on isoelectric focusing to consist of three components. When these were separated by preparative isoelectric focusing, two of the three produced beautiful single crystals.

If good crystals still cannot be grown, the next thing to do is to change the source of the material. If the *E. coli* protein does not crystallize, the *Salmonella typhimurium* protein or the yeast protein or the rat liver protein may very well do so. Many biochemists in pharmaceutical companies balk at this step, partly because they are sceptical that a small change in amino acid sequence can make so big a difference in crystallization and partly because they really want the human enzyme or the malarial parasite enzyme or whatever the actual drug target is. Yet the literature abounds in cases where this has made all the difference to crystallization. For example, *E. coli* mercuric ion reductase has never given suitable single crystals despite years of effort. The *Bacillus megatherium* enzyme crystallized overnight in large, well-diffracting prisms (Moore *et al.*, 1989).

So, if the human enzyme is the drug target, is there any point in solving the structure of, say, the yeast enzyme? Indeed there is; if there is any reasonable sequence identity between the human enzyme and the yeast counterpart, it will be possible to use the techniques of homology modelling to construct a model of the human enzyme from the yeast crystal structure, and the model will be good enough for computer-based drug design (see Chapter 8 for a dramatic example).

Data Collection

Once suitable crystals are available, their scattering data must be recorded. Unlike the continuous scattering pattern from a single molecule or a randomly oriented ensemble of molecules, the pattern of X-rays scattered by a crystal consists of a series of discrete waves in specific directions (Fig. 6.3). This effect is a consequence of the molecule having been incorporated into a crystal lattice; the individual molecules in the crystal each scatter, but the scattered waves interfere with each other destructively as well as constructively, giving rise to a series of spots arranged in regular positions in space. The spacing between the spots is related to the reciprocal of the dimensions of the lattice on which the molecules are organized; the distribution of intensities of the spots reflects the continuous scattering pattern of a single molecule. In other words, it is as though someone had placed a mask on top of the scattering pattern of a single molecule, only allowing the underlying Fourier transform to leak through and be observed at positions corresponding to the transform of the crystal lattice.

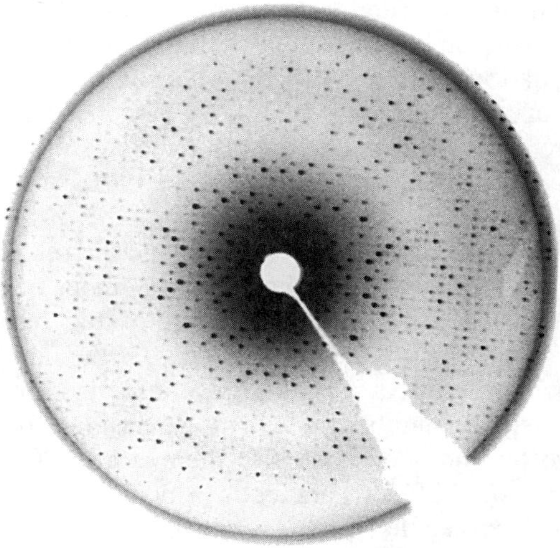

Fig. 6.3 X-Ray precession photograph of a protein crystal diffraction pattern. Note the symmetry in the photograph, which reflects the symmetry in the crystal. Reflections closer to the centre of the photo are at low resolution; those at the edges, high resolution.

Since the pattern of spots resembles what would be observed if light were shone through a diffraction grating, the Fourier transform of a crystal is called the diffraction pattern. Because the crystal is three-dimensional, the diffraction pattern is a three-dimensional array of spots; Fig. 6.3 only shows a section through the complete pattern. The complete three-dimensional diffraction pattern of a protein crystal will have tens of thousands of spots, or more. Crystallographers call these spots reflections although nothing is really being reflected. The structure can be solved by taking the inverse Fourier transform of the diffraction pattern; the fundamental theorem states that such an operation will give an image of the electron density in the molecule.

Diffracted spots are waves, and a complete description of each wave must be fed into the computer before the inverse transformation can be carried out. How does one characterize a wave? If you were standing on a Pacific island and a friend came rushing up to tell you that a tidal wave was coming, you would want to know two things: when it was due to arrive (this is called the 'phase' of the wave) so you would know how much time you had to get to high ground, and how big the wave was (its 'amplitude') so you would know how high you had to climb! The same information is needed for each of the diffracted waves in a crystal structure determination. Phases cannot be measured directly but amplitudes can. Data collection in crystallography is just measurement of the amplitudes of all of the scattered waves (reflections) to a particular resolution.

The resolution of the final structure is determined by how many reflections are measured. If one measures only the strong central region of the diffraction pattern, only a low-resolution picture will be obtained. High-resolution structure determination requires the time-consuming measurement of all observable structure amplitudes, even the weak ones at the limit of the pattern. And there are a lot of reflections to measure.

The number of reflections that must be measured to obtain a structure at a given resolution is inversely proportional to the cube of that resolution (one measures data in a sphere of a certain volume, and the resolution is related to the reciprocal of the radius of that sphere). The number of reflections is also directly proportional to the molecular weight of the basic repeating unit (called the asymmetric unit) of the crystal. Thus, if the number of reflections for a particular size protein to a particular resolution is known, one can easily calculate the approximate number that must be measured for any other protein to any desired resolution. For example, there are 8000 reflections in the diffraction pattern of bovine pancreatic ribonuclease A, a protein of 13 500 Da with one molecule in the asymmetric unit of its crystal form, to 2.0 Å resolution. Therefore, there will be 64 000 reflections to 1.0 Å resolution for ribonuclease A [$1/(1.0)^3$ is 8 times $1/(2.0)^3$, so the number of reflections increases eight-fold]. Chymotrypsin, on the other hand, which is twice as big as ribonuclease A, will have 16 000 reflections to 2.0 Å resolution if there is a monomer in its asymmetric unit, and 32 000 reflections if there is a dimer. Large oligomeric proteins and viruses may have hundreds of thousands of reflections that must be measured if high resolution is desired.

The amplitude of each reflection is easy to measure. It is related to the relative blackness of each spot on the film in Fig. 6.3, and can be quantified by optical scanning of the film. Film processing is laborious, and it means that data acquisition must occur in two discrete and time-consuming steps: recording the complete set of spots in the diffraction pattern on many films, and then extracting the amplitude information by scanning them. Normally, it takes weeks to obtain a protein data set by this method, and a large portion of that time is spent in the manual labour of scanning films.

This labour can be eliminated by counting the scattered photons directly. A machine called a diffractometer is designed to do that. It consists of a Eulerian cradle for positioning the crystal and a scintillation counter, similar to a Geiger counter, mounted on a movable arm. Motion of the crystal and detector is under computer control, and the crystallographer can program the diffractometer to measure the number of scattered X-rays in each reflection automatically, one at a time. Unfortunately, it may take a minute or so to count the scattered photons in one reflection, and if one has 32 000 reflections to collect, at least 32 000 min (over 3 weeks) will be required to measure a data set. Few protein crystals will survive in the X-ray beam for that length of time at ambient temperatures, so one usually requires several crystals per data set, and scaling the partial data sets together often does not remove systematic differences between them.

A newer method that has greatly speeded up the process of amplitude measurement is the use of area detectors or image plates. Area detectors are just electronic film: a two-dimensional grid of wires that is sensitive to the positions and numbers of photons in each reflection. Since area detectors count the scattered X-rays directly, but over a larger area of space than a single counter on a diffractometer, an area detector interfaced to a computer can produce the amplitude information for hundreds of reflections per minute, while it is measuring. Area detectors are expensive: the cost for a simple one is well over $100 000 and some of them cost more than twice that amount. But the money is well-spent; with an area detector a complete set of X-ray amplitudes can be measured from most crystalline biomolecules in only a few days.

Phase Determination

Phase determination is much more difficult. X-rays travel at the speed of light, so there is no way to measure directly the relative time of arrival of each diffracted wave at the detector. This loss of phase information in the diffraction pattern leads to the 'phase problem'. The missing phases must be deduced from the only things that can be measured, the amplitudes.

In small-molecule crystallography a number of very sophisticated mathematical and computational techniques have been developed that can produce phases directly from measured amplitudes. These direct methods of phase determination make small-molecule structure determination automatic in most cases. Thus far, technical obstacles have prevented their application to protein crystallography, so one cannot – as yet – simply take the measured reflection amplitudes, input them into a computer program, and compute their phases from relationships between them.

However, if the macromolecules in the crystal can be labelled specifically with a heavy atom (such as might be accomplished by diffusing a solution of mercuric chloride into the crystal and letting it react with any cysteine residue that might be on the surface of the proteins), the diffracted intensities will change because the electron density distribution in the crystal will have changed. Some spots will increase in intensity, some will decrease, and some will remain unchanged. If a second derivative can be made that places a new heavy atom at a different position, the diffraction pattern will change as well, but different reflections will increase and decrease in intensity. These three data sets (two derivative and one native protein data set) can be combined to give an estimate for the phase of each reflection. Phase determination in this way is somewhat analogous to positional location by triangulation from known distances. There will only be a single value for the phase of a reflection that allows one to calculate the correct effects (increase, decrease or no change) on the reflection intensity of placing two heavy atoms at two known, but different, positions in the crystal lattice. At least two different derivatives are needed because phase determination from a single derivative has an ambiguity, just as position location from a few distances would be ambiguous. (Of course, to carry out this calculation it is essential that the positions of the heavy atoms in the crystal be known exactly. A number of methods have been developed to find the heavy atom locations directly from the intensity differences.)

This method of phase determination is called multiple isomorphous replacement (MIR); multiple, because more than one derivative is needed. Isomorphous means that the binding of the heavy atom must not change the protein structure, since the method depends on all of the intensity differences being due solely to the presence of a heavy atom at a particular place.

Proteins are known to come in structural families, so one might think that the knowledge that a protein of undetermined structure is homologous to a protein whose structure has already been solved could be used somehow in phasing. A second method of phase determination, called the method of molecular replacement, is based on this idea. Recall that the diffraction pattern is just the Fourier transform of the molecule sampled at points corresponding to the lattice of the crystal. If two molecules are similar in structure, their molecular Fourier transforms will also be similar. Suppose one wishes to determine the structure of the aspartic protease from the human immunodeficiency virus (HIV). One can use the fact that its structure is likely to be similar to that of the avian myoblastoma virus (AMV) protease because their sequences are similar. From the known crystal structure of the AMV protease one can construct an atomic model of HIV protease by replacing the corresponding amino acids in the known structure with their HIV counterparts. This model will be highly inaccurate, but if it is Fourier transformed to produce only low-resolution data it should be a reasonable approximation to the actual HIV protease transform at low resolution. The model structure can then be moved in a computer through all possible orientations in the lattice of the actual HIV protease crystal until its calculated low-resolution diffraction pattern matches the observed intensity distribution from the actual measured data set for the HIV protease crystal. When a match is found, the rotated and translated model structure provides a set of crude atomic coordinates for the HIV protease, properly oriented in its lattice. Fourier transformation of the electron density distribution calculated from these coordinates provides a set of calculated phases for every reflection; these can be combined with the original measured amplitudes, yielding a new electron density map at higher resolution. If the process was successful, this map can be reinterpreted in terms of an improved atomic model.

Although the molecular replacement method is dependent on having a good starting model, it often fails when the known and unknown structures are somewhat different. It is very convenient because it is purely computational, requires no heavy-atom derivatives and needs only a single data set. As the database of known structures increases, and as protein engineering produces many mutant and hybrid proteins from well-studied old materials, it is likely that molecular replacement will become even more common a phasing tool than MIR.

Electron Density Map Interpretation

Once phased amplitudes are available, the diffraction data can be Fourier transformed to give an image of the electron density in the crystal. Depending on the resolution and the quality of phase determination, this map may be easy or hard to interpret. It is in the map interpretation stage that most of the errors in structure determination occur. If the phases are good, a crystallographically derived electron density map is a completely objective view of the distribution of electrons in the asymmetric unit of the crystal. However, when individual atoms are not resolved, their positions must be inferred from the size and shape of blobs of electron density, a subjective process carried out by fallible human beings. Refinement of the structure can, in principle, correct most, or even all, of the errors introduced during model building, but sometimes the mistakes are hard to detect. The most common error in map interpretation is getting the connectivity of the secondary structural elements wrong. Individual α-helices and β-strands are usually easy to see, but the order in which they are joined together is sometimes ambiguous, especially if two distant portions of the polypeptide chain come together like a letter X. When one sees such a feature, one is not always sure whether two diagonally running segments (\ and /) are crossing, or whether two U-shaped segments are in contact. The wrong choice leads to the wrong connectivity.

How can the medicinal chemist determine that an error is likely, or not likely, to have been made? It helps to have some sense of the quality of the map. If the crystallographer provides a picture of the initial electron density map, one can look for the clarity of separation between the macromolecules and the solvent. The molecular boundary should be clear, since the solvent regions will have lower average density than that of the protein (Fig. 6.4). Unfortunately, many crystallographers employ a computational procedure

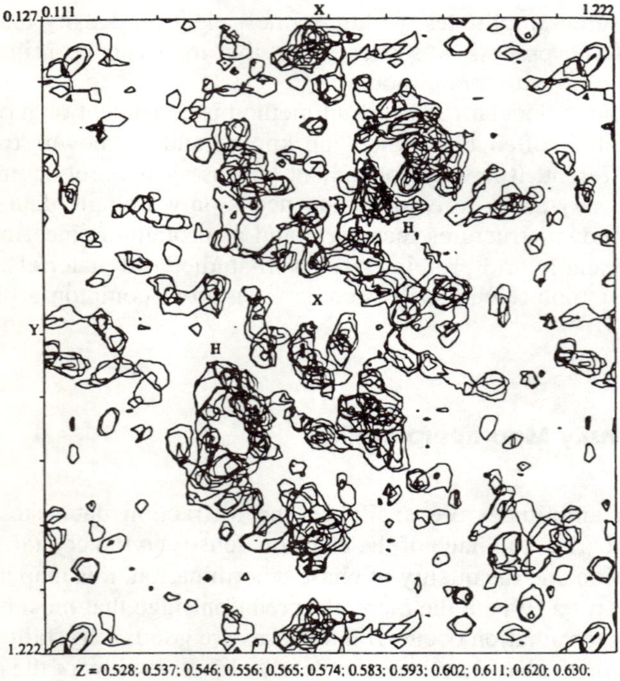

Fig. 6.4 Some sections of an early electron density map in a protein structure determination. Even at this stage the contrast between the molecule and the surrounding solvent is evident, a sign of a good map. Also, this protein is a dimer, and an approximate two-fold symmetry axis can be seen in the map at the position marked by an X. (Data from D.E. McRee, 'Practical Protein Crystallography', Academic Press, Inc., San Diego, 1993.)

called solvent-flattening to improve their phases by enhancing the contrast between protein and solvent. A picture of a solvent-flattened map will always show a spectacularly clear molecular boundary, but this tells the medicinal chemist nothing about the quality of the original map, which is a much better guide to the overall quality of the structure determination.

The path of the polypeptide chain will be discernible as a ribbon of continuous density with branches (the side chains) every 3.8 Å. At low resolution, α-helices may be apparent as rods of high density, but chain connectivity is rarely obvious at 6 or 5 Å resolution. Structures determined at 3 Å resolution should show helices clearly and the strands of β-sheets will appear as twisted ropes of density with side chains pointing alternately in opposite directions. At 3 Å resolution the direction of the chain can be determined, since side chain branching density in helices slants back towards the N-terminus of the helix.

Breaks in the continuity of the polypeptide chain electron density cause problems in the interpretation, since the crystallographer must guess how the discontinuous pieces are joined. Serious errors in connectivity can occur from guessing wrongly! A map that presents no such ambiguities is much more likely to yield a correct final structure.

In a 3 Å resolution map it may be possible to identify bulky side chains such as tryptophan, but in general even at high resolution it is impossible to derive the sequence of the polypeptide or nucleotide from the electron density map alone. Sequence information is essential in generating an accurate atomic model, even from the best maps.

Unfortunately, many sequences contain errors, even those determined by sequencing cloned DNA. (We have hardly ever determined the crystal structure of a protein without detecting at least one sequence error!) After the molecular boundary and chain direction and path have been determined, building of the atomic model usually starts with an attempt to fit part of the known sequence into the map. A segment of polypeptide with a number of aromatic residues is often chosen first, as these large side chains give characteristic large flat electron density at medium to high resolution. Heavy-atom binding sites may provide markers that allow the sequence to be aligned with the electron density. For example, mercury has a high affinity for sulfur and reacts to form a covalent derivative, so mercury binding sites are often the locations of accessible cysteine residues. Computer graphics devices are used to display the map as a basket of lines, with the model superimposed in a different colour in stick representation. Fitting programs allow one to position the model into the density and alter the conformational parameters of the main and side chain groups so as to achieve the optimal fit.

The process is highly subjective and mistakes are likely, especially if the map is poor in quality due to low-resolution, badly measured data, imperfect model structure in the case of molecular replacement phasing, or lack of isomorphism in the derivatives in the case of MIR phasing. Even a good map can have confusing regions if the molecule is flexible and the density in that part of the map represents contributions from more than one conformation. In the end, the crystallographer will try to generate a tentative atomic model with positions for most, if not all, of the residues in the protein or nucleic acid.

Refinement

Once an atomic model has been built, some idea of its quality can be obtained by Fourier transforming its electron density to obtain calculated reflection amplitudes and phases. Comparison of the calculated amplitudes with those actually measured from the crystal by film or area detector yields a quantity denoted R, the crystallographic residual:

$$R = \text{sum} \mid F_{\text{obs}} - F_{\text{calc}} \mid / \text{ sum } \mid F_{\text{obs}} \mid$$

where the F values are the amplitudes and the sums are over all measured reflections. If the model and data were both error-free, R would = 0, but that never happens. A random ensemble of atoms that occupied the same fraction of space as the true structure would give $R = 0.59$. It is somewhat sobering that the crude atomic models obtained from the first fitting of an electron density map usually have $R = 0.45$ or so. An R-factor of this magnitude implies that the average random coordinate error in the structure is close to 1 Å, and that a number of errors of interpretation may exist. Nevertheless, these models are demonstrably better than random and they can be improved. The process of improvement is called refinement.

Structure refinement is based on the comparison of observed and calculated structure amplitudes used in the R-factor. If the reflection amplitudes calculated from the model do not agree well with the measured data, it is possible to define a least-squares function

$$\text{Function} = \text{sum } (F_{\text{obs}} - F_{\text{calc}})^2$$

which should be a minimum for the best model that the data can provide. The sum is taken over all measured reflections. Minimization of this function is a non-linear least-squares problem and therefore cannot be achieved in one step, but some very sophisticated computational methods have been developed to make small changes in the model so that the value of the function is reduced, albeit slowly. Many cycles of refinement are required, and the computer algorithms cannot make very large corrections to the structure, so every so often the process must be interrupted and the model must be rebuilt manually. Monitoring the R-factor is one way to tell when manual intervention is necessary; it will decrease as the function decreases and will level off when the least-squares approach cannot make any further improvements. Manual rebuilding is greatly aided by the refinement, however, since as the *R*-factor decreases the quality of phases calculated from the refined model will increase. New electron density maps calculated with measured data and phases computed from the atomic model should be greatly improved over the original error-filled maps, and better interpretation of problem areas should be possible. Refinement is tedious and time-consuming, but can dramatically improve a structure: the final *R*-factors for most well-refined protein crystal structures are usually 0.20 or lower. Zero is never achieved because the measured data have errors of at least a few per cent, proteins have regions of conformational flexibility that are difficult to characterize, and the large regions of disordered solvent in the crystal are impossible to model accurately.

The precision of a protein crystal structure can be estimated from its *R*-factor and resolution. Unrefined structures at medium resolution can have huge errors and should never be trusted quantitatively, although they may give a fairly accurate picture of the polypeptide chain fold and the relative arrangements in space of the side chains. Refined structures at near 3 Å resolution will still have average positional errors of 0.5 Å or more, and so they cannot be used to decide if two groups are within hydrogen-bonded distance of one another. Refined structures at 2 Å resolution will have coordinate precision of about 0.3 Å and can be used to infer most details of hydrogen bonding. Bound solvent molecules can also be located correctly at this resolution. Structures refined at 1.5 Å resolution or better will have positional errors of 0.2 Å or less and errors in bond angles of only a few degrees.

It is important to remember that all of these error ranges are in precision, not accuracy. Even high-resolution structures with very low *R*-factors may have a few wrongly placed atoms, although gross errors of interpretation are less likely. As protein crystallography becomes more and more a routine tool for structure/function investigation, experimental details are often too tersely reported for even an experienced referee to be certain that no mistakes have been made. We have tried in this chapter to give the medicinal chemist who wishes to use structural information some indication of where problems can arise and what sort of warning signs to watch for, but it is our belief that no number, or set of numbers, can reliably indicate the accuracy of a protein structure determination.

Fortunately, there is a completely reliable indicator that does not depend on any number at all. It is biochemical common sense. The structure must explain and be consistent with the body of experimental data for the molecule in question. If it does, it is probably right in general and also in most of its details. If it does not, it is almost certainly wrong in whole or in part. Every incorrect protein structure, without exception, could have been suspected immediately by this criterion regardless of any of the published experimental details or 'reliability' indices. Of course, if only one or two experiments out of many are inconsistent with the structure, one should probably also question those experiments. But incorrect structures nearly always fail to explain many things, not just one or two. We urge you to try this method of judging structures for yourself, on a structure that was shown to be completely incorrect: Ghosh *et al.* (1981) reports the original, incorrect structure and Antonio *et al.* (1982) and Beinert *et al.* (1983) illustrate how the structure made no sense in terms of the spectroscopic data on the cofactor; Stout *et al.*, (1988) report the correct structure determination, which fits the spectroscopic data beautifully).

The wise medicinal chemist – and the wise crystallographer! – will therefore always check to see if the structure makes sense in terms of what is known about the molecule from experimental data, and if the structure does not explain the results of, say, nearly all of the mutagenesis experiments, the structure should be questioned. In crystallography, as in other things, *caveat emptor* is good advice.

Exploiting the Structure

Protein crystallography provides a large amount of information about a protein which can be exploited rapidly. If the structure of the protein does not change very much when ligands (such as enzyme inhibitors) bind, it may be possible to diffuse them into the crystal lattice and let them form a complex within the active site without having the crystal fall apart. Alternatively, one can co-crystallize the protein in the presence of the small molecule and hope that crystals of the complex will grow under much the same conditions as the native crystals. Co-crystallization is more problematic than diffusing ligands into native crystals, but it does obviate the concern that lattice forces in a pre-grown native crystal might inhibit binding or block important conformational changes.

Ligand binding will cause the intensities in the diffraction pattern to change, but the phases will not change very much if the overall structure has not changed. Thus, for the structure of the protein–ligand complex, the phase problem has already been solved! To determine the structure of the complex, one just measures the amplitudes of the reflections from the crystal of the complex, and computes an electron density map with coefficients ($F_{\mathrm{pl}} - F_{p}$), where F_{p} is the amplitude of the reflection from the native crystal and F_{pl} is the amplitude from the crystal with the ligand bound. The phases for each reflection are just the phases determined experimentally for the native structure, or calculated from the refined atomic model. Such a map is called a difference electron density map and it shows the location of the additional electron density due to the bound ligand and any changes induced in the structure of the protein.

Calculation of a difference map for any ligand complex requires only a few days, most of which time is spent collecting the data. If the map is easy to interpret, one can thus produce a good atomic model for, say, an enzyme–drug complex in less than a week. Mutant proteins produced by recombinant DNA technology can be analysed equally rapidly. This ease of exploitation of a structure is the reward for all of the agony that went before.

Of course, the structure of the protein–ligand complex or of the mutant protein may be sufficiently different from the native structure that the crystals are not isomorphous or even in the same unit cell and space-group. If that happens, the original phases cannot be used and one faces the problem of solving a new structure. However, the path to such a solution is clear: one can usually employ molecular replacement using the refined native structure as the search model, and if that fails, one can simply use the same heavy atom derivatives that worked the previous time.

Some Case Studies

Aldose reductase is an enzyme that has been implicated in complications of juvenile diabetes (Harrison *et al.*, 1994). It uses NADPH to reduce a variety of aldehyde substrates to the corresponding alcohols. Although glucose is not the normal physiological substrate for aldose reductase, when intracellular glucose concentrations are high, as in diabetes, aldose reductase will reduce the glucose to sorbitol. The build-up of sorbitol in, for example, the eye lenses of diabetic patients is thought to be a primary cause of diabetic retinopathy leading to blindness. Thus, inhibition of human aldose reductase is of considerable clinical interest.

Unfortunately, aldose reductase is a member of an extensive family of enzymes with similar amino acid sequences, active sites and catalytic functions. Inhibitors of aldose reductase are likely to inhibit one or more of its family members as well, since all of these enzymes are not very specific. Such cross-reactivity is thought to be the cause of the major side-effects that have prevented the effective use of aldose reductase inhibitors in therapy for juvenile diabetes.

To provide more specific aldose reductase inhibitors, we undertook the refinement of the structure of the human enzyme at high (1.8 Å) resolution. When we examined the active site in the high-resolution electron density map, we saw a region of electron density that could not be explained in terms of either the amino acid sequence of the protein or the structure of the bound NADP cofactor. Apparently, an endogenous ligand for the enzyme had followed the protein throughout the purification and crystallization procedure.

Nature had thus provided us with a lead compound; the only problem was to figure out what it was. Careful refinement of the crystal structure of the protein caused the region to become clearly interpretable as the electron density of a bound citrate molecule (Plate 6.1) (Harrison *et al.*, 1994). Tests on the enzyme in solution confirmed that citrate was indeed an inhibitor of human aldose reductase. Citrate was used as a buffer during the handling of the protein, and bound tightly enough to the active site to survive all the steps in protein crystallography. Further tests revealed that other anionic molecules also bound to the same site; this unexpected 'anion well' in the aldose reductase active site now provides the focus for a drug-design strategy that will produce anionic inhibitors that may be more specific for aldose reductase than any currently available.

This story has parallels in other crystallographic investigations. Endogenous inhibitory peptides have been found in the crystal structures of several proteolytic enzymes, and the discovery of a bound peptide in the structure of the major histocompatability protein led to new insights into how the immune system presents antigens (Bjorkman *et al.*, 1987).

Since proteins come in families of similar structure and often function, the problem for the medicinal chemist is often not one of maximizing affinity but rather of gaining specificity. The two properties are less-closely related than one might hope. It is instructive to see how nature solves this problem. A particularly effective protease inhibitor is the leech protein hirudin, a potent and highly specific inhibitor of thrombin. Analogues of hirudin have considerable clinical importance as anti-clotting agents. Examination of the crystal structure of the thrombin–hirudin complex (Rydel *et al.*, 1990) shows that hirudin interacts with two distinct and widely separated sites on its target protease. Its N-terminal region interacts with the thrombin active site, but other serine proteases such as trypsin have similar active sites. Hirudin gets additional specificity and affinity from the interaction of its C-terminal end

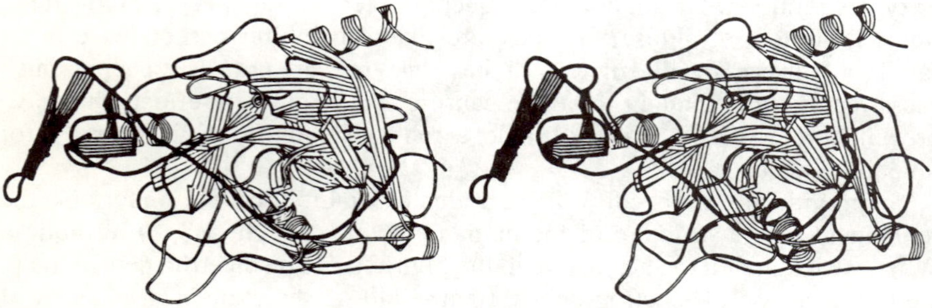

Fig. 6.5 Stereo drawing of the complex of thrombin (light lines) with the leech protein hirudin (thick lines), which inhibits thrombin. Although hirudin binds in the active site of thrombin (left side), it also wraps around thrombin to make another set of interactions at a distant site (right side). This extra site adds specificity and affinity (Rydel *et al.*, 1990).

with another binding site, on the back side of the thrombin molecule from the active site (Fig. 6.5).

Molecules such as hirudin can identify such remote sites. In some cases, crystallographic studies of a series of inhibitor–enzyme complexes may reveal multiple binding modes, for analogous compounds do not always bind analogously (Mattos *et al.*, 1994). These other sites provide regions on the protein surface that are targets for the design of 'Hydra-headed' inhibitors, but very distant sites like the secondary hirudin binding site will be missed by looking at active-site directed inhibitor structures only.

Ringe and co-workers have developed an experimental method to map the complete binding surface of any crystalline protein (Fitzpatrick *et al.*, 1993). The method is conceptually simple: one transfers crystals of the target protein into various organic solvents and determines their structures at sufficiently high resolution that bound solvent molecules can be identified unambiguously (in practice, for most organic solvents employed this means 2.2 Å resolution or higher). The solvents are chosen to probe the binding of various organic functional groups to the protein surface. For example, if one wishes to locate binding sites for hydrophobic aromatic groups, one soaks the crystal in benzene or toluene. If peptide binding sites are desired, *N*-methyl formamide is the solvent of choice. Acetonitrile provides a probe for guanidino side chains, while methanol looks like the side chain of serine, and so forth. About six or seven solvent structures will give a virtually complete map of the protein surface. Medicinal chemists can then 'connect the dots' to make compounds that bridge between any desired sites.

This method has been carried out for several proteins and the results may be summarized as follows: very high concentrations of organic solvents are not required (as little as 20% of the solvent in water by volume will usually reveal the strongest binding sites); all organic solvents bind to the active site region, suggesting that it is generally 'sticky'; most of the ordered water molecules on the surface of the protein are not displaced, even in 100% water-miscible organic solvent; only a few organic molecules (usually < 12) are bound even in 100% organic solvent; and finally, the sites of solvent binding tend to cluster, so that secondary binding sites other than the active site are easy to identify by this technique.

Ringe has examined the binding sites and has formed a conclusion that has profound implications for computer-based drug design. If one examines the surface of a protein, in principle there are dozens of places where functional groups could bind and make excellent interactions. Yet they do not. Why are only a few sites seen? What makes a binding site a binding site? The answer seems to be the ease with which water can be displaced from that site. Computational approaches to site identification that ignore the contribution of water would seem to be limited in efficacy.

These case studies illustrate the power of protein crystallography as a tool in drug design. Although protein crystallography is a tedious and time-consuming technique, it can provide information of a detail and importance that few other methods can approach.

Two useful articles on the subject are those by Branden and Tooze (1991) and Moffat (1984).

References

Antonio, M.A., Averill, B.A., Moura, I., Moura, J.J.G., Orme-Johnson, W.H., Teo, B.K. and Xavier, A.V. (1982). *J. Biol. Chem.* **257**, 6646–6649.

Beinert, H., Emptage, M.H., Dreyer, J.-L., Scott, R.A., Hahn, J.E., Hodgson, K.O. and Thomson, A.J. (1983). *Proc. Natl Acad. Sci. USA* **80**, 393–396.

Bjorkman, P.J., Saper, M.A., Samraoui, B., Bennett, W.S., Strominger, J.L. and Wiley, D.C. (1987). *Nature* **329**, 506–512.

Branden, C.I. and Tooze, J. (1991). 'Introduction to Protein Structure'. Garland, New York.

Fitzpatrick, P.A., Steinmetz, A.C.U., Ringe, D. and Klibanov, A.M. (1993). *Proc. Natl Acad. Sci. USA* **90**, 8653–8657.

Ghosh, D., Furey, W., Jr., O'Donnell, S. and Stout, C.D. (1981). *J. Biol. Chem.* **256**, 4185–4192.

Harrison, D.H., Bohren, K., Ringe, D., Petsko, G.A. and Gabbay, K.H. (1994). *Biochemistry* **33**, 2011–2020.

Kuriyan, J., Kong, X.P., Krishna, T.S.R., Sweet, R.M., Murgolo, N.J., Field, H., Cerami, A. and Henderson, G.B. (1991). *Proc. Natl Acad. Sci. USA* **88**, 8769–8773.

Mattos, C., Rasmussen, B., Ding, X., Petsko, G.A. and Ringe, D. (1994). *Nature Struct. Biol.* **1**, 55–58.

Moffat, K. (1984). Macromolecular crystallography. *In* 'Structural and Resonance Techniques in Biological Research' (D.L. Rousseau, ed.). Academic Press, New York.

Moore, M.J., Distefano, M.D., Walsh, C.T., Schiering, N. and Pai, E.F. (1989). *J. Biol. Chem.* **264**, 14386–14388.

Rydel, T.J., Ravichandran, K.G., Tulinsky, A., Bode, W., Huber, R., Roitsch, C. and Fenton, J.W. II (1990). *Science* **249**, 277–280.

Stout, G.H., Turley, S., Sieker, L. and Jensen, L.H. (1988). *Proc. Natl Acad. Sci. USA* **85**, 1020–1022.

Discussion

R.A. Lewis

In the last example, you were talking about designing ligands which will bind to two discrete binding sites on the enzyme. One of the problems with designing such ligands, however, is that the positions of protein side chains have to be known accurately to avoid steric clashes. You have described designing ligands which will span the surface of the protein. In my experience, protein side chains on the surface tend to have the largest *B* factors and, therefore, the largest uncertainties in the positioning of the side chains. How do you get around the problem of designing, trying to thread your way through a forest of side chains when the precise position of the chains is not known?

G.A. Petsko

To be frank, I do not think it is as big a problem as many people believe, and that the surface of the protein will give more help than might be thought. Most sites in proteins have considerable ability to adjust themselves to the size and shape of the ligands there. Once it has been recognised that a particular type of ligand is needed with roughly certain functional groups that fit to a site that can shed its solvent easily, the plasticity of protein structure will help.

There will certainly not be an optimal fit with the first experiments, but that does not matter because the real power of X-ray crystallography is not so much in lead compound discovery but in second generation design. If something can be found that bridges to that site, even if it binds relatively poorly, it will help us see what to do next when that structure is done. This is the strategy I would advocate. It is rapid; such a structure takes only a day or two to solve, and is also incredibly informative.

With elastase, for example, things can be put into the elastase P_1 pocket, and peptides will still bind perfectly well to the surface of the elastase. Other sites can be picked out: a peptide that would normally go into P_1 and P_2 will go into P_1' and P_2', for example.

E. Westhof

In the case of the TIM barrel proteins, are there methods of guessing from the sequence that they indeed fold into a TIM barrel?

G.A. Petsko

There are several methods. One way is to do secondary structure prediction. Secondary structure predictions, like Chou and Fasman, give limited information, but if there is a pattern, such as sheet–helix–sheet–helix – repeated four times, it is quite likely that there is a TIM barrel protein, even though the exact ranges of those secondary structure elements may be predicted incorrectly.

An even better, and very powerful, method was developed by David Eisenberg and his associates at UCLA, and almost simultaneously by Janet Thornton at University College, London. This method involves taking a sequence, threading it on to many different protein stuctures, and seeing which threading – which fitting – of the sequence on to the structure produces hydrophobic residues on the inside, hydrophilic residues on the outside, reasonable packing and environments for the various side chains, and so forth. It can take the entire sequence database and pick out roughly two-thirds of the known TIM barrel enzymes. It misses some, but it gets an astonishing number of them right.

E. Westhof

What about the active site? Is it always at the same position within the topological fold?

G.A. Petsko

In TIM barrel enzymes the active site is always in the same place. If the structure of a TIM barrel is known, the exact position of the active site is known. This is not true of all other enzymes, but it is true, for example, of nucleotide-binding folds. There, too, the active site is always in the same place.

A.R. Leach

As you know, various computational methods, such as GRID or multiple conformation simulation search (MCSS) can now try to find regions within a protein binding site where functional groups such as the ones you showed are bound. Have you compared these to experimentally observed, bound ligands?

G.A. Petsko

Professor Ringe is working closely with Martin Karplus to improve the MCSS method. She has looked at predictions for elastase. What happens is fascinating. Both the GRID and the MCSS methods find a lot of the sites that I showed, but they also find about 100 more that are *not* binding sites for organic solvents. These computational methods are not sufficiently discriminatory. The energy functions do not provide enough discrimination between where the molecules do and do not bind. A reason may be that those methods – those calculations – do not really take into account the fact that the competition with water is the key to whether or not something can bind.

The good news is that the binding sites will be found. The bad news is that we will not know which ones they are amongst all the sites that are found.

Those methods will now be improved because there is now a database of protein structures with bound organic solvent molecules.

K. Zakrzewska

We have heard a lot about hydrogen bonds and their importance for specificity. In many complexes there are water-mediated hydrogen bonds. What is their importance? Are they important as an artefact of crystallization?

G.A. Petsko

Much has to do with where we are. On the surface of a protein, to make or not to make a hydrogen bond may be more or less equal, but if it is slightly buried away from contact with the solvent, although I cannot predict what a hydrogen bond will be worth, I can say that it is very bad not to make one. It seems worth going to a lot of trouble to avoid having an unsatisfied hydrogen bond donor or acceptor that is buried away from contact with solvent.

K. Zakrzewska
I think the complex between Trp repressor and DNA was famous in that there were no direct hydrogen bonds between DNA and protein, and everything was mediated through water. The question arises because in all these programs like CAVEAT the possibility is never taken into account that binding via water molecules may be important.

G.A. Petsko
In most of the crystal structures of enzyme substrate complexes there are usually at least one or two water molecules that remain in the active site and bridge between one part of the substrate and the protein. I think we are just beginning to understand how important this can be. We certainly know in some cases that it costs us quite a lot if those interactions are taken away.

C.G. Wermuth
I understand that for a given enzyme, for example, if a crystallographic study is done with one inhibitor there is one result, with another inhibitor the docking may be different, and with a third inhibitor different again. How can this be handled with pharmacophore identification and molecular modelling?

G.A. Petsko
In a situation like this where something seems to be going against us, it always seems to me that it should be taken as an opportunity. What I think is happening with something like this is that, without intending to do it, the complete binding characteristics of the active site region are being mapped. Those characteristics will be different between different related members of the family of enzymes. So, if some of those multiple points of contacts can be exploited in the building of the molecule, it may or may not buy affinity – but it should buy quite a lot of specificity.

Proteins are known to behave like this when they interact with each other. When a protease inhibitor interacts with its target protease, it does not make interactions only with the P_1, P_2 and P_1' sites but also makes some additional interactions with sites slightly removed from the active site. These may or may not contribute much to the overall affinity, but they probably contribute considerably to helping that inhibitor be specific for its target protease.

I.D. Kuntz
I think the various analysis schemes should be approached with caution. We need to remind ourselves that there may be alternative binding modes, and ask

whether a strategy can be adopted that searches for them and brings them forward at whatever level we are working.

J.S. Mason
Pharmacophore models generally are just a distillation of known information, they are not precise. Therefore, with different binding modes the distances between the key groups may well be similar. I would always advocate doing a search with a widish tolerance, and then those different compounds will be found. They then need to be docked into the active site by simulation or, better still, by crystallography.

I do not think the pharmacophore models are necessarily invalidated by multiple binding modes; it just needs to be taken into account that they are a general model containing a lot of information – but they *do* contain that information. Even if the model is wrong in one aspect, inherent in that model is a lot of true data. Our experience is that a hit from a particular pharmacophore model may well be found, but it may not dock quite how we expected – but the information is in there, in that model.

G.A. Petsko
I am often asked about outstanding examples of the success of structure-based or computer-aided drug design. I am never quite sure how to respond. What is the most striking success of this procedure *vis-à-vis* the more traditional approach?

J.S. Mason
I think the word 'success' is difficult. This was a subject of discussion with regard to the Computational Chemistry List about three months ago. A lot of examples were discussed there. It depends whether we mean success in terms of finding a lead now or in terms of a compound that is on the market.

G.A. Petsko
The latter.

P. Potier
I am very pleased that this question has been raised, and will try to define it more precisely. I would like a list of successes, first, successes in finding binding etc. – and finally successes in finding a drug.

J.S. Mason
A success to me is finding a lead quickly when we start to screen, on which the medicinal chemists can work and apply all their many years of knowledge to turn into a drug on the market. We have lots of successes because we are finding leads – which I think is true worldwide across all the groups.

It is difficult to list products on the market whose success is due to rational drug design, because of the very long time lag between a compound we find now in screening and bringing it to the market. I say, yes, these methods are successful, but success should not be counted in terms of whether the compound we have found or have designed is now on the market.

C.G. Wermuth
Asking what is done with computers is like asking an organic chemist to publish which successes are due to NMR – it is a tool.

P. Potier
Yes, but it is important to know how successful is NMR.

C.G. Newton
We have to remember, first, the time lag in the pharmaceutical industry between the design of a molecule and getting it on to the market-place; second, that the first protein to be solved by X-ray crystallography was in about 1962 or 1963 (Dr Petsko will correct me if I am wrong), and even by 1968 the structure of only four proteins had been solved. We are now solving structures at the rate of one a day. In the next 10 years I think there will certainly be drugs on the market whose success in research and development has been due to that technique.

The same is true in organic chemistry. It has been said at organic chemistry meetings, for example, that ranitidine, the most successful drug of all time, is currently synthesised by a sequence of types of reactions many of which date to the last century. There is a time lag in organic chemistry as well as in the techniques used in drug design.

I should like to ask Dr Petsko for three predictions:

1) How many families of proteins does he think will be found?
2) By what date does he think it will be possible to assign a new protein to one of those families without having to conduct the X-ray?
3) Dr Ashton talked about a number of polycycles in some of the compounds that are designed by rational design. Taxol or taxotere probably has as many cycles as anything that comes out of Dr Dean's SKELGEN program. Can Dr Petsko predict when he thinks the X-ray crystal structure of taxol bound to its receptor protein might be found? I would be very interested to see it.

G.A. Petsko

1) *How many families of proteins will be found?* If the number of proteins in different families is plotted as a histogram, we can get the beginnings of a distribution function. If some assumptions are made about the shape of this distribution function – which a couple of clever people have done – we

come up with an estimate of 1000 or less protein structural families, which is not a big number. My opinion is that it will be less than 500 – but it is all within the same order of magnitude. There are about 100 now, so we are either 10% or 20% of the way there, if the distribution is an accurate reflection of the number of families. This does not of course include membrane proteins, which remain an uncertain aspect of this calculation.

2) *By what date will it be possible to assign a new protein to one of those families without having to conduct the X-ray?* Because of what I have just said we can do quite a good job now, in many cases, of predicting protein structures based on the sequence. Almost as often as not, a sequence of a newly cloned and sequenced gene turns out to be similar to another gene whose sequence is known. We are rapidly approaching the stage when it will also be similar to a protein whose structure is known. When that happens, the folding problem will become of purely academic interest: there will be no need to predict the folding of a protein from its sequence because it will be possible to get the structure by homology with another protein. I think we will be there for most sequences by the end of this decade.
3) *Can it be predicted when the X-ray crystal structure of taxol bound to its protein might be found?* The receptor for taxol is tubulin. Serge Timashev and Dagmar Ringe have tried for 4 years, thus far without success, to get a preparation of tubulin that is sufficiently monodisperse even to try to crystallize it. I would not care to make a prediction on this. I think it will need really good biochemistry before the crystallography can be done.

P. Potier
In terms of protein structure, of course the situation probably becomes more difficult as soon as the proteins are dimeric or trimeric.

G.A. Petsko
That used to be so, but it is no longer true.

P. Potier
Tubulin is certainly the major target of compounds like taxol, vinblastine and so on, but the problem is more complicated than it appears. Take the micro-tubular-associated proteins for example. I am sure their nature depends on the nature of the cell and on the cell cycle, so there is a large variety of them. Perhaps as interesting as the structure of tubulin – when it is known – is the nature of the microtubular-associated proteins, possibly including oncogenes, proto-oncogenes and growth factors (which, by the way, are sometimes the same), anti-oncogenes, etc. I think a lot of work has yet to be done.

7

Molecular Modelling of the Adenosine A_1 Receptor

A.P. IJZERMAN, P.J.M. VAN GALEN and E.M. VAN DER WENDEN

Leiden/Amsterdam Center for Drug Research, Division of Medicinal Chemistry, PO Box 9502, 2300RA Leiden, The Netherlands

Introduction

Computer-assisted molecular modelling (CAMM) is a relatively new and rapidly developing tool in drug design. Computer graphics techniques allow the transformation of complex data sets obtained from theoretical chemical calculations into a picture on a computer screen. Calculated chemical structures and their properties may thus be visualized, manipulated and matched with other relevant molecules. It thus becomes possible to expand the perspective of conventional molecular models, such as Dreiding or CPK. With regard to drug design it is often possible to delineate qualitative and quantitative features of ligands specifically or selectively interacting with a receptor (subtype) or other biologically relevant proteins. CAMM may help to further understand drug action and lead to a more rational approach towards drug design.

In this chapter CAMM techniques will be applied to the adenosine A_1 receptor. Adenosine receptors belong to the large family of G-protein coupled receptors. There are at least four adenosine receptor subtypes: A_1, A_{2A}, A_{2B} and A_3. All subtypes have been cloned, and have been implicated in various physiological and pathophysiological conditions. The adenosine A_1 receptor is rather ubiquitous in the body, and appears to be involved in cardiovascular and renal function, as well as in the CNS. Some marketed

New Perspectives in Drug Design
ISBN 0–12–208070–X

drugs, such as adenosine (agonist), theophylline and enprofylline (both antagonists), target adenosine receptors. Adenosine receptors also play an important role in the pharmacology of caffeine.

Two complementary approaches will be dealt with. First, a series of ligands (both agonists and antagonists) will be examined to extract three-dimensional information from their structure–affinity relationships (SAR). Second, this information will be used in the construction of a receptor model, based on the atomic coordinates of a related protein, bacteriorhodopsin.

Computational Methods

All methods have been described extensively (Van Galen *et al.*, 1989; Van der Wenden *et al.*, 1991; IJzerman *et al.*, 1992). Ligand modelling was mainly done with the Chem-X package (Chemical Design Ltd.), although all energy calculations were done with the semi-empirical molecular orbital program MOPAC. The software program BIOGRAF (Molecular Simulations Inc.) was used to generate the receptor model, based on the atomic coordinates of bacteriorhodopsin, as retrieved from the Brookhaven Protein Databank (reference code 1BRD). Transmembrane domains in the adenosine receptor were predicted from standard routines available in the Sequence Analysis Software Package (Devereux *et al.*, 1984).

Results

Ligand Modelling

Literature survey

A search of the available literature yielded the affinities (averaged K_i values) of a range of adenosine receptor ligands. Tables 7.1 and 7.2 show a selection of N^6-substituted adenosine derivatives (all agonists) and C8-substituted xanthines (all antagonists), respectively. The total number of compounds examined to map the adenosine receptor was 62.

Conformational analysis

Because of the mutual interaction between receptor and ligand, the receptor-bound conformation of the ligand is not necessarily the lowest energy conformation when not bound. This implies that a survey of energetically acceptable conformations is warranted rather than a search for the unique conformation in the absolute energy minimum. In this study we chose an

Table 7.1

pK_i values of 26 N^6-substituted adenosine derivatives, in order of decreasing affinity at adenosine A_1 receptors

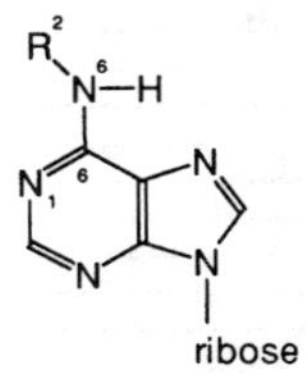

		pK_i			pK_i
R-1-Phenyl-2-butyl	(*R*-PBA)	9.28	*R*-1-Phenyl-2-propyl	(*R*-PIA)	8.62
Cyclopentyl	(CPA)	9.19	1-Methylcyclopentyl		8.44
Endo-2-norbornyl		9.17	*R*-1-Phenylethyl		8.17
7-Norbornyl		9.02	*R*-1-(1-Naphthyl)ethyl		7.74
3-Fluorophyl		9.00	*S*-1-Phenyl-2-butyl	(*S*-PBA)	7.59
Cyclobutyl		8.89	2-Adamanthyl		7.04
Exo-2-norbornyl		8.85	*S*-1-Phenyl-2-propyl	(*S*-PIA)	6.98
Cyclopropylmethyl		8.82	1-Methylcyclohexyl		6.85
Dicyclopropylmethyl		8.82	1-Adamantyl		6.84
3-Pentyl		8.82	Benzyl		6.60
S-2-Butyl		8.80	*S*-1-(1-Naphthyl)ethyl		6.20
Cyclohexyl	(CHA)	8.77	2-Phenyl-2-propyl		5.92
2-Methyl-1-propyl		8.70	2-Methyl-4-phenyl-2-butyl		5.84

Table 7.2

pK_i values of 12 1,3-dipropylxanthines with mainly non-aromatic substituents at the C8-position, in order of decreasing affinity for adenosine A_1 receptors. Values between parentheses are the pK_i values of the corresponding 7-methyl derivatives

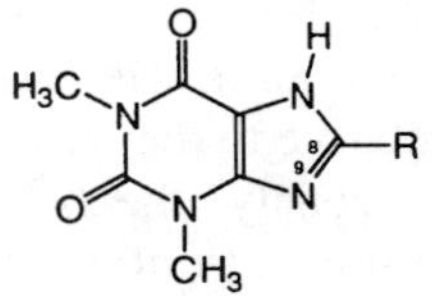

		pK_i		pK_i
Cyclopentyl	(DPCPX)	9.21 (5.64)	Cyclopropyl	7.38
Cyclohexyl		8.70 (5.57)	Cyclopent-3-ene	7.35
Cyclohex-3-ene		8.00	1-Piperazinyl	6.16
Cyclopentylmethyl		7.80	H	6.15 (5.28)
1-Piperidinyl		7.66	4-Piperidinyl	6.06
Cyclohexylmethyl		7.41	Benzyl	6.05

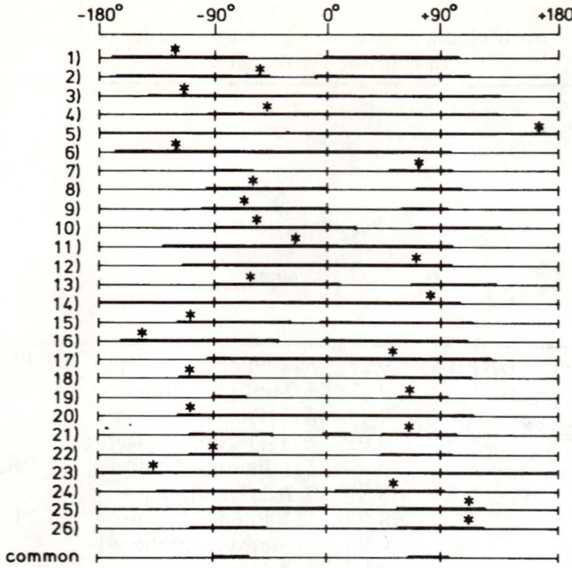

Fig. 7.1. Energetically allowed conformations for all N^6-substituted adenosine derivatives on rotation of the C6–N^6 bond. Thin lines stand for rejected conformations (5 kcal/mol or more from the minimum energy conformation, indicated by an asterisk). Thick lines indicate accepted conformations (less than 5 kcal/mol). The compounds are represented by numbers and follow Table 7.1. (Reproduced with permission from van Galen *et al.*, 1989, Elsevier Science.)

upper limit of 5 kcal/mol above the global minimum. Although this is an arbitrary choice, it has been accepted by many workers in the field.

The adenosine N^6-region

Analysis of the conformational flexibility of the various N^6-substituents was performed in two steps. The torsion angle N1–C6–N^6–C^2 defining the orientation of the N^6-substituent relative to the purine ring system, was rotated with an increment of 5°. Simultaneously, the N^6–C^2 bond was rotated with an increment of 20°, in order to prevent unfavorable steric interactions between the purine moiety and the N^6-substituent. Investigated in this way, most compounds in Table 7.1 appeared to have large rotational freedom. However, some compounds, including very potent ones, such as *R*-PBA (Table 7.1), are largely constrained around the C6–N^6 bond. The combined results of these efforts are shown in Fig. 7.1. Apparently, every single structure can adopt a common torsion angle N1–C6–N^6–C^2 of either between +60° and +90° (mean: +75°) or between −60° and −90° (mean: −75°). The bulk of the high-affinity ligands have a minimum energy conformation not far from the −75°

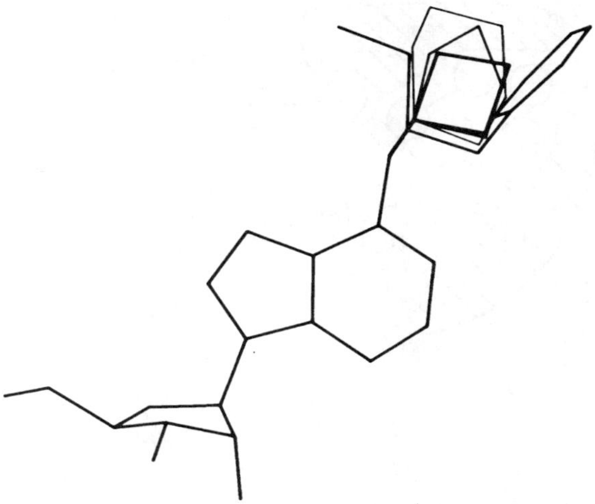

Fig. 7.2 Fit of *N*^{6}-cyclobutyladenosine, *N*^{6}-cyclopentyladenosine, *N*^{6}-cyclohexyladenosine and *R*-PBA. (Reproduced with permission from van Galen *et al.*, 1989, Elsevier Science.)

orientation. Therefore, the N1–C6–N^6–C^2 torsion angle was kept at this latter angle in the next step, viz. the calculation of the possible orientations of the remaining parts of the *N*^{6}-substituents. Again, most ligands have great rotational freedom again, except for the very bulky substituents.

Subsequently, the matching of all substituents (at the expense of some intramolecular energy) was aimed at. Several sets of compounds were analysed in this respect, in each case going from the minimum energy conformations of the set members to a more coincident fit. As an example, the superposition of four high-affinity derivatives is shown in Fig. 7.2.

Of all possible fits with varying numbers of compounds, one fit emerged in particular, since the average increase in intramolecular energy per ligand was 1.5 kcal/mol only. Moreover, the highest expenditure in energy to achieve this conformation (4 kcal/mol) was computed for two low-affinity ligands, viz. *N*^{6}-*R*-1-(1-naphthyl)ethyladenosine and *N*^{6}-2-phenyl-2-propyladenosine. Based on this fit, a comparison was made between the total volume of the first 14 more potent ligands in Table 7.1 and the space occupied by the remaining 12 less potent ones. This yielded a map (Fig. 7.3) of areas that contribute to affinity and other regions that diminish affinity (so-called forbidden areas). The subregions S1(A), S2, S3(A) and A had been defined before by Kusachi *et al.* (1985).

The xanthine C8-region

Analogous to the procedure described for the *N*^{6}-substituents in the adenosine receptor agonists, a conformational search was applied to C8-substituted

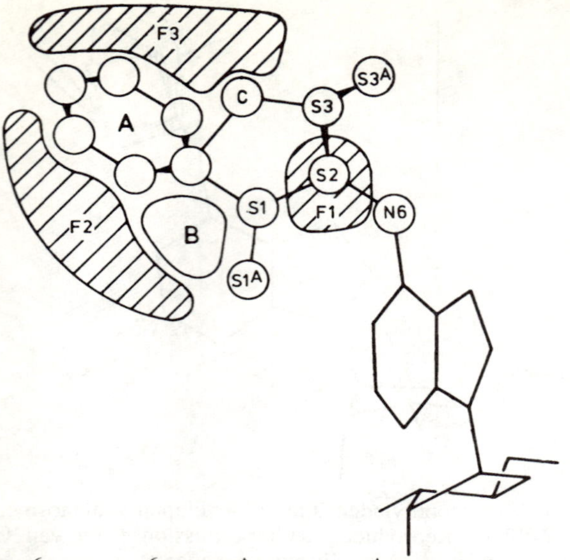

Fig. 7.3 Map of the N^6-region. N^6, S1, $S1^A$, S2, S3, $S3^A$ and A indicate the subregions defined by Kusachi *et al.* (1985). B and C indicate two new subregions: a **B**ulk and a **C**ycloalkyl subregion, respectively. F1, F2, and F3 indicate **F**orbidden areas. (Reproduced with permission from van Galen *et al.*, 1989, Elsevier Science.)

adenosine receptor antagonists. The compounds in Table 7.2 (with no methyl group present on N7) were rotated around the C8–C1′ bond, starting with the minimum energy conformation, varying the N9–C8–C1′–C2′ dihedral angle in 5° to 15° steps. In this way the only feasible dihedral angle was −30°.

From Table 7.2 it is evident that N7-methylation of adenosine receptor antagonists is inherently detrimental for affinity. Large differences in C8-substituents do not affect affinity as much as the introduction of a methyl group at an adjacent atomic position, which is also true for other C8-substituted derivatives not shown in Table 7.2. The energy cost to reach the torsion angle of −30° was 4.5 kcal/mol higher for 7-methyl-8-cyclopentyl-1,3-dipropylxanthine than for DPCPX (Fig. 7.4).

Similarly, this energy cost was 5.0 kcal/mol for the pair of C8-cyclohexyl substituted xanthines (data not shown). A receptor map for the cycloalkyl region, based primarily on the volume of the substituents and the energy cost to reach the dihedral angle of −30° is shown in Figure 7.5.

Receptor Modelling

Adenosine A_1 receptor topology

A two-dimensional model for the human adenosine A_1 receptor is shown in Fig. 7.6, based on the published amino acid sequence (Libert *et al.*, 1992). It is

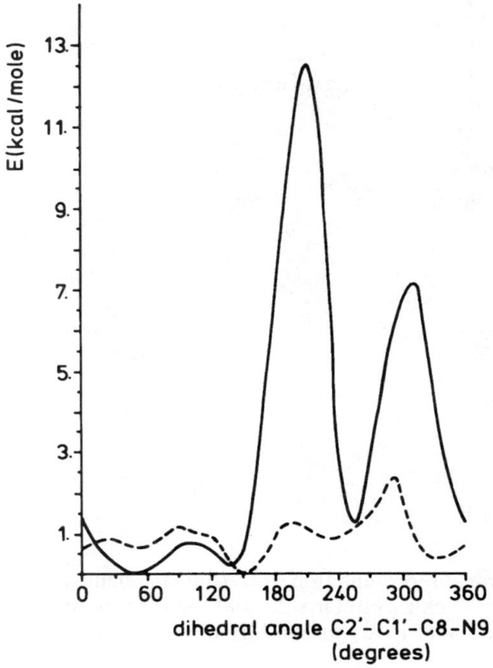

Fig. 7.4 The conformational energy cost vs. dihedral angle of DPCPX (dashed line) and 7-methyl-8-cyclopentyl-1,3-dipropylxanthine (solid line). (Reproduced with permission from van der Wenden *et al.*, 1991, Elsevier Science.)

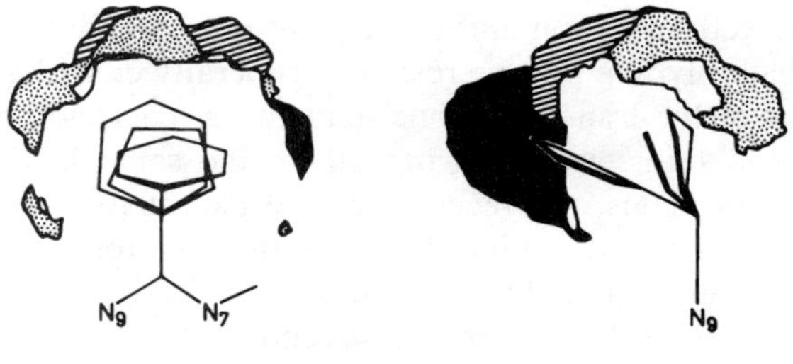

Fig. 7.5 The volume of some C8-substituents in order of decreasing affinity, fitting in the cycloalkyl region in the plane of the xanthine core (right) or 90° rotated (left). The volumes are coded as follows: white, cyclopentyl; dotted, cyclohexyl; shaded, cyclopentylmethyl; black, benzyl. (Reproduced with permission from van der Wenden *et al.*, 1991, Elsevier Science.)

typical of all G-protein coupled receptors, corresponding to a membrane-bound protein with seven relatively hydrophobic transmembrane domains of α-helical nature.

For the construction of a three-dimensional model of the adenosine A$_1$

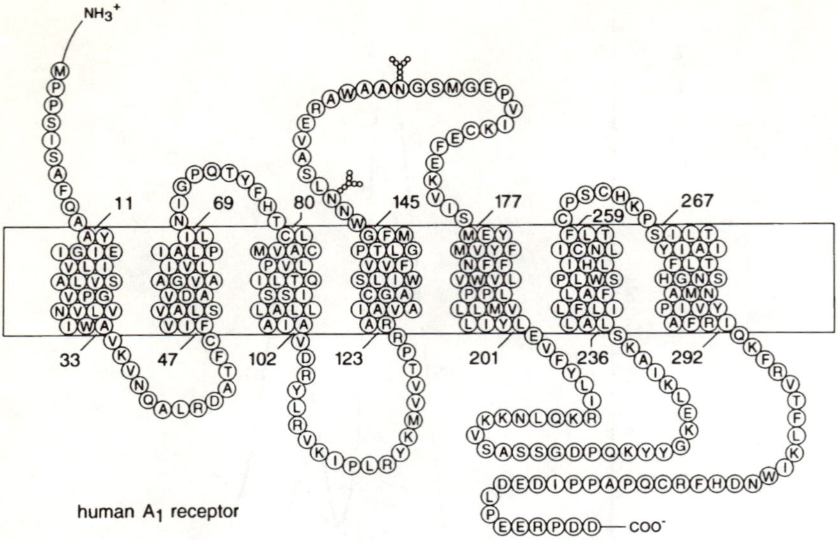

Fig. 7.6 Two-dimensional representation of the human adenosine A_1 receptor. The N-terminus is located on the extracellular side, and the C-terminus on the cytosolic side. Each amino acid is represented by the single letter notation.

receptor we used the atomic coordinates of bacteriorhodopsin (IJzerman *et al.*, 1992). Since no data for the non-membrane parts of this protein are available, only the transmembrane α-helices were modelled. The overall architecture of the receptor model is virtually identical to that of bacteriorhodopsin, due to the procedure followed: mutation and subsequent minimization. It should be mentioned here, that only five proline residues, generally considered as 'helix benders', form part of the transmembrane domains of bacteriorhodopsin, vs. eight in the corresponding parts (but not all on the same location) of the adenosine A_1 receptor. Thus, the receptor model can at its best be a crude approximation of biochemical reality. The two histidine residues (in helices VI and VII, respectively), thought to be important for ligand binding (see Discussion), faced the pore formed by the seven α-helices.

Docking of CPA, DPCPX and other ligands into the receptor model

CPA was docked in several orientations into the pore formed by the seven α-helices. As a starting point the histidine residues mentioned above were used as anchors for the interaction with CPA. Those possibilities with CPA entirely within the pore gave the highest, but not identical, interaction energies. The most favourable orientation was with the cyclopentyl substituent pointing to the extracellular side of the protein, close to helices IV, V and VI. Figure 7.7 is a graphical representation of this orientation.

Upon closer examination of the putative ligand binding site (Fig. 7.8) it can

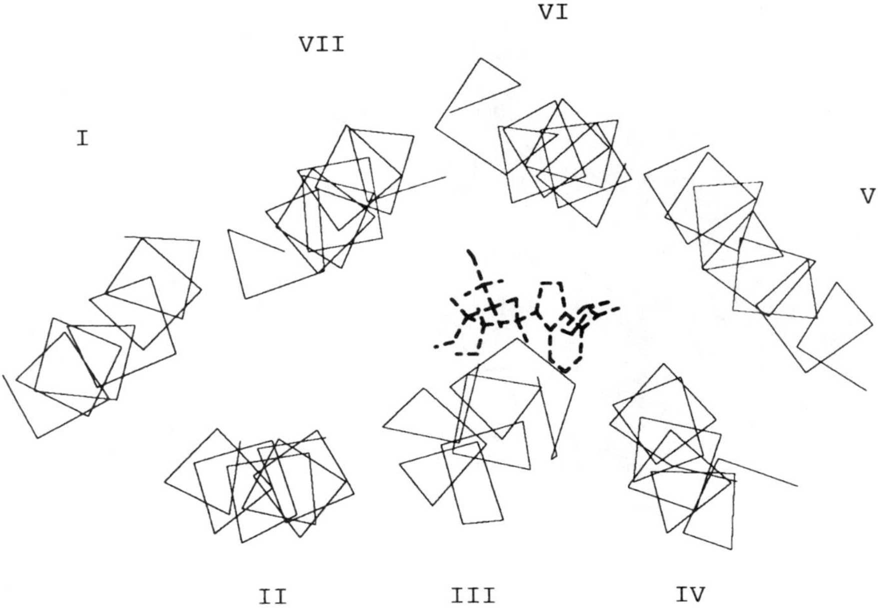

Fig 7.7 The binding of N^6-cyclopentyladenosine (CPA) to the human A_1 adenosine receptor (view from the extra- to the intracellular side). CPA is dashed. The receptor α-helical structure is represented by traces (connected Cα backbone atoms), without amino acid side chains.

be seen that CPA can be positioned to interact with the two histidine residues. The *cis*-diol group in the ribose moiety can form one (or maybe even two) hydrogen bond(s) with His278 in helix VII, whereas N^6–*H* may have a similar interaction with His251 in helix VI. The dihedral angle: N1–C6–N^6–C^2 of CPA in its receptor-bound conformation is −89°. The hydrophilic purine and ribose moiety (in an *anti* conformation) appear to be in a polar receptor region with several serine and threonine residues present (not shown). The hydrophobic cyclopentyl substituent, in contrast, is surrounded by two hydrophobic amino acids, viz. Val138 and Phe185.

The proposed binding site suggests that longer, i.e. more extended, N^6-substituents could also be accommodated. Indeed, derivatives with such characteristics can have high affinity (Van Galen *et al.*, 1987). In Fig. 7.9 a typical example, α,ω-di-(adenosin-N^6-yl)dodecane, has been docked, showing the relative freedom of large substituents by using the entire pore.

The potent antagonist DPCPX could also be docked in the region otherwise occupied by CPA. Three ways of superimposing agonists and antagonists can be discerned (Van der Wenden *et al.*, 1992). From the receptor modelling studies the mode in which both cyclopentyl substituents of CPA and DPCPX

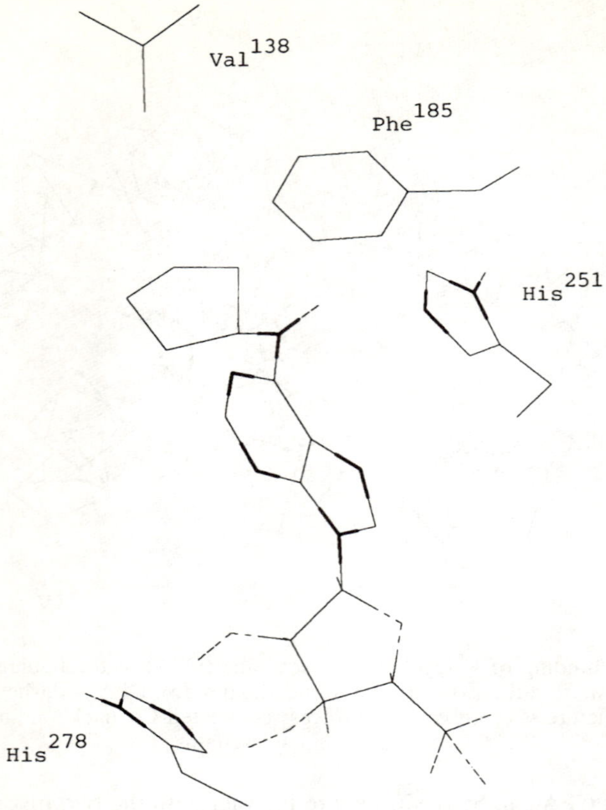

Fig. 7.8 Detail of the binding site of CPA in the human adenosine A_1 receptor. Shown are only four of the amino acid side chains that make up the entire binding site, for reasons of clarity. Thick atoms: nitrogen; dashed atoms: oxygen and hydrogen.

are overlapping is the more convincing (Fig. 7.10). This particular orientation appears to have more general validity, since longer C8-substituents, such as in XAC (xanthine amine congener), can also be accommodated in a way similar to the extended N^6-substituents in agonists. The dihedral angle over the N9–C8–C1′–C2′ bond in DPCPX is −6°.

Discussion

Ligand Modelling

In the 'active analogue' approach (Marshall and Motoc, 1986) pharmacophore patterns are postulated within a set of compounds that share a unique

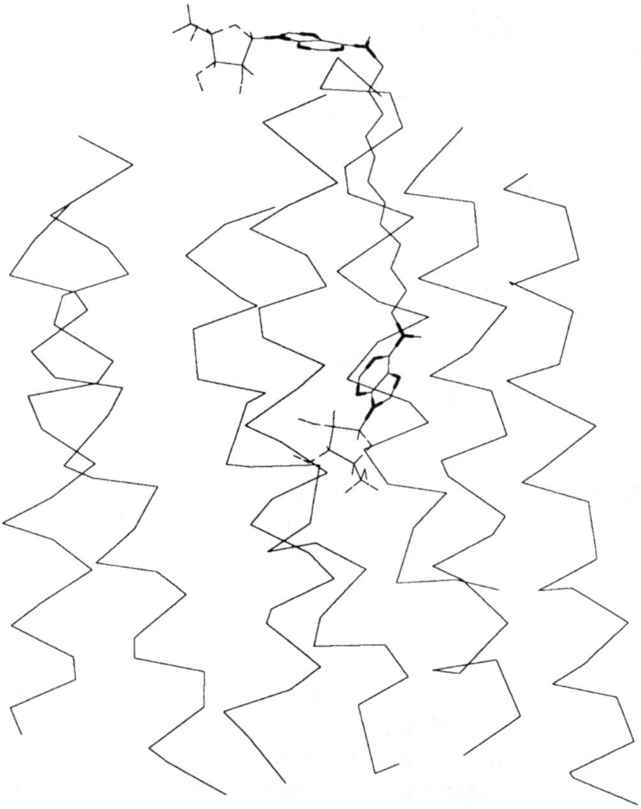

Fig. 7.9 The binding of α,ω-di-(adenosin-N^6-yl)dodecane to the human adenosine A$_1$ receptor (overview). Atoms in the adenosine analogue are represented as in Fig. 7.8, the helices as in Fig. 7.7. Top of figure represents the extracellular side.

biological activity. Comparison of the conformers of each individual compound that are sterically acceptable, may yield areas that are common to every single active analogue. The resulting pattern is indicative for the prerequisites for receptor interaction. Further analysis of closely related, but inactive or less active compounds may lead to the definition of 'forbidden' areas, that are exclusively occupied by the not (very) active ligands. In this particular study we have applied this approach to only small parts of the studied molecules, viz. the N^6-region of adenosine receptor agonists and the C8-region of adenosine receptor antagonists.

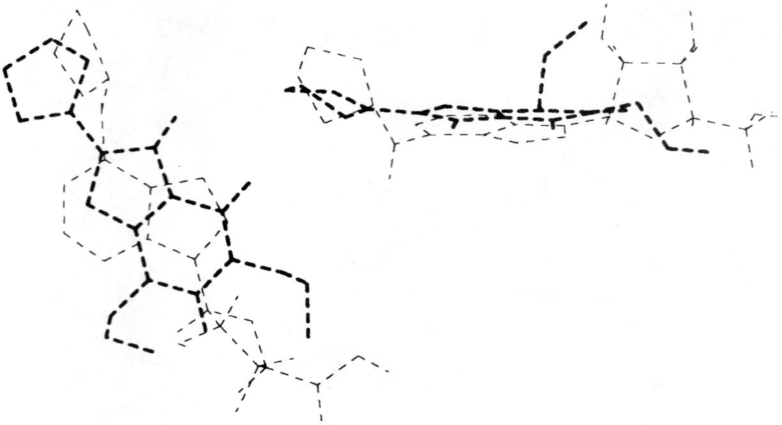

Fig. 7.10 Receptor-bound conformations (from two different viewpoints) of N^6-cyclopentyladenosine (CPA, thin) and 1,3-dipropyl-8-cyclopentylxanthine (DPCPX, thick).

The adenosine N^6-region

Qualitative map of the N^6-region

Figure 7.3 can be regarded as an extension of a model described previously (Kusachi *et al.*, 1985). Additional subregions have been defined, viz. a C (cycloalkyl) and a B (bulk) region. Three further areas (F1, F2 and F3), the so-called forbidden areas that contribute negatively to affinity when they are occupied by a ligand, have also been identified. These could very well be part of the receptor 'wall'. As an example, the presence of a C subregion becomes clear when the affinities of CPA (pK_i = 9.19) and N^6-2-propyladenosine (pK_i = 8.43) are compared. The latter compound occupies the S1, S2 and S3 subregions as readily as CPA, but it cannot fill the proposed C region. Similarly, forbidden area F1 is based on the large differences in affinity between the *R* and *S* isomers of PIA and PBA. This area is also occupied by the methyl groups of N^6-1-methylcyclopentyladenosine and N^6-1-methyl-cyclohexyladenosine, both being less potent than their analogues CPA and CHA. In fact, F1 is identical to the $S3^A$ subregion with C^2 in the *S*-configuration.

Validation and quantification of the map

The model can also be used to rationalize the affinities of compounds that were not used for the construction of the map. As an example, N^6-*R*-indanyl-adenosine, a compound with low affinity (pK_i = 6.89), interacts with the S1/$S1^A$, S2, S3 and C subregions, but it also hits the F2-area (Fig. 7.11). The

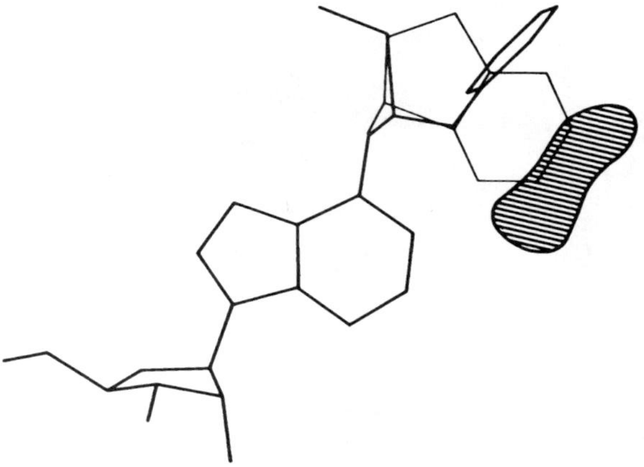

Fig. 7.11 *N^6-R*-indanyladenosine occupies space in forbidden area F2 (shaded), which accounts for its low affinity. *R*-PBA is also shown. (Reproduced with permission from van Galen *et al.*, 1989, Elsevier Science.)

division of the receptor volume in the N^6-region into well-defined subregions also allows a quantitative evaluation of the model according to Motoc and Marshall (1985a,b). In this approach, the contribution of each region can be calculated by a comparison of the affinities of ligands that differ in the occupation of only one subregion, yielding ΔpK_i values. The S3 region is a representative example. It is occupied by *R*-PIA ($pK_i = 8.62$) and not by N^6-2-phenylethyladenosine ($pK_i = 8.09$, not in Table 7.1), yielding a ΔpK_i value of 0.53. Except for the S2 and B subregions, all regions could thus be quantified (Van Galen *et al.*, 1989), and subsequently used for the prediction of affinities of compounds not used for deriving the map. An excellent correlation between experimentally determined and calculated values emerged (Van Galen *et al.*, 1989).

Finally, the model can be used for the design of novel ligands with predicted high affinity. One such compound should be a spirodecene derivative, as shown in Fig. 7.12.

The xanthine C8-region

The differences in membrane perturbation and ordering of water (and other) molecules between two closely related molecules, such as the xanthine congeners DPCPX and 7-methylDPCPX, may be relatively small. As a consequence, the difference between the entropy changes of two congeners may also be relatively small or even negligible in receptor binding. If so, the differences in affinity between DPCPX and 7-methyl DPCPX ($\Delta pK_i = 9.21 - 5.64 = 3.57$, corresponding to approx. 5 kcal/mol) should resemble the energy barrier between the two compounds to reach the receptor-bound conformation. This value was 4.5 kcal/mol (see Fig. 7.4) according to

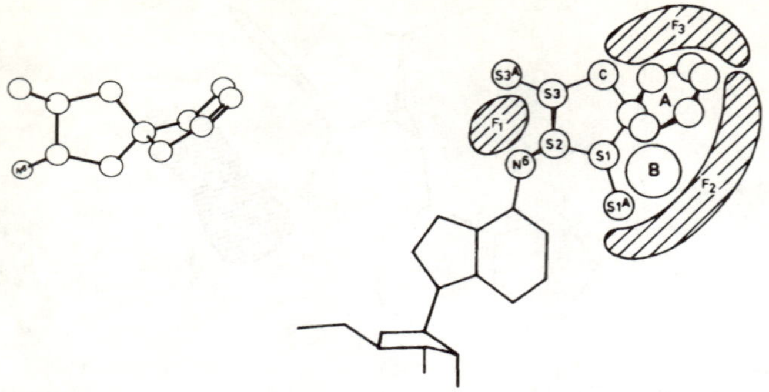

Fig. 7.12 N^6-Spirodecene derivative (left, N^6-substituent shown only) with supposedly high affinity for adenosine A_1 receptors, as derived from the map (right).

semi-empirical calculations. A similar relationship was found for the corresponding 8-cyclohexyl derivatives.

The structure–activity relationship of the C8-region is mainly dependent on the volume of the derivatives. The differences in affinity (see Table 7.2) are mainly due to differences in Van der Waals volumes of the substituents, increase in energy required to reach the dihedral angle of $-30°$, and some influence of polarity.

Is there a common binding site for the N^6- *and C8-substituents of adenosine and xanthine derivatives, respectively?*
Similar substituents in the agonist and antagonist series seem to lead to comparable affinities (see, e.g. Tables 7.1 and 7.2). Also, the dihedral angles discussed above are compatible with a superimposition of adenosine and xanthine derivatives that allow the N^6- and C8-substituents to overlap. This important issue will be discussed below.

Receptor Modelling

Adenosine A_1 receptor topology
Experimental data on structural aspects of membrane-bound proteins is scarce. Recently, Schertler *et al.* (1993) determined a projection map of rhodopsin, the mammalian G-protein coupled visual pigment, at 9 Å resolution. It confirmed the existence of seven transmembrane domains, as had been evident from the atomic coordinates of bacteriorhodopsin, a similar bacterial protein, although not coupled to a G-protein. The three-dimensional structure of the transmembrane segments of bacteriorhodopsin had been determined before (at a better resolution), and served as the first indication of the nature of the general architecture of G-protein coupled receptors (Henderson *et al.*, 1990). There is now considerable debate as to how similar these two protein structures are (Baldwin, 1993; Hoflack *et al.*, 1994). In this study we have

used bacteriorhodopsin as a template for a three-dimensional model of the membrane-spanning parts of the adenosine A_1 receptor. This model can only be approximate at best. Hopefully though, it could serve as a starting point for site-directed mutagenesis and other experiments.

The ligand binding site of the adenosine A_1 receptor

The binding site for the highly hydrophobic ligand retinal in bacteriorhodopsin has been shown to be buried in the membrane, just above the centre of the cavity formed by the seven transmembrane domains (Henderson *et al.*, 1990). Much more hydrophilic ligands, such as adrenaline, may interact with an aspartic acid residue on helix III, present in all receptors for biogenic amines, again suggesting that the binding site for these ligands is also somewhere within the cavity (Strader *et al.*, 1988).

How do adenosine and its derivatives bind to the adenosine A_1 receptor? Unlike the biogenic amines, adenosine is uncharged at physiological pH, and the aspartate on helix III is substituted by a hydrophobic residue (valine or leucine) in all adenosine receptor subtypes. From chemical modification and site-directed mutagenesis studies two histidines (in helices VI and VII, respectively) appear particularly important for ligand binding (Klotz *et al.*, 1988; Garritsen *et al.*, 1990; Olah *et al.*, 1992). Thus, His251 (helix VI) and His278 (helix VII) were used as anchors, leading to the model proposed above. Upon relaxation of the receptor-bound conformation of N^6-cyclopentyladenosine, the reference agonist, the purine–cyclopentyl torsion angle was $-89°$, not very different from the value of $-75°$ determined in the ligand modelling study. The hydrogen bond formed between His251 and N^6-H may well explain the fact that N^6-disubstitution of adenosine derivatives is detrimental for affinity. The ribose moiety, in an *anti* conformation, interacts with His278 via the *cis*-diol moiety. This is compatible with the SAR known for the ribose group. As an example, removal of both hydroxyl groups as in 2′,3′-dideoxy-N^6-cyclohexyladenosine, yielded an antagonist with only moderate affinity (Lohse *et al.*, 1988).

From Fig. 7.9 the relative freedom of large N^6-substituents becomes apparent. The affinities of other adenosine derivatives with N^6-alkyl (hydrophobic), and N^6-alkylamine as well as N^6-alkyladenosine (hydrophilic) substituents are in excellent agreement (Van Galen *et al.*, 1987). Up to alkyl chain lengths of 8 or 9 carbon atoms (the length necessary to reach the extracellular boundaries of the receptor helices) affinities increase, whereas larger chains lead to less active compounds. The hydrophobic alkyl chains in particular (now being in a more aqueous environment) are not well tolerated. As an example, N^6-dodecyladenosine is almost 100-fold less active than the corresponding N^6-12-aminoalkyladenosine, and 25-fold less active than α,ω-di-(adenosin-N^6-yl)dodecane, the ligand shown in Fig. 7.9. The general concept of ‘functionalized congeners’ appears to have its biochemical correlate here.

If this is also true for the xanthine receptor antagonists with long C8-substituents, this imposes the xanthine core structure in the 'N^6/C8' orientation, as represented in Fig. 7.10 for CPA and DPCPX. The dihedral angles determining the position of the N^6- and C8-substituents relative to the core of the molecule in agonists and antagonists, respectively, correspond between the ligand and receptor modelling results, also indicative for the 'N^6/C8' model. This orientation would explain the similar increases in affinity for very bulky, such as adamantyl, and other substituents in N^6-substituted agonists and C8-substituted antagonists (Van der Wenden *et al.*, 1992). It remains, however, possible that antagonist structures adopt other orientations, thereby still impeding the binding of the endogenous agonist adenosine, and thus acting as competitive antagonists.

Conclusion

The interaction between the adenosine A_1 receptor and its ligands has been studied through molecular modelling. The thrust of this chapter is the combination of both indirect and direct approaches to visualize and integrate known structure–activity relationships and other biochemical data. The presented receptor model could serve as a starting point for further studies. Combined efforts in seemingly distant fields as computational chemistry, organic synthesis and molecular biology may lead to validation and optimization of the proposed model, eventually enabling the rational design of new chemical entities.

References

Baldwin, J.M. (1993). *EMBO J.* **12**, 1693–1703.

Devereux, J., Haeberli, P. and Smithies, O. (1984). *Nucleic Acids Res.* **12**, 387–395.

Garritsen, A., IJzerman, A.P., Beukers, M.W. and Soudijn, W. (1990). *Biochem. Pharmacol.* **40**, 835–842.

Henderson, R., Baldwin, J.M., Ceska, T.A., Zemlin, F., Beckmann, E. and Downing, K.H. (1990). *J. Mol. Biol.* **213**, 899–929.

Hoflack, J., Trumpp-Kallmeyer, S. and Hibert, M. (1994). *Trends Pharmac. Sci.* **15**, 7–9.

IJzerman, A.P., Van Galen, P.J.M. and Jacobson, K.A. (1992). *Drug Design and Discovery* **9**, 49–67.

Klotz, K.-N., Lohse, M.J. and Schwabe, U. (1988). *J. Biol. Chem.* **263**, 17522–17526.

Kusachi, S., Thompson, R.D., Bugni, W.J., Yamada, N. and Olsson, R.A. (1985). *J. Med. Chem.* **28**, 1636–1643.

Libert, F., Van Sande, J., Lefort, A., Czernilofsky, A., Dumont, J.E., Vassart, G.,

Ensinger, H.A. and Mendla, K.D. (1992). *Biochem. Biophys. Res. Commun.* **187**, 919–926.
Lohse, M.J., Klotz, K.-N., Diekmann, E., Freidrich, K. and Schwabe, U. (1988). *Eur. J. Pharmacol.* **156**, 157–160.
Marshall, G.R. and Motoc, I. (1986). *In* 'Molecular Graphics and drug design' (A.S.V. Burgen *et al.*, eds), pp. 115–156. Elsevier, Amsterdam.
Motoc, I. and Marshall, G. (1985a). *Z. Naturforsch.* **40a**, 1114–1120.
Motoc, I. and Marshall, G. (1985b). *Z. Naturforsch.* **40a**, 1121–1127.
Olah, M.E., Ren, H., Ostrowski, J., Jacobson, K.A. and Stiles, G.L. (1992). *J. Biol. Chem.* **267**, 10764–10770.
Schertler, G.F.X., Villa, C. and Henderson, R. (1993). *Nature* **362**, 770–772.
Strader, C.D., Sigal, I.S., Candelore, M.R., Rands, E., Mill, W.S. and Dixon, R.A.F. (1988). *J. Biol. Chem.* **263**, 10267–10271.
Van der Wenden, E.M., Van Galen, P.J.M., IJzerman, A.P. and Soudijn, W. (1991). *Eur. J. Pharmacol. – Mol. Pharm. Sect.* **206**, 315–323.
Van der Wenden, E.M., IJzerman, A.P. and Soudijn, W. (1992). *J. Med. Chem.* **35**, 629–635.
Van Galen, P.J.M., IJzerman, A.P. and Soudijn, W. (1987). *FEBS Lett.* **223**, 197–201.
Van Galen, P.J.M., Leusen, F.J.J., IJzerman, A.P. and Soudijn, W. (1989). *Eur. J. Pharmacol. – Mol. Pharm. Sect.* **172**, 19–27.

Discussion

B.P. Roques

I am impressed by the analogies between Dr IJzerman's model and the model that we proposed for the interaction of agonists and antagonists with the CCK-B receptors. It seems to me that there is a superimposition of your agonist and antagonist. But, on the antagonist there are additionally two oxygens on the 6-membered ring.

First, have you tried to replace one of these oxygens, for instance, by nitrogen, to come back from an antagonist to an agonist? Second, has your adenosine receptor model been supported by site-directed mutagenesis, for instance, of the histidine by replacing the amino acid by phenylalanine or something else?

A.P. IJzerman

The ribose group is needed for agonist activity, so simply replacing an oxygen by a nitrogen in the antagonist will not yield an agonist – the ribose group is necessary to have the interaction with the histidine in helix 7. This somehow answers the second question because it has been shown from site-directed mutagenesis studies on the bovine receptor that the histidine in helix 7 is particularly important for agonist binding.

Some mutation studies have been done, but more are needed – it is up to other people probably to do the required mutation studies. We have indicated quite a few amino acid side chains that could be important for ligand binding here. To that end, we have had some collaboration with Ken Jacobson at the National Institutes of Health. He is currently trying to make mutants predicted from these models.

P. Potier

For a long time, at least 20 years, some derivatives of adenosine substituted on nitrogen by prenyl type compounds – terpenes and so on – have been known. They have apparently been rediscovered recently for their important role in controlling, for instance, protein synthesis and similar things. Was it deliberate that these sorts of derivatives were not mentioned?

A.P. IJzerman

It was not deliberate. The isoprenyl derivatives to which you refer come from plant medicinal chemistry and are important metabolic factors there. They do show some affinity towards adenosine A_1 receptors. They could be compared with the weakly active compounds shown in the table: around 1 μM affinity. In this case, hydrophobicity itself is not enough. The shape of the substituent is important to gain receptor affinity for adenosine receptors.

8

Challenges in Structure-Based Drug Design

I.D. KUNTZ, E.C. MENG and B.K. SHOICHET*

Department of Pharmaceutical Chemistry, University of California, San Francisco, CA 94143-0446, USA

Introduction

Creating molecules with specific properties has long been a cherished goal of chemists. Finding new drugs, in particular, is the target for many of us. In this chapter, we will consider the discovery or design of molecules that interact with biochemical targets whose three-dimensional structures are known, a field called 'structure-based' design. Of course, highly specific interactions were well described a century ago (Fischer, 1894). We explore the usefulness of this concept by reviewing both general principles of molecular recognition and specific computer programs that pack molecules together. A recent summary has been published (Kuntz *et al.*, 1994).

The drug discovery process is complex, typically taking 10 years. Structure-based design is one of many ways of taking the first step of finding interesting leads (Kuntz, 1992). It is now being tested as a means of generating new pharmaceuticals (Reich *et al.*, 1992). A critical assumption is that our understanding of intermolecular interactions and molecular plasticity is sufficiently advanced so that novel compounds can be proposed and optimized.

We limit this chapter to computational approaches to molecular design (Cohen *et al.*, 1990; Kuntz, 1992), with particular emphasis on the 'docking problem'. We discuss some of the fundamental problems of representing molecular properties and analysing interaction energies and look at the

* Current address, Molecular Biology Institute, University of Oregon, Eugene, OR 97403-1229, USA.

New Perspectives in Drug Design
ISBN 0–12–208070–X

progress to date. Many crucial issues in drug design such as the ease of synthesis or the toxicology or bioavailability of specific compounds are not easily assessed using molecular calculations and will not be considered here.

Methodological Issues

We must recognize that there are serious mathematical issues to address. First, there is no 'best' method for describing molecular shape (Johnson and Maggiora, 1990; Mezey, 1990). Second, packing irregular objects together, the so-called 'knapsack' problem (Salomaa, 1991), has no general solution. Third, the search issues involve the study of isomorphous subgraphs (Ullman, 1976). Fourth, the full conformational space of ligand and receptor involves a search of astronomical proportion. It is unlikely that general algorithmic solutions will be found for all of these problems. Rather, progress depends on the quality of the approximations used to reduce the effort to what is practicable on current computers.

Quality of Structures

What quality is demanded of the structures used for structure-based design? Excellent protein structures derived from X-ray diffraction have an average uncertainty of a few tenths of angstroms for non-hydrogen atoms (Chambers and Stroud, 1979) with the greatest errors arising in occasional regions of very low electron density. There are now estimates of the effects of the infamous 'crystal packing forces' which can introduce differences of about 1.0 Å (Kossiakoff *et al.*, 1992). NMR-generated coordinates have precisions of 0.5–1.0 Å in the backbone region and 1.5 Å or greater in average side chain positions (Billeter, 1992). Homology modelling has *minimum* errors of 0.5–1.0 Å for the backbones of highly similar sequences and much larger (and uncertain) side chain errors in loop regions (Chothia and Lesk, 1986). Structural models accurate to 1.0–2.0 Å have been useful for structure-based design (Kuntz, 1992).

Ligand geometries are normally known to high accuracy, typically better than 0.1 Å (Allen *et al.*, 1979) except for conformational concerns which can be explored through a variety of computer programs including systematic search (Marshall *et al.*, 1979); MM3 (Allinger *et al.*, 1989); WIZARD (Dolata *et al.*, 1987); and COBRA (Leach and Prout, 1990). To obtain approximate three-dimensional coordinates for compounds not included in the experimental database, one can turn to the programs above, or CONCORD (Rusinko *et al.*, 1989). The major uncertainty is identification of the preferred conformation in the receptor environment.

Molecular Juxtaposition of the Ligand and Receptor

The objective of molecular docking is to obtain the lowest free energy structure(s) for the receptor–ligand complex. The most systematic approach is to search through all binding orientations of all conformations of the ligand and receptor. This algorithm requires exponentially increasing resources as the molecules increase in size. It is not practical for docking two macromolecules and has severe limitations even in small molecule searches.

There are two major classes of automated searching. *Geometric* methods match ligand and receptor site descriptors. These procedures reduce the search space by judicious limitation of the number of descriptors and the use of heuristic rules for pruning the search tree. Alternatively, one can align by minimizing the receptor–ligand interaction *energy*. Energy-driven search, based on molecular dynamics (MD) and Monte Carlo (MC) simulations, is well-studied (Karplus and McCammon, 1983; Jorgensen and Nguyen, 1993). Advantages of energy searches are the relatively firm physical basis of force fields (see below) and very general applicability. The disadvantage is the enormous computational resources required for extensive searches.

Force Fields

The quantity of interest for ligand design is the free energy of binding (ΔG_{bind}) in aqueous solution. It can be calculated directly using free energy perturbation methods *if* an accurate geometric model of the complex is available (Straatsma and McCammon, 1992). Accuracy in such calculations depends heavily on the quality of the force field and the extent of sampling of conformational space. It is certainly a curious aspect of molecular simulation that the field moved rapidly from simulations of small molecules in the gas phase to simple liquids to protein and nucleic acid aqueous solutions. It still requires a careful effort to simulate the properties of water or methanol to an accuracy of 1 kcal/mol. Why should we expect a system of thousands of atoms of diverse kinds to be well represented by empirical, truncated force fields? Major force field development projects are underway in the Kollman laboratory at UCSF (Cornell *et al.*, 1993), the Biosym consortium (Dinur and Hagler, 1990) and at Merck (Halgren, 1992). The issues include better representations of radii, bond bending, polarizability and multibody terms. Electrostatics remains a difficult area. Coulomb's law is deceptively simple. The long-range nature of electrostatic forces means that truncation of inter-atomic potentials at fixed distances can lead to difficulties. Ewald sums offer one method of avoiding these difficulties (Schreiber and Steinhauser, 1992). Modelling macroscopic dielectric constants with microscopic dielectric boundaries cannot be the best long-term solution (Warshel and Åqvist, 1991). Appropriate protonation of functional groups during simulations is also a concern. At some level, we have been 'lucky' that empirical adjustments to atomic radii, dipole moments and dielectric properties have generally led to well-bounded problems.

Entropy and Sampling

In most calculations of molecular interaction, entropic considerations are ignored or treated at a much lower level of approximation than enthalpic terms. In principle, if we have an accurate force field, all that is required to obtain a useful measure of entropy is a sufficiently long simulation run, in a large enough vessel, to sample the accessible conformational and configurational states. In practice, we know the sampling is inadequate even in calculations lasting for nanoseconds. What is surprising is that an estimate of the degree of sampling, and hence the accuracy of the calculation, is rarely made. There are some guideposts: comparison with simplified lattice calculations; assessment of the heat capacity of the system; or a Boltzmann distribution among the conformational states. Brünger has shown how effective cross-validation statistical methods can be in assessing the quality of structural refinement (Brünger, 1993). The convergence of directed systems must be determined by using repeated randomized starts or random perturbation methods, and the reversibility of the system should be examined.

The hydrophobic effect requires special attention. It is mainly a statistical entropic effect (Dill, 1990) and its direct calculation requires an ensemble of configurations of explicit water molecules. Empirical models focus on solvent-exposed surface area (Chothia, 1974; Still *et al.*, 1990; Cramer and Truhlar, 1992), with a recent extension to consider surface curvature (Nichols *et al.*, 1991). Surface area contributions to the free energy have been derived from experimental free energies of transfer (Eisenberg and McLachlan, 1986). These empirical values include both the hydrophobic effect and enthalpic interactions of atoms with the solvent. The underpinnings of hydrophobicity theory and solvation effects are still undergoing vigorous evolution (Ben-Naim, 1994; Chan and Dill, in preparation).

Conformational Issues

Methods which employ single rigid conformations and which neglect conformational energy terms depend on the assumption that complexation does not distort molecules very far from their dominant conformations in the unbound state. Many molecular complexes violate this assumption and show 'induced fit' (Koshland, 1971; Schulz *et al.*, 1990; Jorgensen, 1991). A partial remedy is to use a variety of low-energy conformations treated as independent complexes. Alternative conformations for protein side chains can be explored (Ponder and Richards, 1987; Wilson *et al.*, 1991), but variants of the protein backbone are hard to predict.

Accuracy of Calculations

It is surprisingly difficult to determine the accuracy of calculational techniques. Experimentalists can usually detect differences in binding affinity of 10%, equivalent to a free energy determination to within 50 cal/mol! This accuracy is not likely to be seen in calculations for another decade. In the *best* cases, the free energy perturbation method has been reported to agree with experiment within ± 1 kcal/mol. Energy minimization, yielding only an approximation to the enthalpy, is much less accurate. The usefulness of molecular force fields is critically sensitive to solvent representation and the description of the dielectric behavior of the system. Comparisons of a diverse series of molecules would rarely be more accurate than ± 2 kcal/mol, and more often this technique gives semi-quantitative rankings with uncertainties of ± 5 kcal/mol. Force field calculations are expected to be more reliable when a family of quite similar molecules are compared. Even these approximate results can be useful in screening or SAR applications.

Types of Docking Programs

Finding the low-energy states of ligand–receptor complexes presents the fundamental problem that receptor sites have complicated and adjustable shapes and there are many ways of fitting a flexible ligand to them.

Matching Methods

These approaches focus on complementarity. Ligand atoms are placed at the 'best' positions in the site, generating a reasonable ligand–receptor configuration that may require optimization. Descriptor matching methods are rarely exhaustive, but they are fast and can usually provide satisfactory sampling of a particular region of the receptor site. Many of these algorithms use combinatorial search strategies, and small changes in parameter values can sometimes move the problem out of the feasible range of computer time.

DOCK

One of the earliest descriptor matching programs, DOCK uses spheres locally complementary to the receptor molecular surface (Connolly, 1983) to create a space-filling negative image of the receptor site (Kuntz *et al.*, 1982). Site descriptions require 30–150 spheres. Several (4–5) ligand atoms are matched with receptor spheres to generate chiral orientations of the ligand in the site. DOCK uses molecular force fields (Meng *et al.*, 1992), limited conformational searches (Leach and Kuntz, 1992), and chemical labelling of descriptors (Shoichet and Kuntz, 1993). Its most common use is in the discovery of

Table 8.1
DOCK leads developed at UCSF

System	Affinities (μM)		Reference
	1st lead	2nd generation	
HIV protease	100	0.8	(DesJarlais *et al.*, 1990; Rutenber *et al.*, 1993)
B-form DNA	10		(Kerwin *et al.*, 1991)
Thymidylate synthase	900	0.03	(Shoichet *et al.*, 1993)
Haemagglutinin	100	5	(Bodian *et al.*, 1993)
CD4–gp120[a]	5	1	(McGregor, Cohen and Kuntz, 1992, unpublished results)
Malaria protease[b]	10	0.1	(Ring *et al.*, 1993)

[a] Developed in collaboration with Procept, Inc., Cambridge, MA.
[b] Structure obtained from homology model-building.

novel inhibitors (DesJarlais *et al.*, 1990; Kuntz, 1992; Shoichet *et al.*, 1993). Databases of small molecules are searched for candidates which complement the structure of the receptor (DesJarlais *et al.*, 1988). DOCK has found novel, micromolar inhibitors for several receptors of therapeutic interest (Table 8.1). Its limitations are those of all descriptor matching programs: sensitivity to the quality of the negative image; non-exhaustive searches; limited conformational exploration. As with most descriptor matching methods, it is relatively fast (Meng *et al.*, 1992; Shoichet *et al.*, 1992).

CAVEAT
CAVEAT is based on directional characterization of ligands (Bartlett *et al.*, 1989). It searches for ligands with atoms located along specified vectors, typically derived from structural information from known complexes. CAVEAT rapidly searches reformatted versions of the usual ligand databases. The program has been successfully used to design α-amylase inhibitors, as well as non-peptide mimics of somatostatin. CAVEAT focuses on finding templates as starting points for chemical modification.

FOUNDATION
FOUNDATION represents an important attempt to combine models of the crucial ligand atoms (pharmacophore models) and structure-based methods. (Ho and Marshall, 1993). The user identifies atom and bonding types that a candidate molecule must possess. Steric constraints of the receptor binding site eliminate candidates that do not complement the shape of the binding site, and candidates are oriented in the receptor site. FOUNDATION relies heavily on detailed atom-type, bond-type, chain-length and topology constraints to restrict its search. FOUNDATION only considers the steric component of the active site, relying on its matching information to find chemically

complementary ligands. The tight constraints restrict the candidates to one orientation in the site, whereas in DOCK and CLIX, many orientations are sampled.

CLIX

CLIX (Lawrence and Davis, 1992) resembles DOCK by using receptor site features to define possible binding configurations. CLIX relies on an elaborate chemical description of receptor site 'hot spots', using the 23 different classes of receptor environment provided by GRID (Goodford, 1985). It uses fewer receptor–ligand matches than does DOCK. CLIX has been used to search for ligands complementary to the sialic acid binding site of haemagglutinin, returning several interesting structures. The program is fairly fast. It does not allow for ligand or receptor conformational flexibility. CLIX evaluates interaction energies using the GRID potential function.

Connolly presents an interesting and provocative discussion of some of the important issues in protein docking (Connolly, 1985).

Grid Search Methods

Grid searches sample the six degrees of freedom of orientation space. They find the neighborhood of the correct solution(s), which cannot be guaranteed with discrete sampling methods. Accuracy is limited by the step size used in the search, which also determines the time of the search. Methods which use additional sampling in regions of high complementarity can overcome this problem.

Side chain spheres

Wodak and Janin explored protein–protein complexes using simplified sphere representations of side chain atoms and a grid search of four rigid degrees of freedom (Wodak and Janin, 1978). The approach has been extended recently to include more sophisticated surface burial evaluation algorithms (Wodak *et al.*, 1987), full molecular force field evaluation of complexes and simulated annealing to refine initial docked structures (Cherfils *et al.*, 1991).

Soft docking

Soft docking (Jiang and Kim, 1991) divides receptor and ligand surface into cubes to generate the translational part of the search. A pure rotational grid search samples ligand orientations in discrete angular increments. The accuracy is limited by step size, with run time scaling as the cube of the rotational step size and as the product of the number of receptor and ligand surface points. Soft docking has been successful in docking NADPH and methotrexate into dihydrofolate reductase (DHFR), as well as bovine pancreatic trypsin inhibitor (BPTI) into trypsin, and lysozyme into an antibody. Non-crystallographic solutions are occasionally generated.

Fragment Joining Methods

Fragment methods identify regions of high complementarity by docking functional groups independently into receptors. They overcome most of the rigid ligand issues at the expense of adding a combinatorial search over fragment types. These approaches can suggest unsynthesized compounds, but connecting the fragments in sensible, synthetically accessible patterns is a challenging problem. These methods are attractive for chemical elaboration.

GROW

GROW is a well-tested fragment method (Moon and Howe, 1991). It designs peptides complementary to proteins of known structure. A seed amino acid is placed in the receptor site followed by iterative additions of amino acids. Conformations are chosen from a library of pre-calculated low-energy forms. At each addition the energy of the peptide and of the peptide–receptor complex is briefly minimized and evaluated. Only the best 10–100 low-energy structures are kept at any stage. A GROW program for organic molecules is under development.

HOOK

HOOK (Miranker and Karplus, 1991) finds 'hot spots' in receptor sites by seeking low-energy locations for functional groups. HOOK differs from Goodford's GRID program by using random placement of many copies of several functional fragments followed by molecular dynamics. HOOK was tested by reproducing sialic acid derivatives known to bind a haemagglutinin. The most serious drawback of HOOK is shared by all fragment methods: the need to reconnect functional groups to form complete molecules while maintaining the geometric positions of lowest energy.

BUILDER

This program uses a family of docked structures to provide an irregular lattice of controllable density, which can be searched for paths that link molecular fragments. It has been shown to generate chemically reasonable compounds in the HIV protease site (Lewis *et al.*, 1992).

LUDI

A prototypic fragment joining effort, LUDI (Böhm, 1992) proposes inhibitors by connecting fragments that dock into micro-sites on the receptor. The fragments come from a list of approximately 600 molecular fragments such as benzene, adamantane and naphthol. Micro-sites are defined by hydrogen bonding and hydrophobic groups using the author's own algorithm, or using the output of GRID (Goodford, 1985). Ligand pseudo-atom (hot spot) positions are generated within micro-sites based on the appropriate angle and distance minima for various interactions. In this respect the method resembles

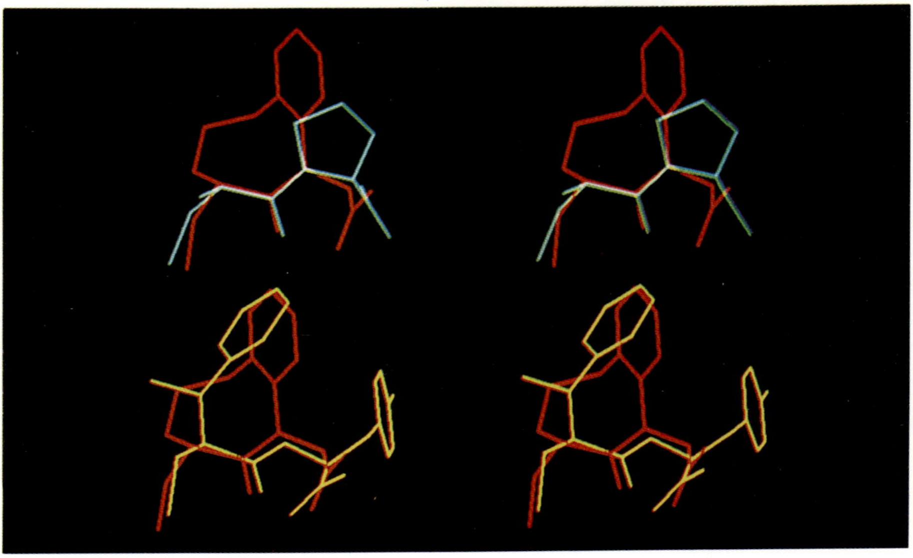

Plate 2.1 (top) ACE pharmacophore defined by the overlap of the biologically active conformation of captopril [(2*S*)-2-mercaptomethyl-3-methylpropanoyl)proline] (in blue) with the most stable conformer of (3-mercaptomethyl)-3,4,5,6-tetrahydro-2-oxo-^{1}H-1-benzazocine-1-acetic acid (in red). (bottom) Superimposition (r.m.s.d. 0.783) of the most stable and populated (41%) conformer of N-[2*S*,3*R*)-2-mercapto-methyl-3-phenylbutanoyl](*S*)-alanine (RB 105) in yellow) and the ACE template (in red).

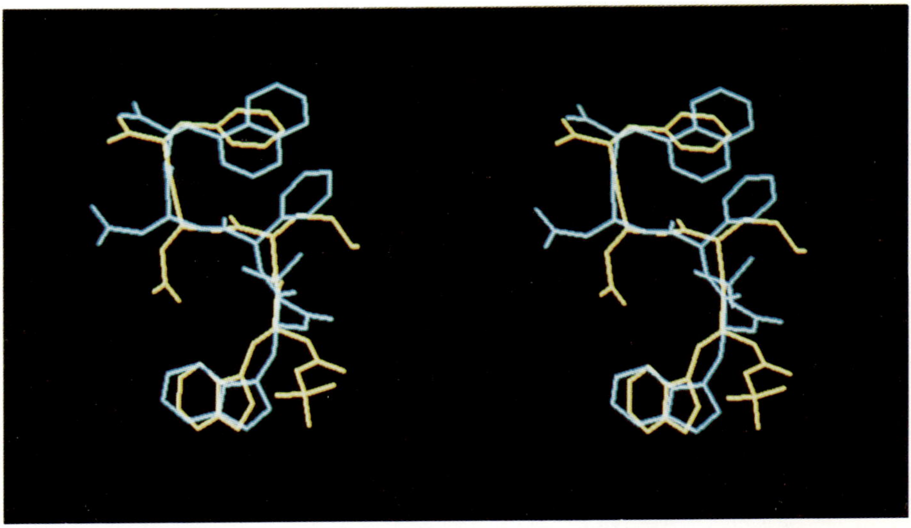

Plate 2.2 Stereoview of the superposition (backbone atoms only) of the NMR-derived structures for the two CCK-B agonists: Boc–Trp–(*N*-Me)Nle–Asp–Phe–NH_2 (yellow) and Boc–Trp–Phg–Asp–(1-Nal)–NH_2 (blue). For clarity, hydrogen atoms are not shown.

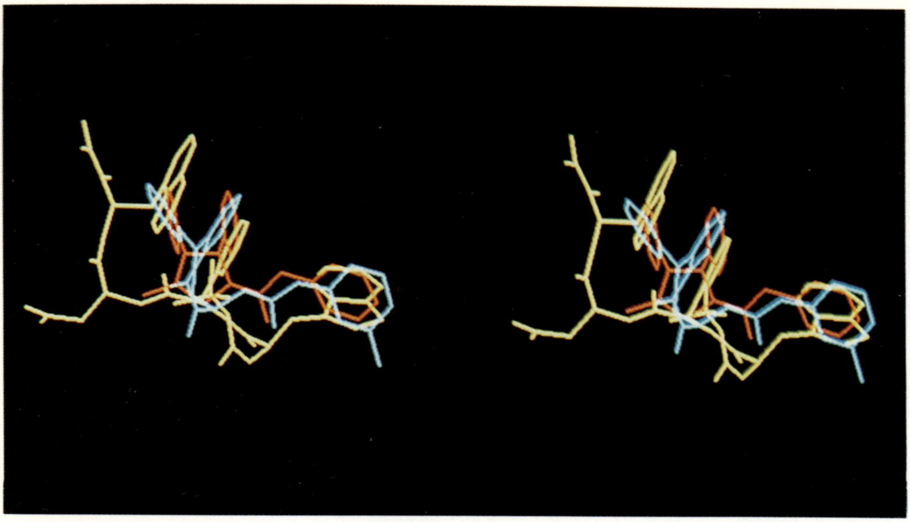

Plate 2.3 Stereoview of the superposition of the NMR-derived structure for Boc–Trp–Phg–Asp–(1-Nal)–*N*(Me)$_2$ (yellow) along with low energy conformations proposed for two other CCK-B antagonists: L-365 260 (blue) and LY-288 513 (red). For clarity, hydrogen atoms are not shown. The superposition was done by selecting the centre of the three aromatic moieties in each molecule.

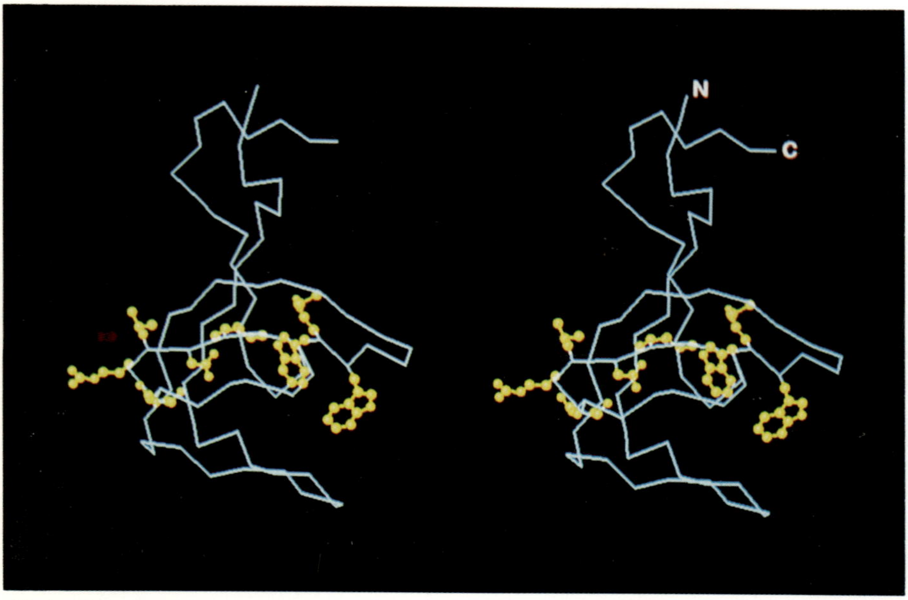

Plate 2.4 Spatial arrangement of the essential Ras signalling 43–52 (317–326) peptide in the 3D structure of GAP SH_3.

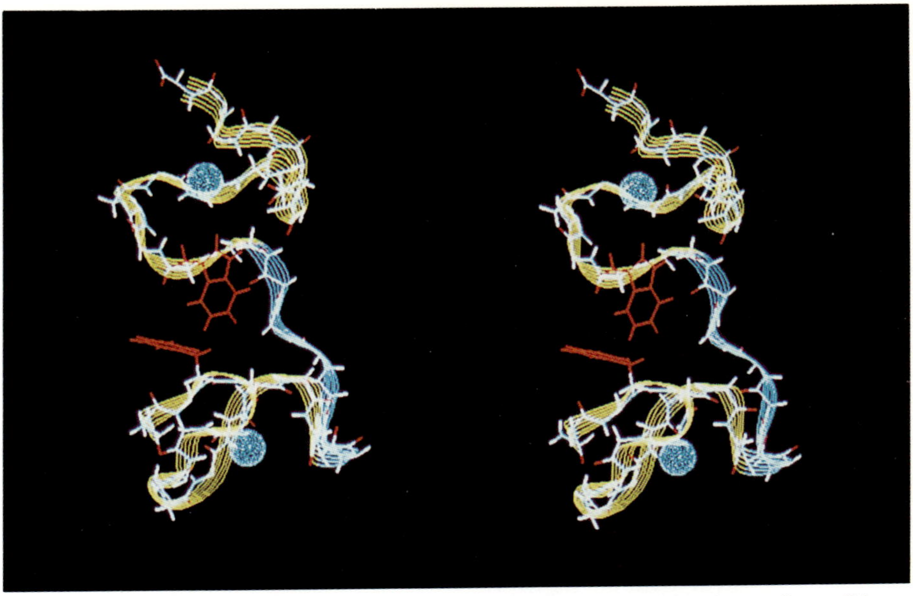

Plate 2.5 Conformational behaviour of (13–51)NCp7. Stereoview of a ribbon representation of the (13–51)NCp7. Only side chain atoms of aromatic residues (red).

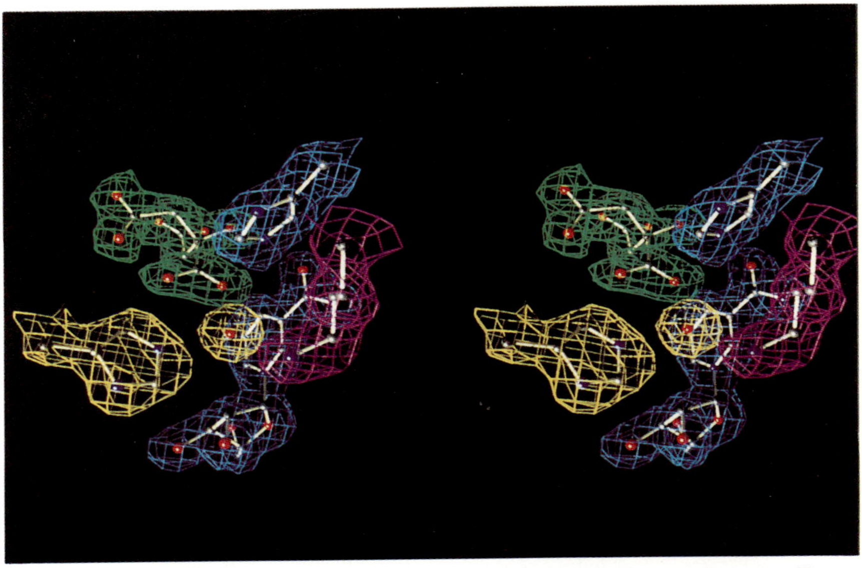

Plate 6.1 Stereophotograph of the active site of human aldose reductase. Enzyme residues are shown with their associated electron density in blue, yellow and purple. Shown in green is a region of electron density that does not belong to the protein. Fitted into this region is the structure of citrate, which was shown afterwards to be a good inhibitor of the enzyme (Harrison *et al.*, 1994).

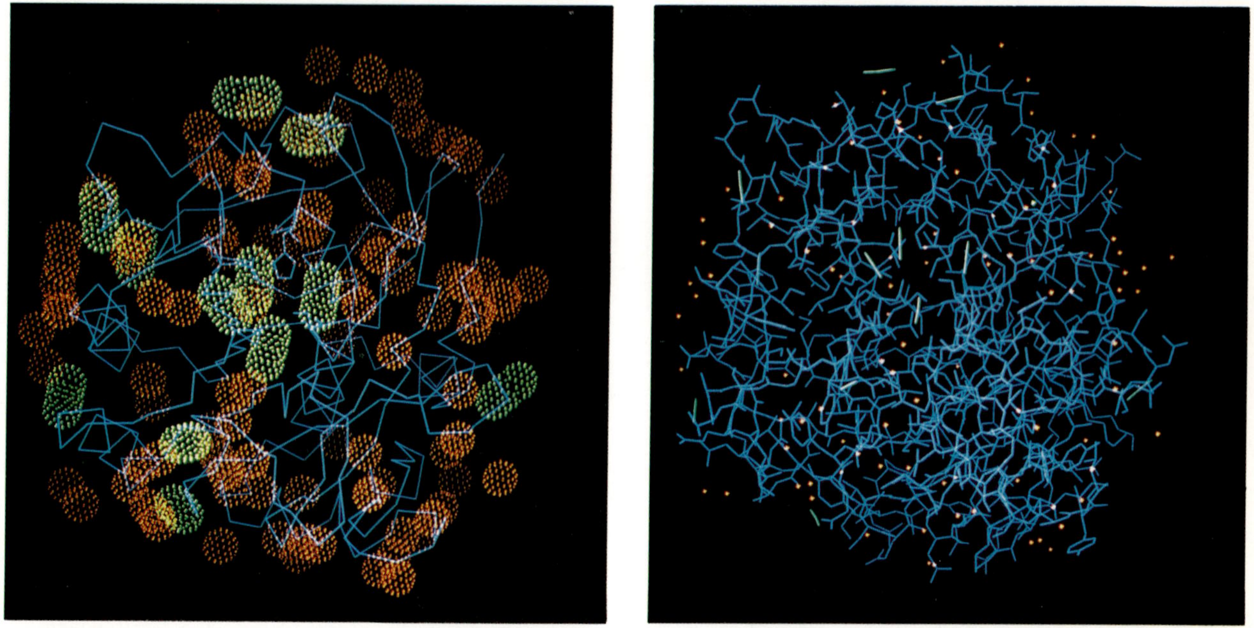

Plate 6.2 Solvent mapping of subtilisin. On the right is the enzyme structure in 100% acetonitrile. Bound waters that remain with the protein under these conditions are shown as red dots. Acetonitrile molecules that bind to the enzyme in specific sites are shown as white lines. The picture on the left is the same view, but now only the backbone of the enzyme is shown. The water molecules are red spheres and the acetonitrile molecules are yellow dumbbells. The cluster of four bound acetonitrile molecules in the centre of the picture define the active site of the enzyme.

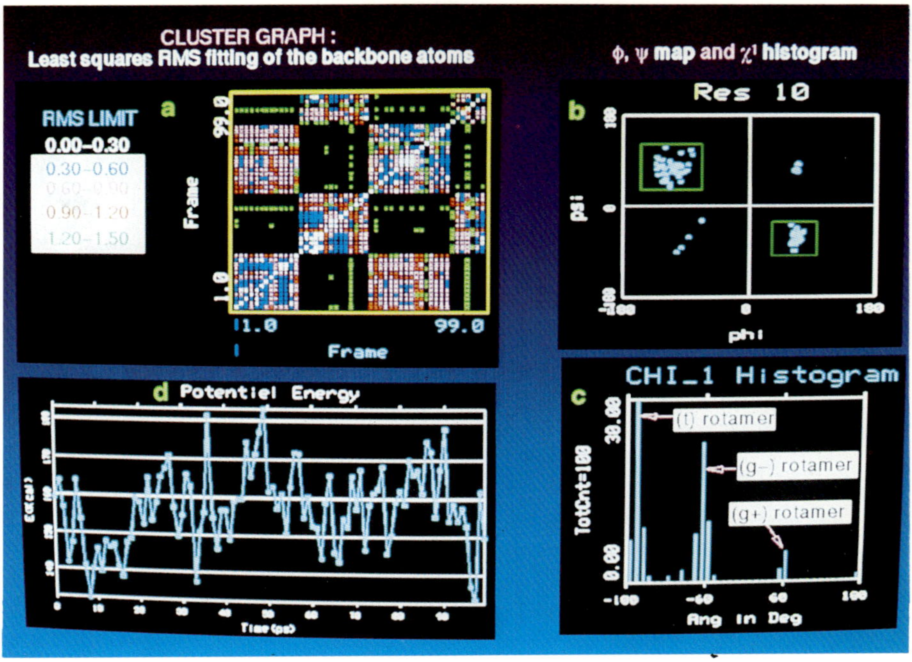

Plate 13.1 Tools for conformational family analysis (see text).

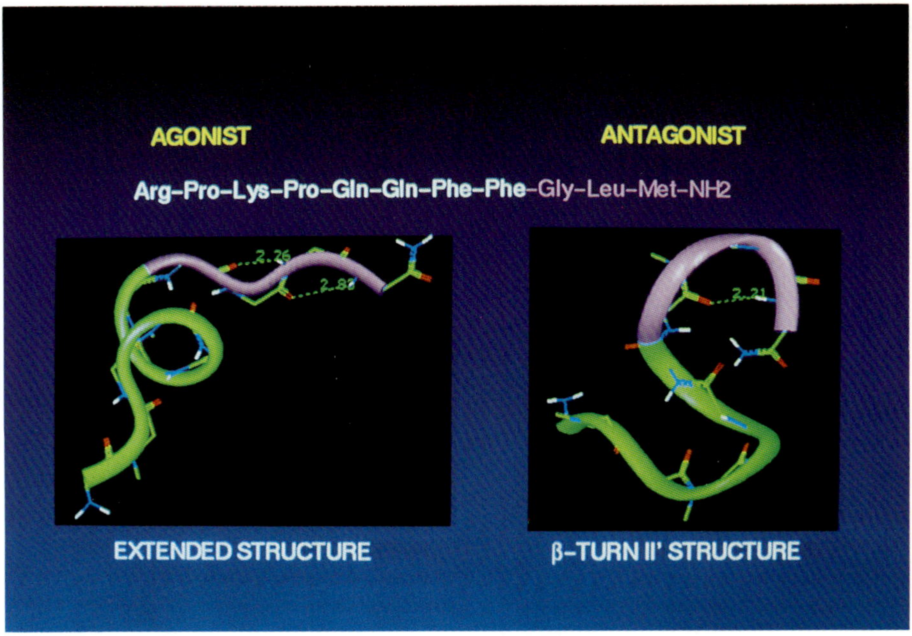

Plate 13.2 Comparison of SP agonist and antagonist conformations.

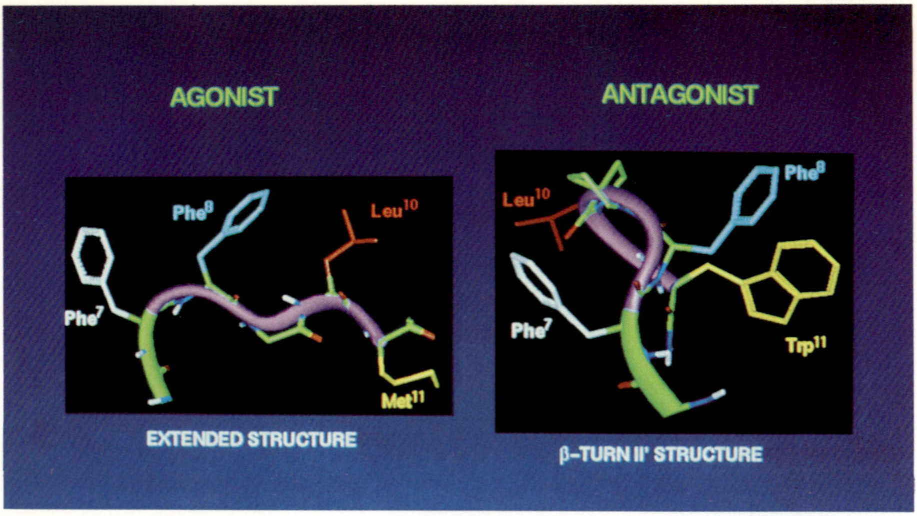

Plate 13.3 Side chain orientations of the important residues for SP agonist and antagonist peptides.

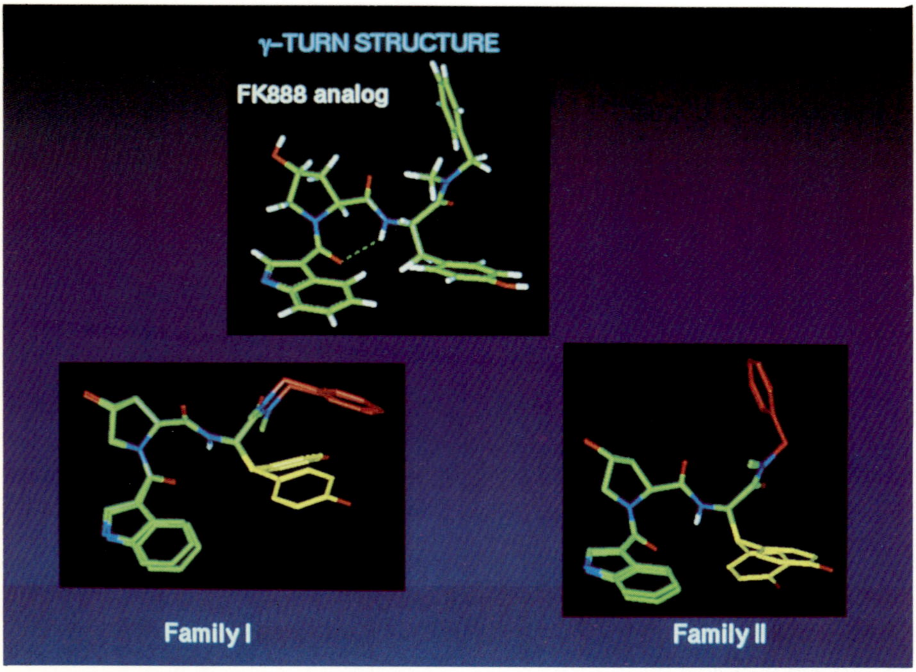

Plate 13.4 Representative structures of the two families obtained from the restrained MD simulations.

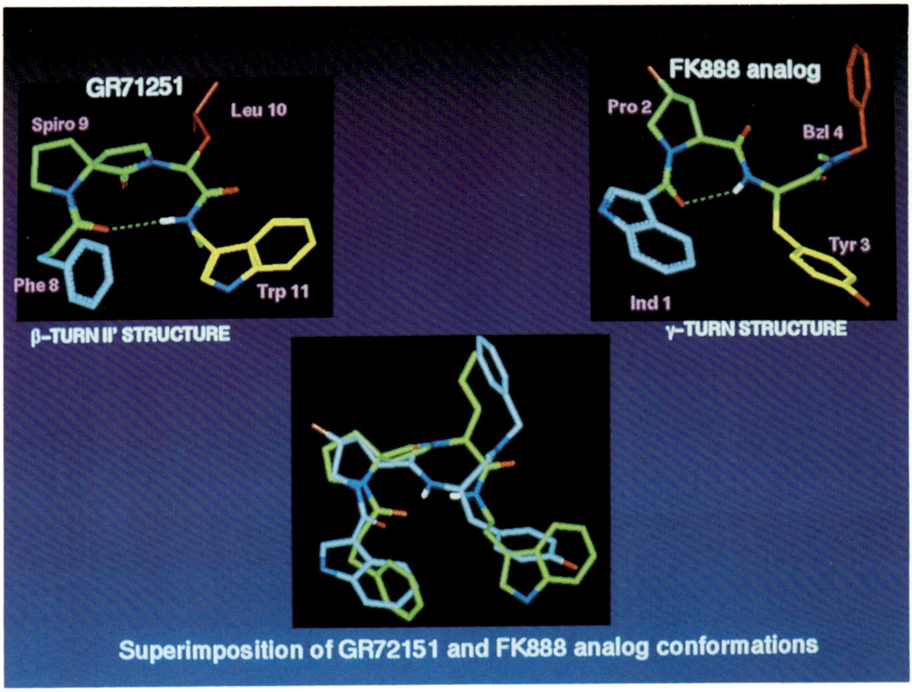

Plate 13.5 Bioactive conformation models.

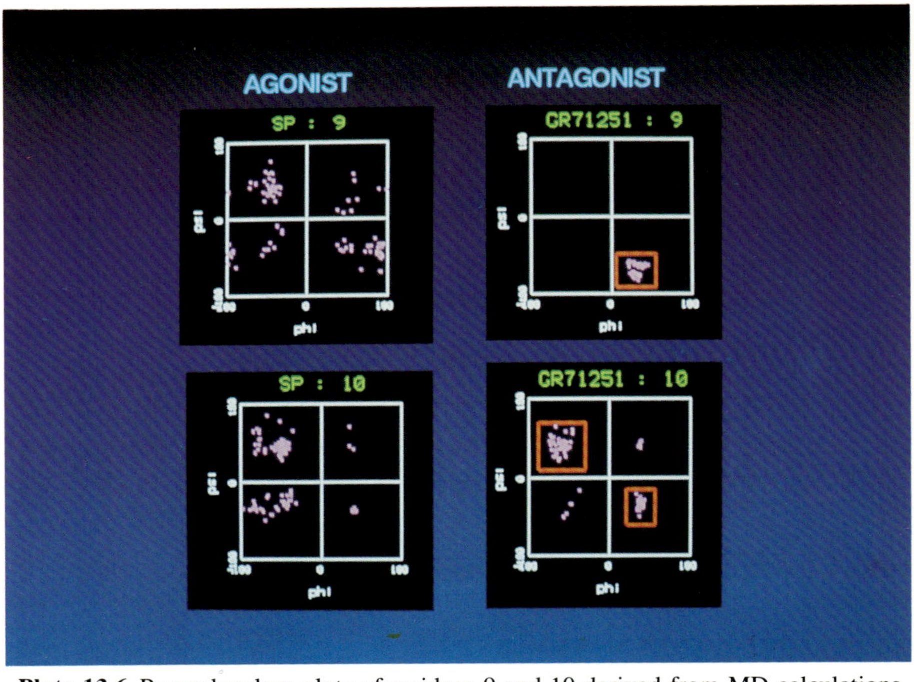

Plate 13.6 Ramachandran plots of residues 9 and 10 derived from MD calculations.

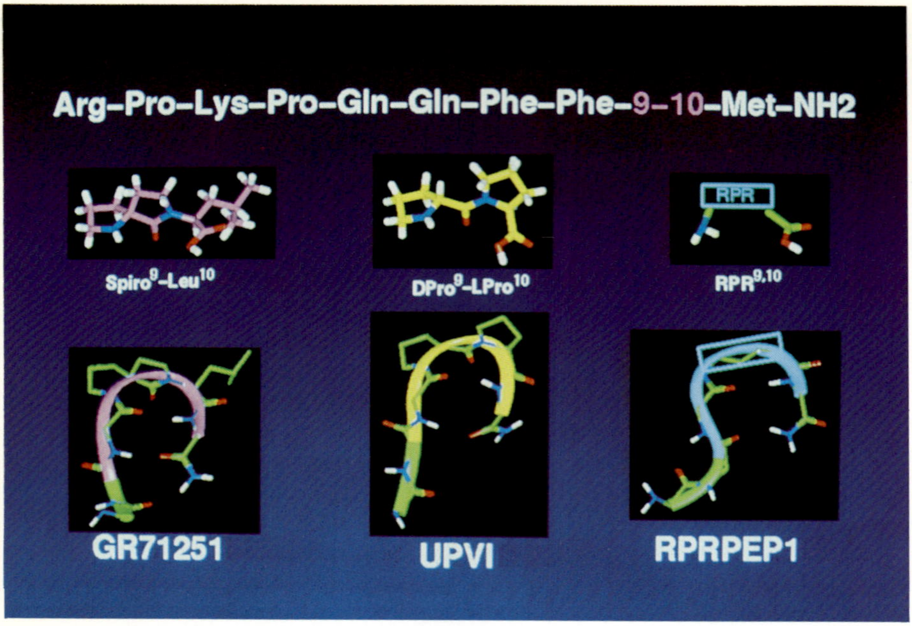

Plate 13.7 Conformations induced by β-turn mimics.

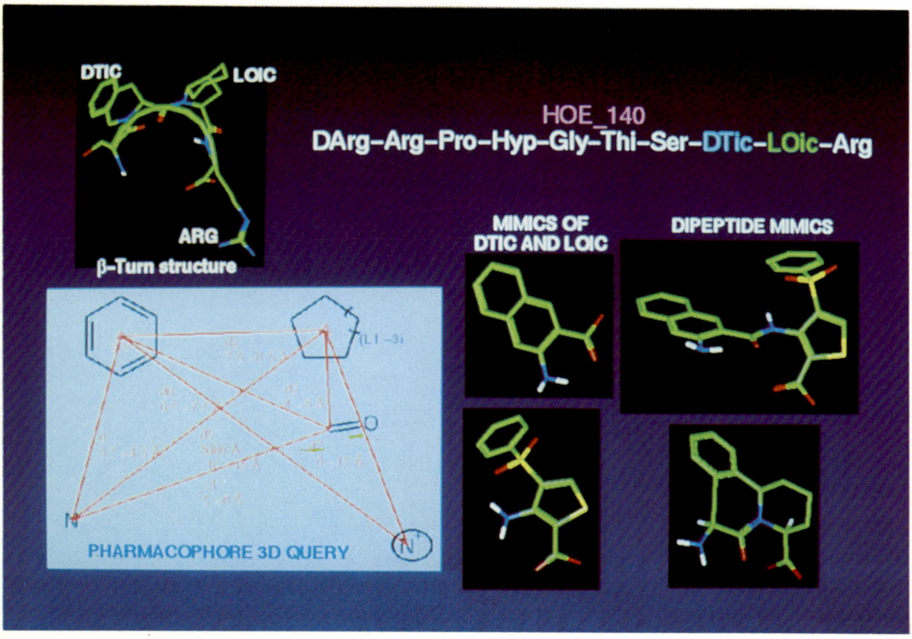

Plate 13.8 Applications to bradykinin antagonist design.

descriptor methods. In the last stage, the fragments are connected together using linear chains composed of one or more of 12 different functional groups, including -CH_2-, -CO-, -CONH-. LUDI, as all fragment methods, will have to cope with synthetic feasibility issues as *de novo* inhibitors are constructed. The program can also be used to add functionality to a known inhibitor.

Energy Search Methods

These docking techniques use molecular dynamics or simulated annealing and employ full molecular mechanics force fields. They smoothly merge the configurational and conformational aspects of docking. However, the complex topography and multiple minima of molecular potential surfaces often lead to relatively long run times.

Autodock

Goodsell and Olson (1990) use the Metropolis algorithm to find low-energy complexes of ligands in receptor sites, searching all configurational and several conformational degrees of freedom. The program was tested by docking phosphocholine into the antibody McPC 603, *N*-formyltryptophan into chymotrypsin, *N*-acetylglucosamine (two anomers) into lysozyme, and sulfate and citrate into aconitase. In most cases, the crystallographic solution was reproduced to better than 2 Å. The program is quite efficient considering the number of degrees of freedom. It is not clear how the run time scales with conformational freedom for larger systems. Stoddard and Koshland (1992) have applied this algorithm to predict the structure of the maltose binding protein – aspartate receptor complex.

Peptide docking

Caflisch and co-workers (1992) use graphics to place peptides in binding sites, followed by energy minimization and then a local search using Monte Carlo simulation. Test cases were a peptidic inhibitor of HIV-1 protease, and, courageously, an undecapeptide recognized by the HLA-A2 protein where the structure was not known at the time of writing. In the HIV-1 case, Monte Carlo refinement yielded a configuration closely resembling the crystallographic complex. In the HLA-A2 case, the peptide was docked in a helical conformation and then subjected to local refinement by Monte Carlo search. The helical complex, while consistent with the mutagenesis work then available, is in conflict with recent crystallographic results in which peptides bind in an extended geometry (Silver *et al.*, 1992).

Table 8.2
Examples of structure-based drug design leading to clinical trials

System	Company	Reference
Thymidylate synthase	Agouron	(Reich *et al.*, 1992)
Purine nucleoside phosphorylase	Biocryst, Ciba-Geigy	(Montgomery *et al.*, 1993)
HIV-1 protease	Merck	(Ghosh *et al.*, 1993)
	DuPont Merck	(Lam *et al.*, 1994)

Conclusions

Certain aspects of the docking problem have been solved. (1) Both known and novel binding sites can be identified through automatic procedures such as the negative imaging approach used with DOCK (Kuntz, 1992). (2) Many of the programs discussed above can reassemble the components of a known complex within 1 Å rms of the experimental structure. Thus, the problem of constructing a 'three-dimensional jigsaw puzzle' from rigid pieces of proper conformation has been solved. However, multiple binding geometries, plausible on steric and chemical grounds, are routinely seen (Shoichet and Kuntz, 1991). The number of alternatives increases when conformational freedom is introduced. To sort among these states requires quite accurate determinations of free energy (e.g. ± 1 kcal/mol).

Calculations serve many purposes in the drug design effort. Four goals of structure-driven design are: (1) screening for new leads; (2) rank-ordering similar and diverse compounds; (3) proposing preferred ligand–receptor geometries; and (4) rapid, semi-automatic optimization of a lead compound. A refinement of this last goal is coupling calculations to combinatorial chemistry (Bunin and Ellman, 1993).

Present programs are relatively successful at lead identification. A brief set of examples of compounds in various stages of clinical review derived from structure-based leads is given in Table 8.2. Lead generation is, of course, the easiest task since false positives are acceptable and false negatives are not recognized. Typical hit rates of 1–10% are competitive with high throughput experimental screens, and computer screening is much less expensive. An important issue is to determine the false-negative rate in computer screening. An appropriate test would be to run a substantial, diverse database of compounds through both computer and experimental screenings.

The task of rank-ordering the binding energies for a diverse set of compounds is more difficult. As noted above, force fields and empirical energy functions can rarely achieve better than ± 2 kcal/mol accuracy except within a family of compounds that have little conformational flexibility and that all bind in a very similar manner. A substantial increase in accuracy of current force fields and entropic estimates is required before one can expect a high correlation between calculated and measured K_i or IC_{50} data spanning several orders of magnitude.

It remains a difficult task to propose accurate (± 1 Å rms) geometric models for novel systems. With DOCK, the best cases have shown displacements of 1–2 Å from the predicted geometry. In the worst cases, the displacements are about 5 Å (Rutenber *et al.*, 1993; Shoichet *et al.*, 1993). Complications include the conformational freedom of the ligand and the receptor, the possibility of alternative binding modes (configurational freedom), and the inclusion of water molecules and ions as part of the binding complex. We have had problems with all of these phenomena. The obvious design/test protocol is to combine structural experiments with computations to provide rapid assessment of the degrees of freedom of a particular system of interest (Shoichet *et al.*, 1993). The most successful efforts at structure-based design have used one X-ray structure per 1–2 compounds synthesized (Reich *et al.*, 1992).

De novo strategies have the potential to assist in the optimization process, especially if coupled to a rule-based approach to what modifications are synthetically feasible. An appropriate challenge for such methods is to recreate known high-affinity inhibitors in the proper conformations, given the relevant binding site (Nishibata and Itai, 1993).

The fundamental limitations of computational methods are in sampling conformational and configurational space (the 'induced-fit' problem) and evaluating the free energy of interaction. Hardware advances, re-parameterization of force fields, and improved heuristics should all contribute to significant improvements in the near future. Opportunities for directed ligand design will increase dramatically as the number of solved structures grows and the molecular mechanisms of disease are clarified. It will be an exicting challenge to make maximal use of this new information to design new molecules.

Acknowledgements

This chapter is based, in part, on a recent review. Many colleagues contributed to the software described here, Drs Renée DesJarlais, J. Scott Dixon, George Seibel, Robert Sheridan and Dale Bodian especially should be thanked. We are grateful for the interactions provided by the UCSF Computer Graphics Laboratory. Support for our work was provided by the National Institutes of Health, the Advanced Research Project Agency, Molecular Design Limited Information Systems, Tripos Associates, Parke-Davis, Smithkline Beecham and Glaxo.

References

Allen, F.H., Bellard, S., Brice, M.D., Cartwright, B.A., Doubleday, A., Higgs, H., Hummelink, T., Hummelink-Peters, B.G., Kennard, O., Motherwell, W.D.S., Rodgers, J.R. and Watson, D.G. (1979). *Acta Crystallogr.* **B35**, 2331–2339.

Allinger, N.L., Yuh, Y.H. and Lii, J.J. (1989) *J. Am. Chem. Soc.* **111**, 8551–8566.

Bartlett, P.A., Shea, G.T., Telfer, S.T. and Waterman, S. (1989). *In* 'Molecular Recognition: Chemical and Biochemical Problems' (S.M. Roberts, ed.), pp. 182–196. Royal Society of Chemistry, London.

Ben-Naim, A. (1994). *Curr. Opin. Struct. Biol.* **4** (in press).

Billeter, M. (1992). *Q. Rev. Biophys.* **25**, 325–377.

Bodian, D.L., Yamasaki, R.B., Buswell, R.L., Stearns, J.F., White, J.M. and Kuntz, I.D. (1993). *Biochemistry* **32**, 2967–2978.

Böhm, H.J. (1992). *J. Comput.-Aided Mol. Design* **6**, 593–606.

Brünger, A.T. (1993). *Acta Crystallogr.* **D49**, 24–36.

Bunin, B.A., and Ellman, J.A. (1993). *J. Am. Chem. Soc.* **114**, 10997–10998.

Caflisch, A., Niederer, P. and Anliker, M. (1992). *Proteins* **13**, 223–230.

Chambers, J.L. and Stroud, R.M. (1979). *Acta Crystallogr.* **B35**, 1861–74.

Cherfils, J., Duquerroy, S. and Janin, J. (1991). *Proteins* **11**, 271–280.

Chothia, C. (1974). *Nature* **248**, 338–339.

Chothia, C. and Lesk, A.M. (1986). *EMBO. J.* **5**, 823–826.

Cohen, N.C., Blaney, J.M., Humblet, C., Gund, P. and Barry, D.C. (1990). *J. Med. Chem.* **33**, 883–894.

Connolly, M.L. (1983). *Science* **221**, 709–713.

Connolly, M.L. (1985). *Biopolymers* **25**, 1229–1247.

Cornell, W.D., Cieplak, P., Bayly, C.I. and Kollman, P.A. (1993). *J. Am. Chem. Soc.* **115**, 9620–9631.

Cramer, C.J. and Truhlar, D.G. (1992). *Science* **256**, 213–217.

DesJarlais, R., Sheridan, R.P., Seibel, G.L., Dixon, J.S., Kuntz, I.D. and Venkataraghavan, R. (1988). *J. Med. Chem.* **31**, 722–729.

DesJarlais, R.L., Seibel, G.L., Kuntz, I.D., Ortiz de Montellano, P.R., Furth, P.S., Alvarez, J.C., DeCamp, D.L., Babé, L.M. and Craik, C.S. (1990). *Proc. Natl. Acad. Sci. USA* **87**, 6644–6648.

Dill, K.A. (1990). *Biochemistry* **29**, 7133–7155.

Dinur, U. and Hagler, A.T. (1990). *J. Comput. Chem.* **11**, 91–105.

Dolata, D.P., Leach, A.R. and Prout, K. (1987). *J. Comput.-Aided Mol. Design* **1**, 73–85.

Eisenberg, D. and McLachlan, A.D. (1986). *Nature* **319**, 199–203.

Fischer, E. (1894). *Chem. Berichte* **27**, 2985–2993.

Ghosh, A.K., Thompson, W.J., Lee, H.Y., McKee, S.P., Munson, P.M., Duong, T.T., Darke, P.L., Zugay, J.A., Emini, E.A., Schleif, W.A., Huff, J.R. and Anderson, P.S. (1993). *J. Med. Chem.* **36**, 924–927.

Goodford, P.J. (1985). *J. Med. Chem.* **28**, 849–857.

Goodsell, D.S. and Olson, A.J. (1990). *Proteins* **8**, 195–202.

Halgren, T.A. (1992). *J. Am. Chem. Soc.* **114**, 7827–7843.

Ho, C.M.W. and Marshall, G.R. (1993). *J. Comput.-Aided Mol. Design* **7**, 3–22.

Jiang, F. and Kim, S.H. (1991). *J. Mol. Biol.* **219**, 79–102.

Johnson, M.A. and Maggiora, G.M. (1990). *In* 'Concepts and Applications of Molecular Similarity', John Wiley, New York.

Jorgensen, W.L. (1991). *Science* **254**, 954–955.

Jorgensen, W.L. and Nguyen, T.B. (1993). *J. Comput. Chem.* **14**, 195–205.

Karplus, M. and McCammon, J.A. (1983). *Annu. Rev. Biochem.* **52**, 263–300.
Kerwin, S.M., Kuntz, I.D. and Kenyon, G.L. (1991). *Med. Chem. Res.* **1**, 361–368.
Koshland, D.E., Jr. (1971) *Pure Appl. Chem.* **25**, 119–133.
Kossiakoff, A.A., Randal, M., Guenot, J. and Eignebrot, C. (1992). *Proteins – Struct. Func. Genetics* **14**, 65–74.
Kuntz, I.D. (1992). *Science* **257**, 1078–1082.
Kuntz, I.D., Blaney, J.M., Oatley, S.J., Langridge, R. and Ferrin, T.E. (1982). *J. Mol. Biol.* **161**, 269–288.
Kuntz, I.D., Meng, E.C. and Shoichet, B.K. (1994). *Acc. Chem. Res.* **27**, 117–123.
Lam, P.Y.S., Jadhav, P.K., Eyermann, C.J., Hodge, C.N., Ru, Y., Bacheler, L.T., Meek, J.L., Otto, M.J., Rayner, M.M., Wong, Y.N., Chang, C.-H., Weber, P.C., Jackson, D.A., Sharpe, T.R. and Erickson-Viitanen, S. (1994). *Science* **263**, 380–384.
Lawrence, M.C. and Davis, P.C. (1992). *Proteins* **12**, 31–41.
Leach, A.R. and Prout, K. (1990). *J. Comput. Chem.* **11**, 1193.
Leach, A.R. and Kuntz, I.D. (1992). *J. Comput. Chem.* **13**, 730–748.
Lewis, R.A., Roe, D.C., Huang, C., Ferrin, T.E., Langridge, R. and Kuntz, I.D. (1992). *J. Mol. Graphics* **10**, 66–78.
Marshall, G.R., Barry, D.C., Bosshard, H.E., Dammkoehler, R.A. and Dunn, D.A. (1979). *In* 'Computer-Assisted Drug Design' (E.C. Olson, and R.E. Christoffersen, eds.) pp. 205–226. American Chemical Society, Washington, D.C.
Meng, E.C., Shoichet, B.K. and Kuntz, I.D. (1992). *J. Comput. Chem.* **13**, 505–524.
Mezey, P.G. (1990). *Rev. Comput. Chem.* **1**, 265.
Miranker, A. and Karplus, M. (1991). *Proteins–Struct. Func. Genetics* **11**, 29–34.
Montgomery, J.A., Niwas, S., Rose, J.D., Secrist, J.A., 3rd, Babu, Y.S., Bugg, C.E., Erion, M.D., Guida, W.C. and Ealick, S.E. (1993). *J. Med. Chem.* **36**, 55–69.
Moon, J.B. and Howe, J.W. (1991). *Proteins* **11**, 314–328.
Nichols, A., Sharp, K.A. and Honig, B. (1991). *Proteins* **11**, 281–296.
Nishibata, Y. and Itai, A. (1993). *J. Med. Chem.* **36**, 2921–2928.
Ponder, J.W. and Richards, F.M. (1987). *J. Mol. Biol.* **193**, 775–791.
Reich, S.H., Fuhry, M.A.M., Nguyen, D., Pino, M.J., Welsh, K.M., Webber, S., Janson, C.A., Jordan, S.R., Matthews, D.A., Smith, W.W., Bartlett, C.A., Booth, C.L.J., Herrmann, S.M., Howland, E.F., Morse, C.A., Ward, R.W. and White, J. (1992). *J. Med. Chem.* **35**, 847–858.
Ring, C.S., Sun, E., McKerrow, J.H., Lee, G.K., Rosenthal, P.J., Kuntz, I.D. and Cohen, F.E. (1993). *Proc. Natl Acad. Sci. USA* **90**, 3583–3587.
Rusinko, A., Sheridan, R.P., Nilakatan, R., Haraki, K.S., Bauman, N. and Venkataghavan, R. (1989). *J. Chem. Info. Comput. Sci.* **29**, 251–255.
Rutenber, E., Fauman, E.B., Keenan, R.J., Fong, S., Furth, P.S., Ortiz de Montellano, P.R., Meng, E., Kuntz, I.D., DeCamp, D.L., Salto, R., Rosé, J.R., Craik, C. and Stroud, R.M. (1993). *J. Biol. Chem.* **268**, 15343–15346.
Salomma, A. (1991). *Theor. Comput. Sci.* **88**, 127–138.
Schreiber, H. and Steinhauser, O. (1992). *Biochemistry* **31**, 5856–5860.
Schulz, G.E., Muller, C.W. and Diederichs, K. (1990). *J. Mol. Biol.* **213**, 627–630.
Shoichet, B.K. and Kuntz, I.D. (1991). *J. Mol. Biol.* **221**, 327–346.
Shoichet, B.K. and Kuntz, I.D. (1993). *Prot. Engng* **6**, 723–732.
Shoichet, B.K., Bodian, D.L. and Kuntz, I.D. (1992). *J. Comput. Chem.* **13**, 380–397.
Shoichet, B.K., Stroud, R.M., Santi, D.V., Kuntz, I.D. and Perry, K.M. (1993). *Science* **259**, 1445–1450.
Silver, M., Go, H., Strominger, J. and Wiley, D. (1992). *Nature* **360**, 367–369.
Still, W.C., Tempczyk, A., Hawley, R.C. and Hendrickson, T. (1990). *J. Am. Chem. Soc.* **112**, 6127–6129.

Stoddard, B.L. and Koshland, D.E. (1992). *Nature* **358**, 774–776.
Straatsma, T.P. and McCammon, J.A. (1992). *Annu. Rev. Phys. Chem.* **43**, 407–435.
Ullman, J.R. (1976). *J. Assoc. Comput. Mach.* **16**, 31.
Warshel, A. and Åqvist, J. (1991). *Annu. Rev. Biophys. BioPhys. Chem.* **20**, 267–298.
Wilson, C., Mace, J.E. and Agard, D. (1991). *J. Mol. Biol.* **220**, 495–506.
Wodak, S.J. and Janin, J. (1978). *J. Mol. Biol.* **124**, 323–342.
Wodak, S.J., De Crombrugghe, M. and Janin, J. (1987). *Prog. Biophys. Mol. Biol.* **49**, 29–63.

Discussion

S. Perez
With regard to the influence of crystallographic resolution on drug design, we have been doing a lot of work in our laboratory trying to design new inhibitors for α-amylase. Starting from a crystal structure which was known at 3 Å resolution, we spent 2 years on this and could not find the proper orientation of the oligosaccharide with this badly resolved structure. For a proper and decent answer we had to wait until we had a highly resolved structure (down to about 2.1 Å resolution). Have you also experienced this problem?

I.D. Kuntz
I would support that completely. Greg Petsko and I have discussed this privately. At 3 Å so many things can be wrong. We have to focus specifically on the fact that almost nothing is known about bound water at 3 Å and also about many of the side chain positions. After all, most of the time, except for protease inhibitors, we are 'talking' to the enzyme through the side chains and not through the backbone. Critical assessment is needed. This is why I believe firmly that this work is a team effort; the structural people must be brought directly in to say that they honestly do not know *that* region well. If that region is the focus of the work, we must either undergo the agonies of model building, molecular dynamics and so on or just use it to test qualitative hypotheses.

I think this will also show up in some of the nuclear magnetic resonance structures because, again, they have many areas that are relatively 'soft'.

On the other hand, if the focus is a well-described active site, sometimes even a low-resolution picture can make use of some of the ideas put forward by Dr Bartlett about transition state analogues, suicide inhibitors – things of that kind which will have to be positioned roughly, and which then can do the chemical 'dirty work' on their own.

J.N. Barton
In, for example, the comparison of the theoretical binding potencies of folate inhibitors to mammalian and bacterial DHFR, do the scoring functions correlate with the activities/selectivities that are seen?

I.D. Kuntz
We did not get a wonderful correlation – over two orders of magnitude – of our force field score and the K_i values. I have seen some fairly good correlations with these force fields, but only within a closely related set of compounds. These compounds were chosen because they had the biggest differential between the human dihydrofolate reductase (DHFR) score and the parasitic DHFR score. The ones with the biggest differential in fact do look like the best selectivity – but only three of them really stand out as very interesting compounds. It is asking a lot of the method to try to compare with a free energy when entropies or solvation terms are not being calculated.

A.R. Leach
Which of the various areas for further development that were mentioned do you think are the most important, and which are most amenable to solution?

I.D. Kuntz
That is a tough question. Many people are focusing on conformation search. Nothing is more embarrassing than to be in direct competition with a high-throughput screen and miss the compound in the computation, because computational chemists have to know more than just putting the compound into the right solvent for the screen. It has to be recognized that there are many different uses of this set of tools. I have often told people that they have the best of all worlds in lead discovery because false positives are expected – every screen has many – and, by-and-large, people do not recognize false negatives. We therefore escape some of the genuine angst that might come otherwise.

I feel that the conformation problem is in relatively good hands. I do not have to focus much of my attention on this because there are programs such as those of Andrew Leach and Dan Dolata. The genetic algorithm is also promising.

I am, however, worried about the solvation issues, much along the lines raised by Greg Petsko. Some waters have to be displaced: some we see, some we do not see. All of them cost enthalpy; some of them benefit us in entropy. It is still not known whether we are better off if no assessment is made than if a first-order assessment is made. This is where most of our effort is going.

I.M. McLay
I am sure DOCK has been tried on a single conformer of one molecule. Could you describe your successes in this area – if it has been successful?

I.D. Kuntz
Success in those kind of systems would generally be measured by the proper structural end-point: put it back in and see what happens. We have done that in an important way only in two systems: human immunodeficiency virus

protease and a project on thymidylate synthase. In other words, I am not allowing for reconstituting other people's complexes when the active site, as Greg Petsko said, has already had the proper induced fit and so on.

In the two examples, the good and bad news is combined in an interesting way. In both cases we seriously missed what we thought from the first round of crystallography was the answer. In the protease case, neither a chloride ion nor a conformation change of the protein had been included, and a single point mutation yielded the exact mode of binding that we had first predicted. My message is that there are alternative modes of binding, and the best that can be done in the computer version is to enumerate these modes and leave it to clever experimentalists to sort them out.

The moral is similar in the case of the thymidylate synthetase. We missed badly – about 5 Å – on our first structure. The nice thing about this procedure is that it is possible logically to backtrack and see whose fault it is. It turned out that the fault again lay in an anion bound tightly to a phosphate binding site not included in the modelling. When this was included in the modelling the results made sense, and the next generation of compounds fell within 1 Å of where we thought they should.

In that sense, these stories have happy endings, but they point to the importance of 'stand-by' information that we might not always be given. I particularly stress that monovalent anions are often included in the inventory of bound water. It would be thought that chloride and oxygen are immediately distinguishable, but this is not so at partial occupancy.

M.J. Ashton

Nature is much more clever than any individual person or combination thereof, and enzymes and receptors construct themselves in such a way as just to do what they wish to do. In active sites there is much redundancy, so when structures are grown in active sites there may be the risk of growing pentacyclic and heptacyclic structures which look like something that has come out of carbon or coal and which are not very useful to the synthetic chemist. If a stopping procedure is put to that to restrict it to perhaps three cycles or a certain number of atoms, the problem then is where to choose our point to start: the left-hand side, in the middle or at the right-hand side?

Secondly, with regard to the placing of atoms upon those skeletons to enable the chemists perhaps to synthesize molecules as rapidly as technology allows us today, perhaps Dr Johnson would comment on how such placement can be linked with an ease-of-synthesis program.

I.D. Kuntz

As to filling the site in some way, I do not think we want to limit the number of rings *per se*, but the number of atoms probably does have to be limited. I think some strategies can be developed, making whatever use we can of our biochemical knowledge as the starting point and the recognition pockets, and going out as far as a reasonable number of atoms takes us – because we learn repeatedly that high molecular weight compounds do not make good drugs even if they are excellent inhibitors.

I do not think there are any generic rules about where to start and stop in placing atoms on to a template that would magically provide the guide every time. We will be governed by trying to get the optimum interactions first out of the problem, and then seeing what else is needed.

I am interested to hear what Dr Johnson says, but my guess is that one good route to synthetic feasibility is to use linkers that we know we can make, then have the fragments – the warhead parts – linked together in any way that is convenient. There are still hundreds of possible linkers, so it may not narrow the field enormously, but it is a good starting point.

A.P. Johnson
First, on the structure generation programs, it is easy to put limits on, for example, the number of fusions. This overcomes Dr Ashton's problem of avoiding making anthracenes and so on.

On the synthetic accessibility, at the moment our system assigns an accessibility number to each molecule individually on the basis of a number of rules. The kind of advances we want to make are, on the one hand, to compare molecules from an answer set. Where there are sufficient similarities between them it might often be possible to use a synthesis which leads to many compounds from a common intermediate. This is a case where the multiplicity – or the clustering – of compounds is important with regard to synthetic accessibility.

Answering the second part of Dr Ashton's question, a medicinal chemist will take a suggested structure and put heteroatoms at suitable points to make it easier to synthesize. Again, a set of rules can probably be applied in a computer system to do precisely that – or by comparison with databases of available starting materials. This would also help to identify points for heteroatom substitution.

In terms of heteroatom substitution, another aspect that has not been considered is that one has not just to consider the binding or the synthetic accessibility but also the transport properties of the compound. The compound has to get to the site of biological action. Again, I think this is something that can be done.

9

Optimization of Combinatoric Problems in Structure Generation for Drug Design

P.M. DEAN, M.T. BARAKAT and N.P. TODOROV

Drug Design Group, Department of Pharmacology, University of Cambridge, Tennis Court Road, Cambridge CB2 1QJ, UK

Introduction

How to optimize lead generation is the fundamental question that has to be tackled by any pharmaceutical company to ensure its future economic success. There are no shortages of pharmacological targets. One has only to consider the explosion in our knowledge of small bioactive peptides in recent years to appreciate the large number of receptors that are specific for the pharmacological actions of these peptides. Mass screening of combinatorial libraries of peptides will undoubtedly yield many tantalizing problems for the medicinal chemist to convert the peptide into a non-peptide peptidomimetic. Crucially important targets for drug design will also come from the Human Genome Project and protein folding studies, either *de novo* folding or by homology modelling. The advent of automated methods for drug design should provide pharmaceutical companies with a powerful new armoury for suggesting novel lead compounds.

Commercial companies are driven by two instincts: desire that they may not be beaten in the race to find a lead, and need in their wish to monopolize on the lead they have designed. The desire to be the first to find a lead is understandable. However, if simple software packages are used to piece

New Perspectives in Drug Design
ISBN 0–12–208070–X

together a putative molecular structure by a set paradigm, there is a danger that the algorithm will design basically similar structures for every company that uses the software on the same target problem. This scenario can be disrupted only if the combinatorial problems of design are tackled rigorously with some element of random structure generation. The problem with structure generation is that it has combinatoric components at numerous steps. This chapter outlines the combinatoric problems and suggests ways of optimizing them. Combinatorial methods offer the drug designer a massive, and potentially far richer choice of putative structures to consider. The size of the combinatorial space is frequently large, $> 10^{25}$, and thus cannot be tackled effectively by iterative procedures.

It is desirable to have design methods that are completely general in their applicability. That is to say they must, where possible, be free from conceptual and site constraints. The methods must be able to cope with all conceivable steric shapes for the site; take into account, but not be dependent on, site-point hydrogen bonds; and be able to cope with any molecular field or combination of fields. Furthermore, and this is probably more important in practice, can the same algorithms that are used for site-directed structure generation also be used for similarity-directed generation when the site structure is unavailable?

Complementarity and Similarity Paradigms

Site-directed *de novo* drug design is based on the complementarity between the generated ligand and its site. The paramount problem that has to be resolved is how to generate structures, and this is purposefully made plural since we are concerned with exploring a wide range of structural diversity, which have steric complementarity with the site surface at their binding faces. A consequence of the simple energetics, for example equation (3) (see page 160) estimated *in vacuo*, for the ligand–site inteaction is that there will be complementarity, or similarity if we are considering the hydrophobicity, in the molecular fields between the generated structure and the site. Can this conceptual equivalence of complementarity be used for ligand structure generation in the absence of any coordinates for the site? In this case it should be possible to use molecular similarity methods to superpose, say, two naturally occurring substrates or inhibitors, and to use the supersurface as the conceptual equivalent of a site. This supersurface we call an envelope, in which structurally diverse ligands can be generated. The combinatoric problems here lie in the definition of the envelopes as well as in the generation step. If the base ligands, that is those which are used to define the envelope, are structurally distinct, then there may be multiple superpositions. These may reflect different binding modes at the site, or may be artefacts of the superposition analysis. However, despite these caveats, it is possible to take the envelope(s) and generate structures *de novo* with close steric fits and with similar surface potentials.

Methods for *de novo* Structure Generation

Structure generation algorithms can be classified by the basic philosophy that underpins their methodology. First, those methods which attempt to reduce drastically the number of possible structures generated. Second, those strategies which allow a less constrained structure generation to create a larger diversity of structures.

Drastic reduction of the combinational problem can be achieved by searching for the largest structure from a database of pieces which will fit the local constraints of the site. These pieces may be a subset of a much larger database such as the Cambridge Structural Database (CSD) or a company database. Two methods for fitting the pieces seem to be in common usage: steric fits of large fragments to fill the available space (DOCK) (DesJarlais *et al.*, 1988; see Chapter 8) and vector procedures to search a database for structures containing specified vectors placed in the site (CAVEAT) (Lauri *et al.*, 1989; Laurie and Bartlett, 1994; see Chapter 4). The principal advantage of either of these methods is that only small numbers of potential structures are generated and need to be inspected to decide which are synthetically feasible. Since the pieces have been obtained from known structures this provides a clear advantage in understanding the synthesis of the dominant pieces. The method works quite nicely for small sites since the site constrains the number of possible fits that may be generated from large pieces. If algorithms are written to constrain heavily the number of generations it is more likely that multiple runs of the algorithm will generate the same small set of structures for a particular site; this reduction in structural variety can be a disadvantage of the philosophy.

In the second case of a weakly constrained generator, making structures from very small fragments, vast numbers of structures may be generated. Some of these will be synthetically difficult with unusual ring combinations and conformations. Hearsay evidence exists where 10^5 structures have been generated to fit a site; subsequent classification shows that up to half are duplicated, but the number of distinctly different structures is still substantial. Clearly, some form of data reduction is necessary in order to inspect manageable numbers of structures. Structural diversity needs to be scanned by cluster analysis of common subgraphs to identify basic families of skeletal frameworks, if they exist, within the generated structures.

Shortcomings of Current Attempts at *de novo* Structure Generation

In essence structure generation is combinatoric; if we have n fragments, or pieces, they can be arranged in $n!$ ways for adjacency of fragments; if each fragment can also be connected to its neighbor by m different ways there is a further possibility of m^n different connections between each combination of fragments. For example, suppose we have six different fragments and for simplicity let each fragment have three structurally distinct ways to connect to its neighbour; then we have 720 permutations of fragments and 729 connection patterns for each combination giving a total of more than 500 000 structurally distinct entities. Conformational differences are neglected. Clearly, any method which relies on fitting large conglomerates into a site must have a massive database to choose from if shape diversity is to be pursued in a rigorous way. A corollary is that methods which are based on generating structures from small fragments must potentially consider massive numbers of structures to generate. If generation programs can be sufficiently optimized it should be possible to handle much larger numbers of structures than can be stored in databases.

Suppose a structure generator suggests a large number of structures to fit the site. How are we to decide on a small number to synthesize? Putative structures need to be ranked in some order of priority. Ranking according to an energy of interaction between the ligand structure and the site is an obvious suggestion. However, the problem is how to scale the different energy contributions. Most computational methods are derived for the *in vacuo* situation but this is not a reasonable picture of the interaction. Scoring methods need to be elaborated which take into account the aqueous environment.

Whatever philosophy is used to generate structures, decisions have to be taken about the synthetic feasibility of the putative structures. Clearly, with methods based on fitting conglomerate fragments together, much of the structure is known to be synthesizable. However for the stronger combinatoric methods, measures of structural complexity are needed to assess the ranked structures for each of synthesis.

This chapter is concerned with defining the combinatoric problems of structure generation so that a sober assessment of each problem can be taken before attempts are made to reduce the problems by optimization methods.

Combinatoric Problems

For a small site, a designer may wish to generate a very large number of possibilities for the site and to decide whether certain structural types are constantly being generated with excellent scores for the fit. However, if the site is large, it may not be feasible to include all the site as a target for structure generation since the resulting structures may be too large to be effective drug molecules. How is the site to be divided?

Subsets of the Site

Division of the site into a subset of regions will often have an element of arbitrariness, especially if the site is predominantly hydrophobic with no clear internal boundaries. However, if the site can be partitioned into subsets of site points then combinations can be selected and structures generated for each subset. The reduction of the site to a set of site points may be achieved by defining regions of maximum hydrogen-bonding probability, dividing the electrostatic potential to regions of maxima and minima and defining the center of hydrophobic regions.

Combinatorics of the site points
The number of combinations of subsets, $C(n,r)$, of site points of size r taken from a set of n site points is given by the equation

$$C(n,r) = \frac{n!}{r!\ (n-r)!} \tag{1}$$

Thus, suppose that four site points are needed for a pharmacophore to be attached and that there are ten possible site points to chose from, then the number of subsets of site points taken four at a time is 210. Which subsets would be a good choice for structure generation? Two features strongly affect the choice: specificity and spatial distribution.

Selection of site points for specificity
One of the goals of drug design is to generate putative ligands which are highly specific for the site. If the site is a member of a family of related proteins then differences between the proteins should be sought which might have an influence on specificity. Ideally one would like to select a set of site points which are characteristic for the target only and not shared by related proteins. If crystal structures are present, these distinguishing features can easily be identified. It is likely that this strategy will reduce the number of combinations drastically. However, in the absence of crystallographic data for multiple sites, it might be possible to take sequences from gene banks and perform consensus sequence alignments. Equivalent residues can then be aligned to identify possible differences in site points.

Sensible sets of specific site points
If by the above procedure, site points can be classified into structurally important subsets, there is still the problem of selecting subsets which are the best for the structure generation problem. Consider two extremes. If the members of the subset are too widely spaced it will be difficult to generate sufficiently inflexible structures to span the site points; furthermore, the generated structures will show little similarity between themselves. On the

other hand, if the site points are too close together only a few rigid structures can be generated. Some compromise is needed. A procedure that can be adopted would be, in the example above of four site points for structure generation, to take a subset of three important site points and allow the algorithm to select the fourth site point randomly for each attempted generation. This procedure ensures that a reasonable variety of site points are sampled for structure generation.

Structure Generation

Ideally it should be possible to develop a structure generator, for site-directed *de novo* design, to give a score for the final structures generated by equation (2) (Moon and Howe, 1990, 1991):

$$\text{SCORE} = -[E_{\text{vdw}} + E_{\text{es}} + E_{\text{conf}} + (E_{\text{solv}})\text{ligand} + (E_{\text{solv}})\text{protein}] \qquad (2)$$

This equation implies that the structure is correctly docked into the site at each step of the generation and that all terms are constantly recalculated as generation proceeds. Atom assignments have been made to the structure. If structure generation is envelope directed a different scoring scheme is necessary. The first two terms can be expanded to:

$$E = \sum_{i}^{I} \sum_{j \neq i}^{J} \left(-\frac{A_{ij}^{\text{ab}}}{r_{ij}^{6}} + \frac{B_{ij}^{\text{ab}}}{r_{ij}^{12}} + \frac{C_{ij}^{\text{ab}} q_i q_j}{r_{ij}} \right) \qquad (3)$$

which is the familiar Lennard Jones potential with a coulombic component but re-expressed with superscripts by Clementi (1980). Molecule I, with atoms i may represent the site and molecule J with atoms j may represent the ligand. A, B and C are fitting constants for atom pairs i and j; the superscripts a and b represent the atom types and the class to which they belong; r_{ij} is the interatomic distance; q_i and q_j represent the charges on each atom.

Equation (3) divides naturally into a geometric component as the denominator and an atomic component in the numerator. The first two terms are short range and are effectively limited to contact atoms, whilst the electrostatic term operates over a longer range. Wherever an equation contains multiple parameters for summation there will be many different solutions with a similar value; thus the equation may be difficult to optimize without a sophisticated optimization procedure.

The questions to be considered in the following account are: can structure generation be divided into two steps: (1) can the generation of different skeletons be to a large extent independent of atom types, and (2) can atom placement be considered as a separate problem on selected skeletons generated? Is it possible to devize a general method of combinatorial optimization for each step in the strategy? Can transferability be used in the electrostatic term to reduce the need to recalculate the electronic distribution for each atom placement attempted?

Fragments of structure

In order to reduce the combinatoric problem of storing large numbers of molecular fragments, the smallest useful set is possibly the set of fragments where a specified atom has its connecting bonds attached to possible atoms. Thus, the smallest set consists of all 3-atom, 4-atom and 5-atom fragments. Aromatic rings are a special case and combinations of them may have to be taken. A useful set of atoms for drug design is {H, C, N, O, halogen} and certain structures containing S and P. All combinations of atoms from the set can be found that fulfil the valence requirements. Searches of the CSD for each combination reveal that only about half the possible combinations are actually found (Chau and Dean, 1992a). The geometrical properties of each fragment can be ascertained (Chau and Dean, 1992b) along with calculations of their electronic charges. About 90% of the computed standard fragment charges lie within 2 standard deviations of those taken from a random set of molecules containing the fragment (Chau and Dean, 1992c). This suggests that the charges in each fragment are transferable. Since these charges are to be used in an optimization process for atom placement on to generated skeletons, one further question has to be satisfied: are the electrostatic potentials computed from fragments comparable to those computed directly from the molecular structure? In general there is a good correlation between the fragment derived potentials and the computed potential, except as one would expect in highly conjugated regions. However, in aromatic regions the electrostatic potential is low anyway and so this problem may not be so important in practice.

Skeleton growing

We have shown that structure generation is highly combinatoric. The number of molecular graphs, G, that can be generated from n geometric fragments, where each fragment has m growing points, is:

$$G = n!m^n\,(m - 1)^{n-2} \qquad (4)$$

although there may be some reduction in numbers through symmetry effects. We will show, later that atom placement onto a molecular graph is also a potential combinatoric problem and can be treated separately for convenience. Our experience is that optimization of atom placement can converge satisfactorily (see later).

If a true combinatoric method of structure generation is to be attempted from geometric fragments, the fundamental problems lie in the choice of starting position, the trajectory for growth and the conformation of the growing skeleton. For a site-point model the starting position should be close to one point. To economize on growth, a directed trajectory from one seed point to another, or from a branch point in the developing skeleton to a seed point, is essential; otherwise the trajectory would be too random. If portions of the structure can be made with sensible torsion angles within the constraints of the site and in the developing skeletal pattern, these are preferred. Two methods for combinatorial skeleton generation are possible: first, chains can be generated over the site surface to optimize the pathway between site points, leaving cycles to be created at a subsequent step (this is our preferred method and is described below); second, combinations of 3-, 4- and 5-atom fragments with some rings can be used in a randomized order. Since this generation step, in either case, will be iterated many times, the objective function has to be as simple as possible. Only crude constraints of the site need to be taken into account at this stage so steric checks are the only necessary ones for the hydrogen atoms and heavy atoms.

How many structurally different chains are there, neglecting conformational differences for the moment, which can connect two site points? The geometry of the chain is determined by the internal coordinates. Consider bonds of a single length and bond angles to be linear, planar or tetrahedral. These can be combined independently, so for k atoms with $k-1$ bonds there are 3^{k-2} possible chains; thus if k varies from 2 to N there are G possibilities where G is defined as

$$G = \frac{3^{N-1}-1}{2} \tag{5}$$

If we consider a further approximation that all the angles are similar and restrict the number of linear geometries to M then

$$G = \sum_{k=1}^{N-2} \sum_{j=0}^{M} C(k,j) \tag{6}$$

$C(k, j)$ is analogous to $C(n, r)$ in equation (1). Thus for $N = 6$ and $M = 2$, $G = 25$.

In order to ensure that the skeleton has a reasonable probability of a snug fit to the site when it is fleshed out with atoms at a later stage, the developing structure should maximize its surface contacts. Other strategies such as creating planar growing systems may be appropriate for bridging across site points provided that sufficient contacts can be made with the site. These strategies might make use of templates of planar rings (Lewis and Dean, 1989a,b) or lattices of atoms (Lewis, 1990).

Chain conformation problems

Two major problems arise in considering the conformation(s) of an evolving skeleton which are hidden in the E_{conf} term of equation (2); they are conformational energy and rotational entropy. The reduction in bond rotational entropy is a complex problem in drug design and is probably more important than conformational energy for *de novo* structure generation. A fixed pharmacophore is a desirable goal for good interactions with the site. However, this stiffening of the ligand in the appropriate conformation by complex ring arrangements is likely to be synthetically difficult. A compromise strategy is needed which allows some flexibility since atom types and different bond lengths can be considered at a later stage.

If structure generation proceeds via chain growth between site points, how many conformations are allowed for each chain? Consider a k atom chain; there are $k-2$ dihedral angles. If $k \leqslant 7$ an exact solution exists (Lewis, 1992). For $k > 7$ the TWEAK algorithm can be used (Shenkin *et al.*, 1987). This algorithm starts from a random conformation and forces the conformation to the nearest one which fulfils the distance constraint. Chains are generated until all conformation clusters are well populated; significantly different conformations can then be counted (Perkins and Dean, 1993).

To give an example, consider two fragments of methotrexate that have to be joined by an 11-atom chain. If approximately 50 angle samples are taken per bond, the brute-force complexity is 5.6×10^{18}. The number of solutions

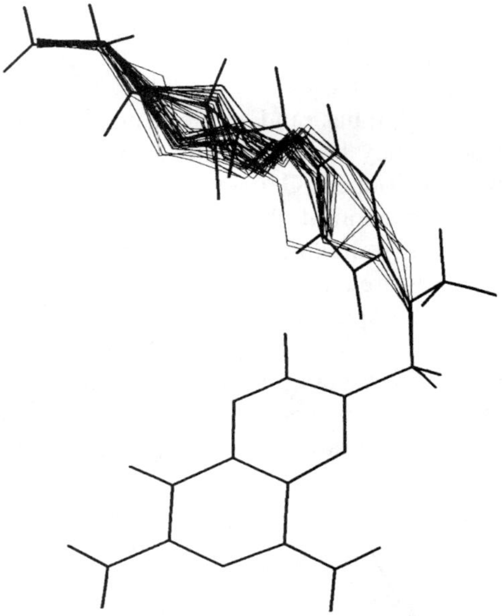

Fig. 9.1 Methotrexate chain growing between two portions of the structure.

without a receptor check is 1.3×10^6, but if receptor checks are included the number lying within 25 kcal/mol is 12 112. An illustration of a small number of chains is given in Fig. 9.1.

Chain bifurcation problems

So far the chain growth has been considered only in terms of a single chain between two points. If we have three site points there are four ways they may be visited (Fig. 9.2). The first three are consecutive visits whilst the fourth uses a bifurcation of the trajectory. A combinatorial explosion occurs with more site points; if we use four site points then there are 41 ways of spanning the site points.

Structure growth proceeds by a random walk and may have branching. A strategy which randomly constrains the conformation during growth is unlikely to allocate optimal constraints since they will occur in random positions. Random walk with a look ahead is too costly on store and time. A sensible strategy would be to minimize the bounds for the distance matrix of the pharmacophore. This can be achieved by placing more emphasis on the need to stiffen parts of the generated skeleton close to its centroid. The stiffening process should not significantly distort the distance matrix of the evolving pharmacophore. Similarly the conformation of the final structure should lie close to the conformational minimum.

These constraints create, in our opinion, the most difficult aspect of *de novo* structure generation. Our strategy is to generate chains within the sites and then stiffen them later.

Examples of chain growing in sites

The chain growing algorithm has random elements. If a site point paradigm is used, an initiation point may be placed close to a site point, otherwise the initiation is randomly positioned. Generation proceeds with chain fragments randomly chosen. The direction of chain growth is vectorial towards a target point with surface contacts maximized. Small movements of the evolving structure are optimized as are small conformational changes along the chain. Simulated annealing is the optimization procedure (described later for atom placement). Structure generation can proceed along many pathways for a given set of site points. Two examples are shown in Fig. 9.3. Only for very small sites are repeated pathways found due to the extreme constraints imposed by the site. In general for most sites there are a multiplicity of

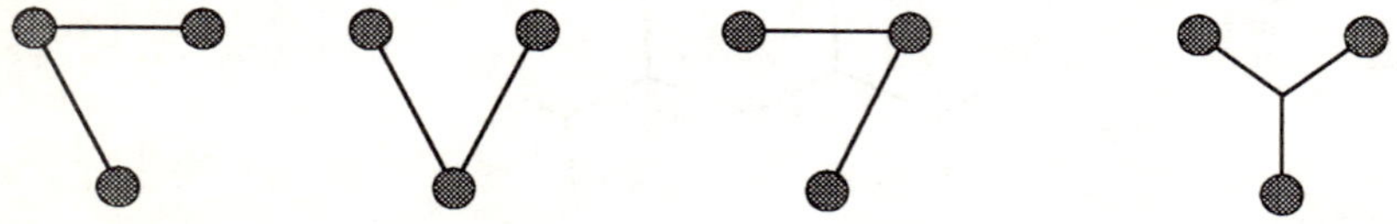

Fig. 9.2 Graphs spanning three site points.

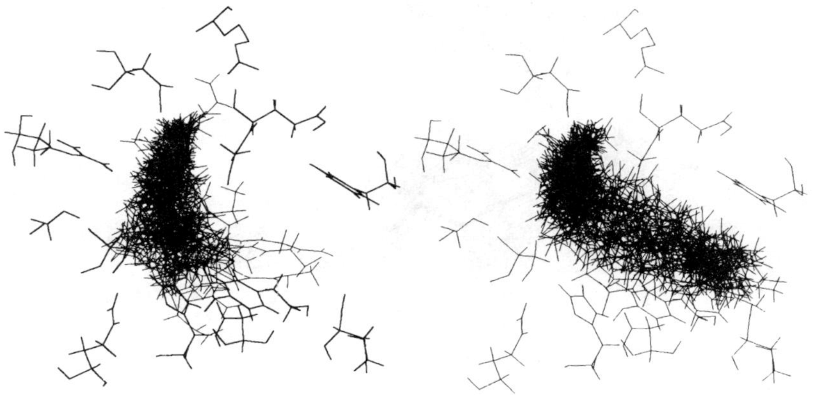

Fig. 9.3 Example of chain growing to three specified site points plus one site point chosen randomly. The drawings show two subsets of site points for structure generation.

pathways which, by inspection of equations (1) and (6), is not surprising. An almost identical procedure can be used for structure generation within a molecular envelope.

Problems of ring bracing

At this step we are still concerned with generating 'atom-free' skeletons so that conformations necessary to stiffen the structure can only be crudely incorporated. A small variety of rings, 5-, 6- and 7-membered, in an appropriate set of conformations form the data set for a ring-bracing algorithm. Bracing has to take place within the constraints of the site. Four types of bracing are possible: (1) weak isolated bracing where two or more rotatable bonds separate two rings; (2) ring bridging where one bond separates two rings; this condition may impose severe restraints on the conformation across the bridging bond and is highly dependent on the final chemical nature of the two rings; (3) ring fusion where a bond is shared; and (4) spiro structures where a single vertex joins two rings. The questions that have to be resolved are: how many rings should be allowed (Fig. 9.4) and what combinations of bracing are synthetically feasible? Stiffening towards the centre of the skeleton will reduce the bounds for the distance matrix of the pharmacophore, therefore a random initiation process for bracing would be a poor strategy; it needs to be centrally directed.

Watching an unconstrained algorithm bracing a chain is highly instructive and is time well spent. It becomes immediately apparent that a weighting scheme is essential to prevent the algorithm from fitting poor ring conformations and from creating unreasonable combinations of rings. Weighting should be sufficiently strong to discourage unwanted results. The problem

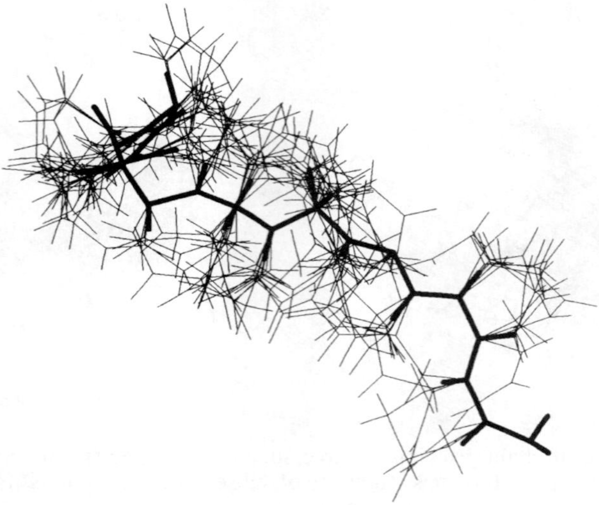

Fig. 9.4 Numerous ring-bracing attempts to stiffen a chain. The bracing is unconstrained by the site.

arises from the need of the algorithm to fit a ring conformation to an identified subset of connected bonds in a locked conformation. If the subset of bonds from the chain is allowed a small conformational tolerance then it is possible that a better choice of ring can be fitted. The conformational tolerance has to be tested for steric clashes with the site. The problem is exacerbated if the algorithm attempts a ring fusion or a spiro join.

Chemical complexity

The complexity of joined rings is a problem that needs to be addressed urgently from the viewpoint of synthesizability. Chemical complexity is related to a collection of features: the number of acyclic bonds, number of rings of a particular size, number of particular ring duplices, number of atoms common to a certain number of rings, number of conformational units with a particular number of rings, number of acyclic chains, number of acyclic chains of a particular length, and number of atoms with a particular number of substituents. We need to define an upper and lower bound for each feature. As the ring-bracing algorithm is run, the structures which satisfy the bounds are kept.

Some guide to what is feasible for a company to make can be gleaned by analysing the historic frequency of ring combinations, multiple ring structures, and all the above features of complexity in the company database. A bracing algorithm can then be tailored to fit only those ring combinations and features which have been frequently handled by the company. Each feature would need a weight (perhaps given by an expert company chemist). The complexity, C, could then be derived from the equation

$$C = \sum_{i=1}^{f} w_i P_i \tag{7}$$

where w_i is the weight of feature i and P_i is its probability of occurrence in the company database, f is the number of features present in the structure. However, ideally we need to create a recognized measure of agreed complexity based on the number of synthetic steps. Conformational bracing would need to be maximized at the same time as minimizing C.

Atom Placement Problems

So far this account has neglected the problem of chemical structure and has concentrated on *de novo* generation of skeletons to fit sites. Skeleton generation has been shown to be strongly combinatoric. Atom placement is also combinatoric on any given skeleton. The rest of this chapter will be devoted to the optimization of atom placement; it is a discrete optimization problem with a satisfactory solution.

When presented with a molecular graph, there are two ways in which atoms can be assigned to the skeleton; atoms may be assigned either by an atom-by-atom or fragment-by-fragment procedure. For both cases, let the set of possible atoms for use on the skeleton be {H, C, N, O, F, P, S, C1}. This set of atoms is associated with the connectivity features shown in Table 9.1 and uses only those fragments taken from Chau and Dean (1992a).

Atom-by-atom assignment

In the atom-by-atom placement method, each vertex of the molecular graph can be assigned any one of the atoms in the allowed atom set. If the simple 16-vertex molecular graph of the 3,4-dihydroxybenzoate molecule is considered, atoms can be assigned to the various vertices. This example is only illustrative of the problem, and the bonding network between the atoms has been ignored. Figure 9.5 shows the ways in which atoms can be placed. It should be noted

Table 9.1
List of the various connectivities associated with each atom

Connectivity of 1	H, N, O, F, S, Cl
Connectivity of 2	C, N, O, S
Connectivity of 3	C, N
Connectivity of 4	C, N^+, P, S

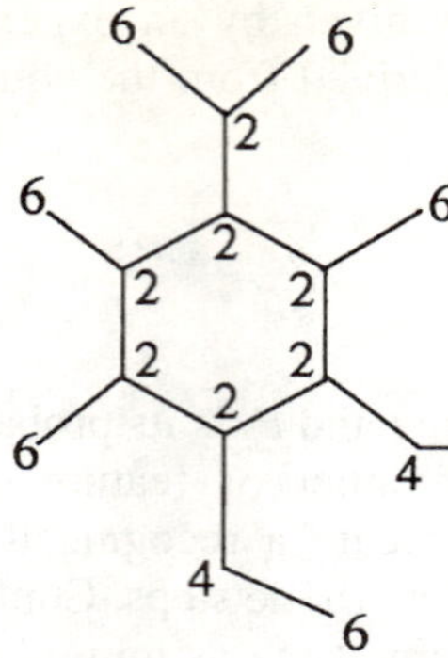

Fig. 9.5 The combinatorics of atom assignation using the atom-by-atom approach. The numbers on the dihydroxybenzoate graph represent the numbers of atom placements at the vertices. Number of possible arrangements of atoms =

$$\prod_{i=1}^{n} m_i$$

where n is the total number of vertices, and m_i is the number of atoms allowed at vertex i. In this example $n = 16$, and possible arrangements $= 5.7 \times 10^8$.

that most of the 570 million arrangements will be rejected because of bonding violations, or chemical instability.

In addition to the very large number of possibilities, each arrangement will require calculation of some properties used to optimize the objective function. If residual charges are necessary, then this will need significant computing effort for each of the many placements. This clearly is a major handicap to the procedure of atom-by-atom placement. For this reason, a different approach can be used.

Fragment-by-fragment assignment

In order to overcome the difficulties with the atom-by-atom approach, a fragment-by-fragment method can be considered in which small, frequently occurring molecular fragments are placed on to a molecular graph. The main advantage of such a procedure is the fact that each of the fragments would have precalculated atomic properties. The properties could then simply be transferred onto the molecular graph each time a fragment was used. Figure 9.6 illustrates the combinatorics of fragment-by-fragment placement.

Again no consideration has been taken for inter-fragment connectivity. The increase in the number of possibilities is due to the existence of fragments in which the atom types are the same, but some property of the fragment is different (e.g. bond order or charge). Since this limitation is small compared

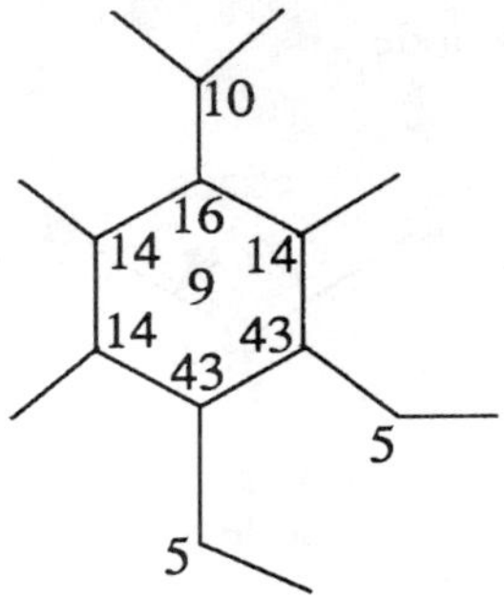

Fig. 9.6 The combinatorics of atom assignment using the fragment-by-fragment approach. The numbers on the dihydroxybenzoate graph represent the numbers of fragment placements at the nodes. Number of possible arrangements of atoms =

$$\prod_{i=1}^{n} m_i$$

where n is the total number of nodes, and m_i is the number of fragments with rotations allowed at node i. In this example, $n = 10$, and possible arrangements $= 1.8 \times 10^{11}$.

to the major advantage of precalculated properties, we use the fragment approach for the placement of atoms onto a molecular graph.

Fragment placement procedure

The molecular graph is made up of vertices and edges, as illustrated in Fig. 9.7. In the approach used here, a node is taken to be a vertex with more than one vertex bonded to it, while a terminus is defined as a vertex with a connectivity of only one. Vertices can therefore be subdivided into nodes (3-, 4- and 5-atom non-cyclical nodes) and termini. This distinction is important in fragment placement, since there is no need to place fragments at termini; fragment placement should occur only at nodes. Similarly, edges, which represent bonds, can be subdivided into chains and cycles. For the purposes of fragment placement, the presence of a planar cycle indicates that an aromatic ring fragment should be placed on to that cycle, and it is pointless trying to place an aromatic ring at a node which is not a cycle.

In the fragment placement algorithm, the perception of nodes is made at the two-dimensional level: *i.e.* in terms of connectivity. So all 3-, 4- and 5-atom non-cyclical nodes are noted, as well as any 5-, 6-, 9- and 10-edged cyclical nodes. Each node must correspond to at least one fragment from the library. However, if there is no fragment which can fit a node, and the atoms of that node can be assigned from the overlap of fragments at adjacent nodes, then there is no need to exit, and execution continues. In addition to connectivity of nodes, certain nodes carry extra information, such as:

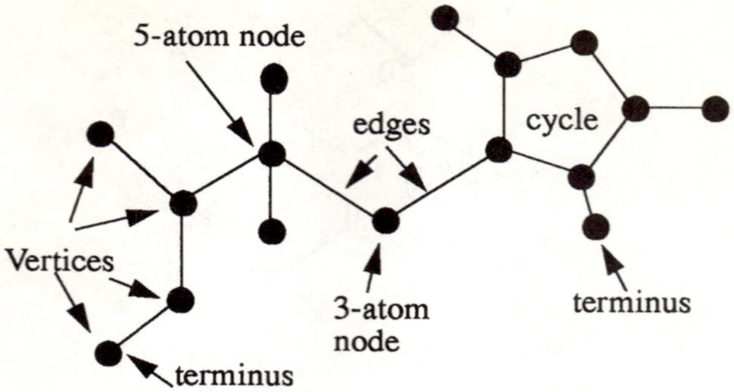

Fig. 9.7 A schematic molecular graph.

1) *Fixed atom type at a certain vertex.* This is an option in the program which is particularly useful when there is an existing lead and only slight modifications are required to the atoms on the graph.
2) *Hydrogen bonding information.* A drug designer may require some hydrogen-bond acceptor (or donor) at a certain vertex.
3) *Three-atom non-cyclical nodes have a central bond angle* (see Fig. 9.7). Depending on the sp/sp^2/sp^3 cut-off criteria (160°, 122°, 114°), the 3-atom node could be treated as an sp, sp^2 or sp^3 node. If the bond angle lies between 114° and 122°, then the node adopts both sp^2 and sp^3 status, since the resolution of the graph is not assumed to be perfect.

Ring perception is a complex but well-understood problem. We use the algorithm outlined by Wipke and Dyott (1975). It makes use of the Welch-assembly-Gibbs algorithm, which first finds the fundamental basis set of rings by Welch's stage 1 algorithm (Welch, 1966); second, ring assemblies are explored by grouping those fundamental cycles with edges in common; and third, all rings are found by the Gibb's algorithm (Gibbs, 1969) by taking the ring sum of all combinations of the associated cycle vectors.

The molecular graph is fixed; the fragments are allowed to rotate on the graph. When only fragment connectivities are considered, a particular fragment may be placed in more than one way on to the molecular graph.

In the example illustrated in Fig. 9.8, fragment m040 could be placed on to the molecular graph as drawn, or with the O and H swapped round. Therefore, in the fragment library, where some repeat patterns of connectivity exist (excluding those rotations in which the atom types and bond orders of the atoms to be swapped are identical), all possible rotations of the fragments are calculated (including stereoisomers for the 5-atom aliphatic fragments). Each rotation gives the identical connectivity pattern of the original orientation of the fragment. The largest number of rotations for each aliphatic fragment is $n!$, where n is the number of outer atoms in that fragment. Thus, for a 4-atom

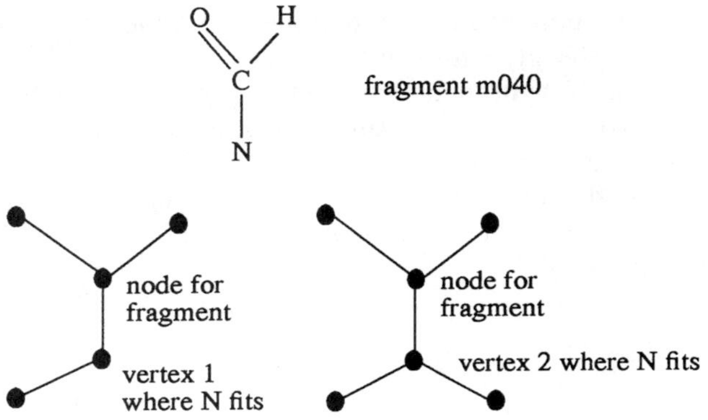

Fig. 9.8 Illustration of how a nitrogen atom in a fragment could be placed at more than one graph vertex.

fragment, the maximum number of rotations is 6, whilst the value of a 5-atom fragment is 24 (including stereoisomers). For the aromatic fragments, the maximum number of rotations is 2 for the 5-, 6- and 9-edged rings, and 4 for the 10-edged duplex.

Properties to be Optimized in Atom Placement

In the preceding section it has been shown that structure generation and atom placement are combinatoric problems. The aim in *de novo* structure generation is the creation of ligands with optimum properties for binding. In the absence of structure generation in solution, we have to be content with a very approximate answer that builds either on notions of complementarity, or on the related phenomenon of molecular similarity.

Optimum electrostatic interactions between the site and the ligand skeleton should show a pattern of complementarity in the spatial disposition of their electrostatic potentials. The distribution of potential is continuous and can be determined readily for every fragment placement. At any point, j, on the ligand surface the potential V_j (in kJ/mol) is given by:

$$V_j = \sum_{i=1}^{n} \frac{q_i}{r_{ij}} c \tag{8}$$

where n is the number of atoms on the skeleton, q_i is the charge of atom i, r_{ij} is the distance between i and the point j, and c = 2626.57 kJ/mol (a.u.)$^{-1}$.

The possibility of using the hydrophobic potential (Fauchère *et al.*, 1988) as a parameter to be optimized can be reasoned from the need to match hydrophobic regions on the site with similar regions on the ligand. However, there are complications if hydrophobicity and electrostatics are to be included together; the two phenomena show a measurable anticorrelation (Chau, 1990). Bearing that caveat in mind, it would be possible to project a hydrophobicity potential from the site on to the ligand skeleton surface and optimize the similarity. The hydrophobicity potential Φ_j (in kJ/mol) can be computed from:

$$\Phi_j = -2.3RT \sum_i^n f_i \mathrm{e}^{-r_{ij}} \tag{9}$$

where n is the number of fragments, f_i is the fragment hydrophobicity potential of the group i, R is the gas constant and T is the temperature.

Hydrogen bonding is a directed interaction but there is some leeway in the direction. This spread in direction can be quantified by constructing probability maps round each hydrogen-bonding group (Danziger and Dean, 1989). However, the hydrogen-bonding maps are confined to specific regions and cannot effectively be considered as a continuous property. They can be included only in a discrete way. A hydrogen-bonding atom, acceptor or donor, complementary to a hydrogen-bonding group in the site may be placed on a skeleton vertex only if the vertex lies within a certain distance of the site atom and within an appropriate angle range with that of the site hydrogen-bonding group. These checks can be carried out during the placement procedure for one of the other properties previously described.

An Objective Function to be Optimized

The strategy adopted here of dividing structure generation into two parts – skeletal generation and atom placement – means that the atom placement problem can be handled in a number of ways for optimization. For economy we have sought a method which is applicable both to site-directed *de novo* structure generation and envelope-directed structure generation. Since in the latter case there is no site structure available, design has to proceed by methods of molecular similarity because energies of interaction with the site cannot be computed. Molecular complementarity is simply the inverse of similarity; thus an objective function which optimizes the atom placement in terms of complementary fields for site-directed design can be used, with trivial modification, for envelope-directed design.

Numerical expression of complementarity

Electrostatic complementarity between a site and a ligand can be studied by projection of the site potential on to the ligand surface and by projection of the ligand potential on to the same surface (Dean, 1990, 1993; Chau and Dean, 1994a,b,c). Complementarity can be correlated either by value using Pearson's correlation, or by pattern using rank correlation. Perpendicular least squares regression analysis provides the slope and intercept for the regression line. For complementarity the slope is negative and should approach -1 for complete complementarity; the correlation coefficient should also approach -1. Pearson's correlation coefficient, r, is given by:

$$r = \frac{\sum_i (x_i - \bar{x})\ (y_i - \bar{y})}{\sqrt{\sum_i (x_i - \bar{x})^2 \sum_i (y_i - \bar{y})^2}} \tag{10}$$

where $\bar{x}$ denotes the mean of x_i values and $\bar{y}$ denotes the mean of y_i values; x_i and y_i are the potentials from the site and the ligand at point i on the ligand surface. This form of analysis of complementarity presupposes a linear relationship between the two projections. Recent analysis suggests that the supposition holds for ideal complementarity (Chau and Dean, 1994c).

Numerical expression for similarity
Molecular similarity can be considered in an analogous way. In this case the correlation coefficient, r, should have a value approaching +1 for perfect similarity, a slope of +1 and an intercept of 0. However, the surface to be considered in the case of envelope-directed design would be a supersurface onto which are projected the properties of the lead structure and the evolving molecular structure for comparison.

Thus the objective function for optimization is r. It is minimized for complementarity in site-directed design and maximized for similarity in envelope-directed design.

Optimization Methods

Fragment placement has been shown to be combinatoric. Furthermore, the potential at any point i on the ligand surface is a through-space phenomenon derived from a summation procedure. If one fragment is replaced by another, the potential is altered by a discrete amount. Thus, we need a discrete optimization method to generate an optimum molecular structure on the molecular skeletons. Brute-force and iterative placements are inadequate to cope with the size of the placement problem. Since part of the objective function is derived from a summation process it is likely that for a particular value of the objective function there will be many closely similar solutions. This is the multiple minima problem that plagues combinatorial optimization. A number of strategies for combinatorial optimization problems of a similar type are available. They include: neural networks, genetic algorithms, simulated annealing and multicanonical algorithms. Neural networks are ideal for problems where parallel processing is possible. Genetic algorithms are generally slower than simulated annealing (Ingber and Rosen, 1992), and multicanonical algorithms are at the moment less understood than any of the other techniques. Therefore, simulated annealing has been chosen to optimize fragment placement.

Simulated Annealing

Simulated annealing is essentially a serial optimization procedure which is thermodynamically motivated. The method reduces an exponential increase in computing time to only small powers of a measure of the size of the problem. The mathematical tool of the heuristic relies on the Monte Carlo condition as modified by Metropolis *et al.* (1953). This simulates a collection of physical particles in thermal equilibrium at a constant temperature. Kirkpatrick *et al.* (1983) adapted this condition for use in the minimization of any objective function in discrete space by incorporating a cooling schedule. The minimization problem is transformed into a statistical physics problem, with the objective function becoming the thermodynamic quantity, E. This procedure is therefore termed optimization by simulated annealing, since it mimics slow cooling of an ensemble of particles from higher temperatures.

The ensemble starts at a high temperature, T, and the objective function for the system is calculated (E_1). A random perturbation is then applied to the system, and the new value for E is found (E_2). The difference, ΔE, is calculated, where $\Delta E = E_2 - E_1$. If ΔE is negative, the perturbation is accepted unconditionally, and the new state E_2 is maintained.

The acceptance of a perturbation with a positive ΔE, on the other hand, depends on the Metropolis condition, which makes use of the Boltzmann probability distribution (equation (11)).

$$P\ (s'|s) = e\ (-\Delta E/kt) \tag{11}$$

where $P(s'|s)$ is the probability of accepting a state s' which has an energy greater than the energy of the existing state, s, by an amount ΔE; k is the Boltzmann constant; and t is the temperature in Kelvin scale. The annealing 'temperature', T is defined in equation (12).

$$T = kt \tag{12}$$

and is in the same units as E. If a random number generated between [0,1) is less than $P(s'|s)$, then the new state s' is accepted. After several perturbations and when equilibrium is reached, the temperature is reduced, and the cycle is repeated. In this way, the system is given the opportunity to escape from a local minimum at high temperatures. The lower the temperature, the smaller the likelihood of surmounting uphill 'energy' barriers. Eventually, when there is no longer any significant decrease in E, the system is said to be 'frozen'. If the cooling rate were optimal, then the frozen state would be at the global minimum, corresponding to perfect crystal formation. Therefore, one of the major hurdles to overcome with simulated annealing, is the design of a cooling schedule which is slow enough to allow crystal formation, but not so slow that the algorithm would take hours of cpu time. In earlier work (Barakat and Dean, 1990a,b, 1991) a dynamic cooling schedule for optimization has been suggested for combinatoric molecular matching problems. The algorithm is controlled by scaling the objective function to make the method independent of the size of the molecular skeleton on to which placement is attempted. The transition mechanism is derived from a random selection of a node and an appropriate random placement of a fragment at that node. The new potential is computed from the charges (or atomic hydrophobic parameters in the case of hydrophobic potential optimization) of the fragment atoms. All rotations of the fragment are examined. The initial temperature is set to 2.0 and decremented dynamically. The length of the Markov chain depends on the size of the graph, but is around 200 for a 40-vertex graph. The stop criterion is set to 5×10^5 Markov chains or a limit of 2 h cpu.

Fragment placement by simulated annealing

The annealing step is divided into two stages. First, at the start of annealing no account is taken of bond order in attempting to place a fragment randomly. This procedure prevents the placement from becoming locked by bond patterns which once set up are difficult to change whilst the potential is optimized. Second, at a later stage once the potential appears to be optimized, the algorithm seeks a placement which checks inter-fragment bond orders by a further reannealing procedure. Furthermore, at this second stage the charges are averaged between connected fragments and the total charge adjusted to an appropriate integer value. Bond lengths on the original skeleton are readjusted for the atom placement that is finally produced. The molecular skeleton is repositioned in the site by the McLachlan (1982) algorithm.

One further annealing run is performed using the current geometry and fragment placement. The aim is to take 25% of the atoms on the skeleton, which show the poorest local surface potential, and try again to optimize them. After this final placement and skeleton geometry adjustment, the charges of the putative molecular structure are computed semi-empirically and the electrostatic potential is correlated with that of the site. Multiple runs of the placement are performed for each initial skeleton used as input to the program; correlations for the final output are ranked for each skeleton.

Self-placement Tests

The convergence and ergodicity of the algorithm described for fragment placement can be tested unambiguously by taking a known molecule and matching its electrostatic potential. This process exactly mimics the case of envelope-directed design. A less rigorous, but more realistic test, is to take a ligand/protein co-crystal where the electrostatic potential shows a strong correlation in complementarity, and examine whether the placement method can produce a molecular structure reminiscent of the original ligand. Cyclic AMP (cAMP) complexed with the gene activator protein (Weber and Steitz, 1987) provides a useful example.

Envelope-directed placement

The electrostatic potential of cAMP(a) in the conformation bound to the site (gene activator protein, 3GAP) is computed semi-empirically on the van der Waals surface. The atoms are removed from the molecule and the skeleton is retained. The algorithm is challenged to find the best placement on the skeleton which correlates with the original electrostatic potential. Repeated runs of the program using different random number sequences show that the algorithm correctly assigns the atoms in proportions given in Table 9.2. The value for r as output by the program is the similarity between the electrostatic potential generated using the fragment charges of the final placement and that generated from the semi-empirical charges of cAMP. The method used is either placement according to electrostatic potential only, or placement by electrostatics with a hydrogen-bond signifier option. It can be seen that the algorithm consistently places the atoms on the skeleton correctly.

Site-directed placement

A very similar test can be performed using the electrostatic potential of the 3GAP site projected onto the surface of cAMP(a). Table 9.3 shows that the algorithm consistently places all but one of the atoms exactly as they are found in cAMP(a). The one difference is the replacement of the hydrogen atom attached to C2 of the adenine moiety with a chlorine atom. The resultant structure has a higher electrostatic complementarity to the 3GAP site ($r = -0.72$) than does the native ligand cAMP(a) itself (where $r = -0.66$). The

Table 9.2
Self-placement of cAMP(a) from its own electrostatic potential

Method	r	Recalculated r	Perfect runs	Incorrect atoms	cpu (s)
cAMP(a)	+0.96	+1.0	10/10	0	70
cAMP(a) + H-bonds	+0.96	+1.0	10/10	0	82

Table 9.3
Placement of the cAMP(a) skeleton using the 3GAP electrostatic potential

Method	r	Recalculated r	Perfect runs	Different atoms	cpu (s)
cAMP(a)	−0.76	−0.72	0/10	1	47
cAMP(a) + H-bonds	−0.76	−0.72	0/10	1	52

fragment placement procedure is therefore able to find a structure which is more electrostatically suited for binding in the 3GAP site.

Conclusions

Site-directed *de novo* structure generation is strongly combinatoric for two reasons: first, the generation of structures likely to be in contact with the site surface is potentially massive for large sites, and second the possible combination of atoms that may be placed on those structures is a product relationship between the number of nodes and the atoms that can be placed at each node. Methods which attempt to place large known molecular pieces within a site reduce the combinatoric problems drastically but make little attempt to optimize structure generation. Those methods offer very little structural diversity. This chapter has attempted to pinpoint each combinatorial problem and to assess whether the steps can be optimized.

The great difficulty in attempting to optimize combinatoric structure generation is that many diverse structures have closely equivalent scores in the final objective function. This landscape optimization difficulty is common to many combinatorial optimization problems. Few studies are available on how structures, generated by *de novo* methods, may be classified for potential use. The notion of structural complexity, although often talked about, has not been tackled rigorously. A number of factors are important in trying to assess complexity: (1) the number of chiral centres needs to be minimized; (2) the conformation of the generated structure needs to be readily accessible; (3) ring aggregates need to be easily synthesizable. Two strategies can be adopted to reduce these problems. First, it might be possible to reduce these factors in the structure generation and atom placement steps; this would be ideal but may lead to the generation of non-optimal structures. Second, it may be simpler to take the output from current algorithms and post-process the structures to eliminate these unwanted features. The last approach is probably the easier option. Classification of structures at each subset of site points is desirable, but not simple, for a combinatoric generation procedure; only if the site is very small is this possibility expected to be successful. In general, for larger sites, structure generation is so diverse that detailed visual inspection of every structure is essential but impracticable if more than a few hundred structures have been generated.

Simulated Annealing Development

In principle, simulated annealing is ergodic. However, in practice it is not always ergodic given time limits for the algorithm to complete. Multiple runs are necessary to gain insight into regions of structure which are frequently reproducible. From our observations with electrostatic potential optimization, ergodicity seems to be related to the electrostatic potential distribution. In strongly electrostatic self-matching studies it appears that the algorithm gives consistent placements; in weakly electrostatic cases the algorithm behaves poorly by providing many alternative placements. This problem arises from the fact that the potential values are close to zero, consequently the differences in potential between alternative placements are very small; thus there are many solutions close to the global optimum solution. However, this may not be a difficulty in usage since the structures generated in the self-match are still weakly electrostatic.

Two new improvements for simulated annealing have recently been described: very fast simulated annealing, VFSA (Ingber and Rosen, 1992) and annealing with simplex optimization (Press *et al.*, 1992). VFSA makes use of smart generator functions which restrict the width of choice of random generations as the algorithm proceeds. If this were to be incorporated into the placement algorithm, fragments would need to be classified in terms of their electronic charges. Selection would have to be restricted from electronic subclasses within each fragment class. In our judgement, after testing on related structure matching problems, VFSA is not worth the effort of exploration. The inclusion of simplex optimization along the annealing trajectory would be simple to code and may well be beneficial. Essentially this approach involves exploring local minima by a downhill simplex at frequent intervals along the Markov chain. This technique finds the global, and near global minima, very well and should lead to improvements in the ergodicity of the algorithm.

Hydration and Drug Design

Current *de novo* structure generation methods ignore the presence of solvent in the generation process. However, *in vacuo* molecular interactions are a poor representation of the energetics of drug–receptor interactions and the neglect of hydration is probably the Achilles' heel of structure generation. Detailed crystallographic studies of water molecules in ligand binding sites reveal complex structural and mechanistic roles for bound water (Prive *et al.*,

1992; Lewendon and Shaw, 1993). Water appears to bridge between ligands and the site and to other water molecules. This stabilizes the complex possibly by reducing the movement of the side chains in the site. Two features seem to be involved: regions in the site with many hydrogen bonds seem to form water bridges to the ligand and vice versa; water molecules are sometimes held tightly in crevices and can link to the ligands (Levitt and Park, 1993). Currently we are surveying many crystal structures of ligand/protein complexes in an effort to identify principal hydration features which might be used in an automated design strategy.

One can only speculate on how water molecules might be incorporated in a design program. First, we might consider them to be fixed, for example in positions where they appear to be conserved in crystal structures. In this case the water would function very much like a site point and may be treated as such. Second, water might be added after a structure generation run to examine where it might bind and then incorporate a 'water score' into the algorithm. Neither of these approaches is in any sense dynamic since water is considered only at the start or end of structure generation. A more interesting approach would be to consider water bridging as an integral part of structure generation. Every time a terminus node is generated on the ligand it should be marked as a potential hydrogen bond to be considered for water bridging. The local region of the site can then be searched for appropriate hydrogen bonds to a water molecule located in that vicinity. The water molecule then behaves rather like a special fragment which can be added or discarded whilst generation proceeds. The success of this strategy will be dependent on whether rules for hydration in ligand/protein crystal complexes can be defined and whether effective scoring schemes can be derived. The inclusion of water molecules would add a further combinatorial step to design.

In summary, on careful scrutiny drug design is plagued by combinatoric elements which creep in at many stages and the whole process is ripe for optimization. Our experience is not yet strong enough to decide on an optimal stragegy for the automated *de novo* design of novel ligands. However, these newly evolving methods are exciting and point towards powerful developments in drug design which should reveal a wealth of sensible alternative structures for assessment, synthesis and testing.

Acknowledgements

The authors are indebted to their sponsors for financial support: to the Wellcome Trust for the award of a Principal Research Fellowship for P.M.D. and for a Wellcome Prize Studentship for M.T.B; N.P.T. is indebted to Rhône-Poulenc Rorer for a research studentship. Part of this work was carried out in the Cambridge Centre for Molecular Recognition.

References

Barakat, M.T., and Dean, P.M. (1990a). *J. Comput.-Aided Mol. Design* **4**, 295–316.
Barakat, M.T., and Dean, P.M. (1990b). *J. Comput.-Aided Mol. Design* **4**, 317–330.
Barakat, M.T., and Dean, P.M. (1991). *J. Comput.-Aided Mol. Design* **5**, 107–117.
Chau, P.-L. (1990). Creation of a molecular fragments database for ligand point prediction from properties of the drug-binding site. PhD dissertation, University of Cambridge.
Chau, P.-L., and Dean, P.M. (1992a). *J. Comput.-Aided Mol. Design* **6**, 385–396.
Chau, P.-L., and Dean, P.M. (1992b). *J. Comput.-Aided Mol. Design* **6**, 397–406.
Chau, P.-L., and Dean, P.M. (1992c). *J. Comput.-Aided Mol. Design* **6**, 407–426.
Chau, P.-L., and Dean, P.M. (1994a). *J. Comput.-Aided Mol. Design* **8**, 513–525.
Chau, P.-L., and Dean, P.M. (1994b). *J. Comput.-Aided Mol. Design* **8**, 527–544.
Chau, P.-L., and Dean, P.M. (1994c). *J. Comput.-Aided Mol. Design* **8**, 545–564.
Clementi, E. (1980). *In* 'Lecture Notes in Chemistry', vol. 19. Springer-Verlag, Berlin.
Danziger, D.J., and Dean, P.M. (1989). *Proc. R. Soc. Lond. B* **236**, 115–124.
Dean, P.M. (1990). *In* 'Concepts and Applications of Molecular Similarity', (M.A. Johnson and G.M. Maggiora, eds), pp. 211–238. John Wiley & Sons, New York.
Dean, P.M. (1993). *In* '3D QSAR in Drug Design. Theory, Methods and Applications' (H. Kubinyi, ed.), pp. 150–172. ESCOM, Leiden.
DesJarlais, R.L., Sheridan, R.P., Seibel, G.L., Dixon, J.S., Kuntz, I.D., and Venkataraghaven, R. (1988). *J. Med. Chem.* **31**, 722–729.
Fauchère, J.-L., Quarendon, P. and Kaetterer, L. (1988). *J. Mol. Graph* **6**, 202–206.
Gibbs, N. (1969). *J. Assoc. Comput. Machinery* **16**, 564–568.
Ingber, L. and Rosen, B. (1992). *Math. Comput. Modelling,* **16**, 87–100.
Kirkpatrick, S., Gellatt Jr., C.D., and Vecchi, M.P. (1983). *Science* **220**, 671–680.
Laurie, G., and Bartlett, P.A. (1994). *J. Comput.-Aided Mol. Design* **8**, 51–66.
Lauri, G., Shea, G.T., Waterman, S., Telfer, S.J., and Bartlett, P.A. (1989). CAVEAT: A Program to Facilitate the Design of Organic Molecules. Version 2.0. University of California, Berkeley.
Levitt, M., and Park, B.H. (1993). *Structure* **1**, 223–226.
Lewendon, A., and Shaw, W.V. (1993) *J. Biol. Chem.* **268**, 20997–21001.
Lewis, R.A. (1990). *J. Comput.-Aided Mol. Design* **4**, 205–210.
Lewis, R.A. (1992). *J. Comput.-Aided Mol. Design* **10**, 131–143.
Lewis, R.A., and Dean, P.M. (1989a). *Proc. R. Soc. Lond. B* **236**, 125–140.
Lewis, R.A., and Dean, P.M. (1989b). *Proc. R. Soc. Lond. B* **236**, 141–162.
McLachlan, A.D. (1982). *Acta Cryst. A* **38**, 871–873.
Metropolis, N., Rosenbluth, A., Rosenbluth, M., Teller, A., and Teller, E. (1953). *J. Chem. Phys.* **21**, 1087–1092.
Moon, J.B., and Howe, W.J. (1990). *Tetrahedron Comput. Methodology* **3**, 681–696.
Moon, J.B., and Howe, W.J. (1991). *Proteins* **11**, 314–328.
Perkins, T.D.J., and Dean, P.M. (1993). *J. Comput.-Aided Mol. Design* **7**, 155–172.
Press, W.H., Teukolsky, S.A., Vetterling, W.T. and Flannery, B.P. (1992). Numerical recipes in C. Cambridge University Press, Cambridge, U.K.
Prive, G.G., Milburn, M.V., Tong, L., de Vos, A.M., Yamaizumi, Z., Nishimura, S., and Kim, S.-H. (1992). *Proc. Natl Acad. Sci. USA* **89**, 3649–3653.
Shenkin, P.S., Yarmush, D.L., Fine, R.M., Wang, H. and Levinthal, C. (1987). *Biopolymers* **26**, 2053–2085.
Weber, I.T., and Steitz, T.A. (1987). *J. Mol. Biol.* **198**, 311–326.
Welch, J. (1966). *J. Assoc. Comput. Machinery* **13**, 205–210.
Wipke, W.T., and Dyott, T.M. (1975). *J. Chem. Inf. Comput. Sci.* **15**, 140–147.

Discussion

C. McCarthy
You have described growing structures that are able to pick up hydrogen bonding interactions. Why choose hydrogen bonding, which is energetically a relatively small part of the ligand receptor interaction?

P.M. Dean
If hydrogen bonds are present, we want to be able to get the vectors correct. If we want to use seed points for generating growth, this is a useful way of doing it.

C. McCarthy
Why not use a hydrophobic point?

P.M. Dean
There is no real reason why structures cannot be grown *ad hoc* within any amorphous volume. It just makes the structure more sensible at the end of the day if it has an appropriate set of hydrogen bonds – if there is a hydrogen-bonding site.

C. McCarthy
If you had, say, a competitor's compound and, using your technique, came up with an alternative structure to mimic it, what are the major advantages of your technique compared to that of traditional medicinal chemist operating with models?

P.M. Dean
Models always have problems, specifically because we look at models with eyes and have a preconceived notion of how these models should be superposed. If models that are based on some form of molecular similarity are superposed, our human bias is reduced, and it ought to be possible to get superpositions which are based on surfaces. It is not easy to do this; despite there being a number of methods in the literature, it is quite a difficult problem. My feeling is that if an envelope has been described, and the properties of that envelope are known, it should be possible to design many hundreds of structures which fit it. It is up to *you* in the drug industry then to look at these structures and make assessments of them.

M.N. Palfreyman
Medicinal chemists in general are rather impatient creatures. In the end, the proof of the pudding is not just designing the compound but in synthesizing it

and seeing whether it has activity. Has this been done and, if not, when do you expect to do it?

P.M. Dean

Trying to create something which can be synthesized is an interesting problem. We tend to let *you* look at the algorithm to make that decision yourself. I do not know *what* you can do, but I know you can do something that your competitors cannot: they do not necessarily have the skills that you have in-house. Although trying to elaborate some algorithm which attempts to give some idea of ease-of-synthesis is a nice goal, it is possibly not necessarily the best way of proceeding. Someone like Jon Mason or yourself would be able to say from looking at these structures which are possible and which are not – 5–10% might be worth looking at.

C.G. Newton

Ease-of-synthesis obviously varies from chemist to chemist. I am sure Professor Nicolaou operates on a different scale to most of the rest of us.

I would also echo Dr McCarthy's earlier comment. We heard that shape complementarity is most responsible for effective binding, and in one case, earlier, that it could be alone responsible for nanomolar potency of a steroidal motif binding to a protein. Do you not think that we are trying to run before we can walk, by trying to map electrostatics and hydrogen bonding on to a surface or a volume – when perhaps with a steroidal motif it might be possible to design the first non-steroidal steroid with a purely carbon framework?

P.M. Dean

If we go back to the Lennard–Jones equation, the important interactions are the atoms at the interface – short-range forces interacting. They far outweigh the rest. Shape, therefore, is pre-eminent. How the rest of it is scored is a matter open to debate. We have simply looked at the other aspect of placing atoms on the skeleton as another part of a problem to be optimized.

There are all sorts of ways of looking at this problem and attempting a design. During this meeting, a number of completely different approaches have been considered. We cannot necessarily yet say which will be best.

I.M. McLay

I do not think any pharmacophore model has been designed without having in it a hydrogen bond acceptor or donor point. It does not make any sense to try to design molecules which do not have hydrogen bond acceptor points. It is true that there can be strong binding without those points, but there cannot be specificity without them. We must have hydrogen bonding points first, and then hydrophobic interactions will give very high potency.

K. Zakrzewska
There are ligands which are specific in their binding to AT sequences of DNA, for which we do not have the possibility of hydrogen bonds – just positive charges.

I.M. McLay
I would include positive charges and polar interactions in my claim for specificity requirements.

A.P. Johnson
As you know, we have a program that also works by first generating graphs, and then by substituting heteroatoms on it. One area in which we have been careful not to do this is in connection with sulphur or phosphorus. You seem to be including sulphur and phosphorus in the second phase, yet the bond angles, bond lengths and so on are sufficiently different from carbon to carbon to make this difficult.

P.M. Dean
That is a fair comment. We use it simply because our test model contains it, so we could not *not* use phosphorus – and if phosphorus is there, sulphur ought to be there too. But you are right: bond lengths and bond angles vary. However, sites can accommodate small movements because there are millions of ways in which these things are able to fold and adjust themselves within the site.

A.P. Johnson
In connection with the heteroatom substitution, as I understand it, you are substituting in order to fulfil the right hydrogen bonding or whatever. Have you considered also making substitutions to increase synthetic accessibility?

P.M. Dean
No, we have not looked at that aspect. It is something that you are much more able to handle than we are. We are simply concerned with combinatorial optimization, looking at landscapes, seeing what variability can be obtained from these generators. The variability intrigues us.

A.P. Johnson
Lastly, the reason for developing the synthetic accessibility assessor is that while we can go to a medicinal chemist and ask him to evaluate 10 or even 50 compounds, if we have 1000 compounds I think we would want some kind of a screen put in front of that. [*P.M. Dean assented.*]

10

Free Energy Calculations in Drug Design: A Practical Guide

A.E. MARK and W.F. VAN GUNSTEREN

Department of Physical Chemistry, Swiss Federal Institute of Technology, ETH Zentrum, CH 8092 Zurich, Switzerland

Introduction

From a physical perspective, drug design is primarily concerned with the estimation of the difference in free energy of specific compounds in different environments. This is because, thermodynamically, the extent to which each of the binding, transport and processing events (which together give rise to a specific biological activity) occur is directly dependent on the associated change in free energy. Historically, drug design studies have relied primarily on empirical estimates of free energy differences. More recently, the availability of structural data on specific biological targets has led to free energy estimates based on a variety of energy-based scoring functions. Free energy is, however, a statistical property. It reflects a thermal average over microscopic configurations and cannot be reliably deduced from a single structure. Thus, to estimate reliably free energy, one must resort to statistical mechanical approaches. A number of such methods have been developed to estimate differences in free energy based on molecular simulation techniques (Beveridge and DiCapua, 1989). The theory underlying these calculations is straightforward. The change in free energy is determined either from the relative probability of finding the system in a given state or from the work required to go from an initial to a final state via a reversible path. Despite this inherent simplicity, efficient implementation is non-trivial. Protocols developed for trivial test cases are frequently inappropriate in biochemical

New Perspectives in Drug Design
ISBN 0–12–208070–X

systems where simplifying assumptions in terms of sampling properties do not hold.

This chapter is intended as a practical guide to the use of free energy calculations in drug design. It aims to do two things. First, to enable the reader to distinguish between the various implementations of what is essentially the same basic methodology and second, to highlight the main factors that determine the reliability of a given calculation.

Theory

In terms of the canonical partition function, $Z_{N,V,T}$, the Helmholtz free energy, F, of a system of N particles in a volume V at a temperature T, is given by

$$F_{N,V,T} = -kT\ln Z_{N,V,T}$$

$$= -kT\ln[(h^{3N}N!)^{-1} \int\int e^{-H(\mathbf{p},\mathbf{q})/kT}\mathrm{dpdq}] \tag{1}$$

where k is Boltzmann's constant, h is Planck's constant and the Hamiltonian, $H(\mathbf{p},\mathbf{q})$, expresses the total energy of system in terms of the coordinates, $\mathbf{q} = (\mathbf{q}_1,\mathbf{q}_2,...,\mathbf{q}_N)$, and conjugate momenta, $\mathbf{p} = (\mathbf{p}_1,\mathbf{p}_2,...,\mathbf{p}_N)$ of the N particles in the system. The absolute free energy is dependent on a double integral over all the coordinates and momenta which are accessible to the system and for realistic systems cannot be determined. It is also not possible to estimate reliably the absolute free energy from a minimum energy configuration or from a molecular simulation. This is because the dominant contributions to the absolute free energy do not necessarily come from the low energy configurations. This can be seen by re-expressing (1) as

$$F_{N,V,T} = +\,kT\ln < e^{+H/kT} >_{N,V,T} \tag{2}$$

where the angle brackets < ... > indicate an ensemble average. The positive sign of the exponent implies that rarely sampled high-energy configurations may in fact dominate the ensemble average.

Although the absolute free energy cannot be determined, the relative free energy between two closely related states can be determined. Using the so-called coupling parameter approach the difference in free energy between two states of a system, X and Y, characterized by the Hamiltonians H_X and H_Y can be determined if the Hamiltonian of the system is made a function of a coupling parameter λ, such that $H(\lambda_X) = H_X$ and $H(\lambda_Y) = H_Y$. As the Hamiltonian, $H(\lambda)$, is a function of λ, the free energy, $F(\lambda)$, also becomes a function of λ. The difference in free energy $\Delta F_{YX} = F_Y - F_X$ may then be determined using either of two standard expressions commonly referred to as the perturbation and integration formula. The perturbation formula is normally expressed as

$$\Delta F_{YX} = F(\lambda_Y) - F(\lambda_X)$$

$$= \sum_{i=X}^{Y-1} -kT\ln < e^{-[H(\lambda_i+\Delta\lambda)-H(\lambda_i)]/kT} > \lambda_i \qquad (3)$$

$$= \sum_{i=X+1}^{Y} +kT\ln < e^{-[H(\lambda_i-\Delta\lambda)-H(\lambda_i)]/kT} > \lambda_i$$

where $< ... >_\lambda$ indicates an ensemble average generated with a Hamiltonian $H(\lambda)$. In order to improve convergence of the ensemble average, the interval (λ_X,λ_Y) is normally split into a number of subintervals using intermediate λ values: λ_X, λ_{X+1}, ..., λ_{Y-1}, λ_Y separated by $\Delta\lambda = \lambda_i - \lambda_{i-1}$. The change in free energy using the integration formula is given by

$$\Delta F_{YX} = \int_{\lambda X}^{\lambda_Y} \langle\frac{\partial H}{\partial\lambda}\rangle_\lambda \; d\lambda \qquad (4)$$

To evaluate the integral in (4) the coupling parameter may be made a function of time and slowly changed throughout a simulation. This procedure is commonly referred to as slow growth, and the integral is approximated by a continuous sum. Alternatively, ensemble averages can be evaluated at specific values of λ and the integral evaluated by numerical quadrature.

Perturbation versus Integration

Determination of the change in free energy using either the perturbation or integration formula depends on the evaluation of an ensemble average. Occasionally in the literature the perturbation formula is misleadingly described as exact whereas the integration formula is described as approximate. This is because the integration in (4) must be performed numerically. The perturbation formula is, however, only exact in the limit of infinite sampling or perfectly overlapping ensembles for $H(\lambda)$ and $H(\lambda + \Delta\lambda)$. In practice either method can be used to determine a given change in free energy to any desired precision. The sampling and convergence properties of the two approaches do, nevertheless, differ and which method is the most appropriate will depend on the nature of the problem. The perturbation formula performs well if the ensembles for the initial and final states overlap closely. If the ensembles do not overlap closely, very small λ increments and long simulation times are required to avoid significant systematic errors. This can be illustrated by considering the case of an isolated particle of mass, m, in a one-dimensional harmonic well. The potential energy, V, in this case is given by

$$V = \tfrac{1}{2}K(x - X_0)^2 + C \tag{5}$$

where K is the harmonic force constant, X_0 is the equilibrium position and C is simply an offset of the potential. The free energy can be analytically shown to be given by

$$F = -kT\ln\,[2\pi h^{-1}kT(m/K)^{\frac{1}{2}}] + C \tag{6}$$

The free energy is independent of X_0. No work is required to move the equilibrium position of the oscillator and the change in free energy for the mutation A illustrated in Fig. 10.1 is zero. This mutation is analogous to changing a bond length in a vacuum or changing the position of a restrained atom in a homogeneous environment. The average of the derivative $\partial H/\partial X_0$ is zero. Thus, the change in free energy calculated using the integration formula for any change in X_0 will also be zero. Using the perturbation formula the calculated free energy will always be positive and dependent on the amount by which X_0 is changed in each window. The free energy will only approach zero, for finite sampling, as $\Delta\lambda$ approaches zero. In contrast, to estimate the free energy difference associated with a change in the offset C (mutation B in Fig. 10.1), use of the perturbation formula is highly efficient. The ensembles for the initial and final states overlap exactly. Only a single window is required and the calculated difference in free energy for any change in C

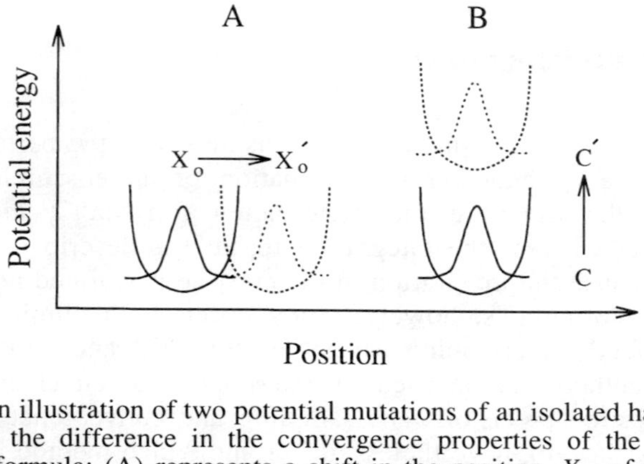

Fig. 10.1 An illustration of two potential mutations of an isolated harmonic oscillator to illustrate the difference in the convergence properties of the perturbation and integration formula: (A) represents a shift in the position, X_0, of the oscillator and (B) a shift in the offset, C, of the potential energy. The parabolic curves correspond to the potential energy, $V(x)$ (equation (5)) and the Gaussian curves the probability distribution of the particle.

will converge rapidly. Using the integration formula the derivative at intermediate λ values may still need to be evaluated in order to perform the integration.

These examples illustrate the danger of using methods such as the 'dynamically modified windows' approach proposed by Pearlman and Kollman (1989). Dynamically modified windows attempts to optimize free energy calculations based on the perturbation formula by relating the window size to the calculated change in free energy. The maximum allowed change in λ does not, however, depend on the free energy change as assumed, but on the degree of overlap of the ensembles.

In the limit of infinite sampling the perturbation and integration formulae are equivalent. However, because the convergence of the ensemble average does not depend on the magnitude of the change in λ, the integration formula offers the better opportunity to reduce and monitor errors in practice.

Slow Growth versus Numerical Quadrature

Using slow growth, only one configuration is sampled for each value of λ. The ensemble average in (4) is approximated by the set of configurations over a small range of λ. As λ is continuously changed throughout the simulation the system is never truly in equilibrium, but lags behind the changing Hamiltonian (Wood, 1991). This results in excess work being done on the system and a systematic overestimation of the free energy. Attempting to correct for this overestimation by averaging results for the forward and reverse mutation from short simulations is an unreliable procedure. A minimum prerequisite to obtain a reliable free energy is that the difference between the forward and reverse processes or hysteresis is small. A small hysteresis, however, indicates only the degree of reversibility. It indicates neither that the system is in equilibrium nor that a representative ensemble has been sampled for each value of λ. Thus, if a mutation is performed much faster than the system can respond, the system will remain trapped in a local state. If this state can be adequately sampled during the simulation, the mutation will appear reversible and a small hysteresis will be observed. The calculated free energy will, however, be dependent on the precise starting configuration. As the length of the simulation is increased, the apparent hysteresis will also increase (Mark *et al.*, 1994).

In practice, slow growth calculations perform well in rapidly equilibrating systems where a single configuration approximates an equilibrium ensemble, e.g. a single ion in water or the simultaneous mutation of a large number of molecules. Where the mutated molecule can adopt multiple configurations, the method converges slowly and the calculated free energy depends strongly on both the starting configuration and the length of the simulation.

By performing different simulations at discrete λ values and integrating numerically, effects due to the equilibration of the system with respect to the change in Hamiltonian and sampling of a representative ensemble can be largely separated. One (or a series) of independent simulations can be followed until the average of the derivative $< \partial H/\partial\lambda >_\lambda$ converges with the desired precision. To perform the integration it must be assumed that the derivative is a smooth and continuous function of λ. However, when atoms are created or destroyed the change in free energy as a function of λ may, depending on the choice of the λ dependence of the Hamiltonian, be highly non-linear or contain singularities. The derivatives of different terms within the Hamiltonian may also exhibit a different dependence on λ. Therefore, the convergence of the integration must be tested independently of the convergence of the derivatives, if significant systematic errors are to be avoided (Mark *et al.*, 1994). The use of higher order derivatives will improve the estimation of the integral with a smaller number of λ values (Smith and van Gunsteren, 1994). Longer simulations are, however, needed to achieve convergence at each point. In summary, though not necessarily the most computationally efficient, use of the thermodynamic integration formula with numerical quadrature of the integral offers the best opportunity to minimize convergence and sampling errors in free energy calculations.

Thermodynamic Cycles

In most free energy calculations the principle of a thermodynamic cycle is evoked. A thermodynamic cycle, as illustrated in Fig. 10.2, is based on the fact that, as a state function, a given change in free energy is independent of the path taken to go from the initial to the final state. The change in free energy for any cyclic mutation is zero. This means that the difference in the free energy of binding for the ligands X and Y ($\Delta\Delta G_{\mathrm{XY}}$) shown in Fig. 10.2 can be calculated by two equivalent pathways. Either the physical process of complexation for X (ΔG_1) and for Y (ΔG_2) can be simulated (horizontal arrows) or the non-physical mutation of X into Y can be performed for X free in solution (ΔG_3) and in the complex (ΔG_4) (vertical arrows). The difference in binding energy is given by $\Delta\Delta G_{XY} = \Delta G_2 - \Delta G_1 = \Delta G_4 - \Delta G_3$. Thermodynamic cycles are primarily used for reasons of computational efficiency. Simulation of the process of complexation between a ligand and a protein with the associated rearrangement of large numbers of solvent molecules is generally not practical. In contrast the non-physical mutation of X into Y involving the conversion of a small number of atoms from one type to another is straightforward. Thermodynamic cycles also allow for the possibility of cancellation of systematic errors in the calculated free energy due to the non-inclusion of quantum mechanical effects, limitations in the force field or

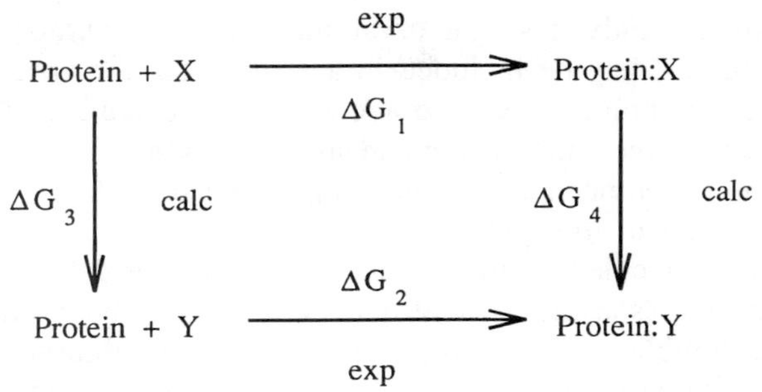

Fig. 10.2 A thermodynamic cycle to determine the difference in free energy of binding of two ligands *X* and *Y* to a protein.

due to the imposition of boundary conditions, cut-off radii, etc. Such cancellation can only occur, however, if simulation conditions in terms of boundary conditions, cut-off radii or constraints on the system are as similar as possible for the two environments (see van Gunsteren and Mark, 1992; Shi *et al.*, 1993).

Within the context of a thermodynamic cycle, terms that make no net contribution to the free energy will cancel and can be ignored. Great care is required, however, when selecting components that can be neglected. The work done creating or destroying a charge during a simulation will depend on the dielectric constant of the medium. Long-range electrostatic contributions can only be ignored if the dielectric properties of the environments on both sides of the thermodynamic cycle are equivalent. This is not the case when one side corresponds to the low dielectric interior of a protein and the other is a high dielectric medium such as water. Whether or not to include internal terms must also be considered. In a number of studies, internal contributions to the free energy have been neglected (Dang *et al.*, 1989; Dang and Kollman, 1991). If, however, the conformational freedom of the ligand is different in the bound and unbound forms, internal terms will make a net contribution to the overall free energy and must be included.

Equilibration and Sampling

A primary, if not the major, source of error in free energy calculations is failure to sample a representative ensemble (Berendsen, 1991). To sample the complete ensemble is not possible, for example, in the case of the folded and unfolded forms of many proteins in equilibrium. Free energy calculations aim not to determine the complete ensemble but rather only to sample a representative ensemble of a specific meta-stable state, e.g. the ligand bound to the folded protein. As only a single or at most a small number of ligand or acceptor molecules may be included in a simulation, the ensemble averages in (3) and (4) are replaced by time averages. The calculated free energy is, thus, correlated in time and may depend strongly on the starting configuration, unless the sampling time, $\tau_{sampling}$, is much longer than the relaxation time of the different modes of the system.

For a single molecule, equilibrium can also only be defined in terms of a time average. The starting structure must not only be a member of the equilibrium ensemble but also represent a common configuration. The equilibration and sampling time required at each λ value will depend on the type of mutation and the properties of the specific system. It cannot be expressed in terms of simulation time. A criterion that can be used is whether the calculated free energy no longer changes as a function of time.

Choice of Pathway

The choice of λ dependence of the Hamiltonian defines the pathway from the initial to the final state. As a state function, the change in free energy is independent of the path. The choice of path, however, strongly affects computational efficiency. The pathway should be chosen such that the relaxation time of the system with respect to the change in Hamiltonian and the time required to sample the ensemble are both minimized. This implies that the most direct path is not necessarily the most efficient (Mark *et al.*, 1991). As only terms in the Hamiltonian that are modified contribute to the change in free energy, the number of changes in the Hamiltonian should be minimized. The introduction of additional degrees of freedom should also be avoided. In most cases involving the creation or deletion of a substituent atom, only the van der Waals and Coulomb interactions should be mutated. Bonded terms such as bond length, angle and dihedral angle terms should be held constant. This avoids the additional work required to modify the associated force constants and the additional sampling required as the atom gains degrees of freedom. Mutations should be designed such that an atom does not become fully uncoupled from the rest of the system. If the bonded terms are held constant, the end state will differ if the force constants are reduced to zero. The calculated free energy for the specific mutation will also be different. This difference will, however, cancel within the context of a thermodynamic cycle. If possible, the mass of the atom should remain unchanged. The contribution to the free energy from the change in momentum is separable from the change in the potential energy and cancels within the thermodynamic cycle.

In most implementations of the coupling parameter approach, a direct correspondence between atoms in the initial state and atoms in the final state is described. Alternatively, two complete functional groups can be defined and interchanged during the simulation. The latter approach is, for example, implemented in the molecular simulation package of CHARMM (Brooks *et al.*, 1983). This has the advantage that changes to interactions between bonded atoms are minimized. The disadvantage is that, for intermediate λ values, effectively both copies exist simultaneously. Though the groups do not interact directly, the conformational space accessible to either group is significantly restricted by the presence of the other. The highly non-linear nature of the van der Waals interaction as a function of interatomic distance means that the effective volume of the other group is only negligible very close to the end states. If a linear coupling of the initial and final states is used, the derivative at the end states may contain singularities, and simulations close to the end states may be numerically unstable. In practice such problems have been avoided by limiting sampling to the interval λ = 0.1–0.9 and extrapolating to the end states (Kuczera *et al.*, 1990; Tidor and Karplus, 1991). The reliability of results based on such an approach is, however, questionable.

Creation and Deletion of Atoms

The Lennard–Jones and Coulomb potential energy terms standardly used in atomic force fields contain a singularity when the interaction distance, r, between two atoms is zero. For fully interacting atoms this singularity is never sampled due to the repulsive term in the Lennard–Jones interaction and does not contribute to an ensemble average of the potential energy. The singularity in the potential energy function when $r = 0$ means, however, that there is a singularity in the derivative of the potential energy function when $r = 0$ for atoms that are created or destroyed. If a linear coupling between the Hamiltonian of the initial and the final states is used, the singularity in the associated derivative may be sampled in the initial or the final state when the effective van der Waals radius of the mutated atom is zero. In this case the ensemble averages in (3) and (4) are indeterminable. In practice, sampling of the singularity may easily be avoided by creating (or deleting) an atom within the effective van der Waals radius of an atom to which it is bound. In some cases the bond length must be reduced to avoid sampling of the singularity. It is, nevertheless, ill-advised to attempt to reduce the bond length to zero. As the bond length is reduced, the vibrational frequency of the associated angle terms increase and an ever smaller time step is required to accurately integrate the equations of motion.

An alternative approach that has been proposed by a number of workers is to choose the dependence of the Hamiltonian on λ such that the derivative of the potential energy function at the end states is zero or finite. Such approaches are applicable where a single atom is removed and the ensemble is generated using a Monte Carlo simulation (Beutler *et al.*, 1994). Using molecular dynamics to generate the ensemble, linear or non-linear coupling of the Hamiltonian will lead to numerical instabilities in the simulation as exposed atoms are created or destroyed. This is because a finite step size is used to integrate the equations of motion. Thus, when the effective radius of the mutated atom is small compared to length of flight of an atom per time step, high energy regions of the potential, including $r = 0$, may be sampled. To avoid such numerical problems a form of potential energy function that does not contain a singularity at $r = 0$ may be used (van Gunsteren *et al.*, 1993; Beutler *et al.*, 1994).

Constraint Corrections

If constraints are used, such as to maintain fixed bond lengths during a simulation, the Hamiltonian of the system is different from the unconstrained case. This will, in turn, lead to a (slightly) different ensemble being generated. To allow for the effects of such constraints a so-called metric tensor correction can be applied (see van Gunsteren *et al.*, 1993 and references therein). In practice the magnitude of such metric tensor corrections in cases relevant to drug design are small and can be safely ignored.

Metric tensor corrections arise directly from the application of constraints. Recently, however, a number of papers have appeared which refer to a contribution or correction to the free energy due to the application of bond length constraints (Straatsma *et al.*, 1992; Pearlman, 1993). In this case, the 'correction' is not due to the imposition of the constraints as such but due to the manner in which the thermodynamic integration or perturbation formula has been implemented. When using the coupling parameter approach, only parts of the Hamiltonian that change as a function of λ contribute to the change in free energy. Thus, if we do not change a bond length parameter, it does not contribute to the free energy change. However, if we do change a bond length parameter, it will contribute to the free energy change, whether or not the bond is treated as a constraint or as a harmonic oscillator. This is irrespective of the method used to generate the ensemble. Whether this bond is automatically included in the calculation will, however, depend on the implementation. For example, in GROMOS (van Gunsteren and Berendsen, 1987) the thermodynamic integration formula is used in conjunction with an analytical derivative $\partial H/\partial\lambda$. If a bond length constraint is changed, the derivative of the potential along the direction of the bond must be determined. This is equal to the force from the environment along the direction of the bond which is resisted by the constraint. This force can be readily calculated during the constraint resetting using the SHAKE procedure (Ryckaert *et al.*, 1977; van Gunsteren *et al.*, 1993) and hence has been referred to by some as a SHAKE contribution. It has, however, nothing intrinsically to do with SHAKE and the same bond length contribution to the free energy must be included irrespective of the method used to reset the constraints. Using the perturbation formula a numerical derivative is calculated. $H(\lambda)$ and $H(\lambda + \Delta\lambda)$ are evaluated for an ensemble generated at $H(\lambda)$. When using constraints, the geometric parameters (i.e. bond lengths) form part of the Hamiltonian. Thus, when evaluating $H(\lambda + \Delta\lambda)$ the bond lengths must have the value corresponding to $H(\lambda + \Delta\lambda)$ and not the value at $H(\lambda)$ used to generate the ensemble. If only the interaction function parameters and not the geometric constraints are changed when evaluating $H(\lambda + \Delta\lambda)$, as is the case in the AMBER simulation package, the contribution to the free energy associated with the change in bond length is in effect neglected and an additional correction is required (Pearlman, 1993).

Free Energy Components

A meaningful separation of the free energy into specific components is, in general, not possible. The total free energy of the system can only be expressed in terms of a sum of components in so far as the total system can be separated into a series of independent subsystems. This is a direct consequence of the basic statistical mechanical definitions of free energy and entropy (e.g. see van Gunsteren *et al.*, 1993; Mark and van Gunsteren, 1994).

In a number of recent studies, however, analysis of a breakdown of free energy components based on free energy calculations using the integration formula have been presented (Kuczera *et al.*, 1990; Tidor and Karplus, 1991; Simonson and Brunger, 1992; Miyamoto and Kollman, 1993; Prod'hom and Karplus, 1993). It may be easily shown that if the Hamiltonian H can be expressed as a linear combination of terms; we may rewrite the integration formula (4) in the form (Gao *et al.*, 1989):

$$\Delta F(X \to Y) = \int_0^1 \left\langle \frac{\partial H_1}{\partial \lambda} \right\rangle_\lambda \mathrm{d}\lambda + \int_0^1 \left\langle \frac{\partial H_2}{\partial \lambda} \right\rangle_\lambda \mathrm{d}\lambda + \ldots + \int_0^1 \left\langle \frac{\partial H_n}{\partial \lambda} \right\rangle_\lambda \mathrm{d}\lambda$$
$$= \Delta F_1(X \to Y) + \Delta F_2(X \to Y) + \ldots + \Delta F_n(X \to Y) \quad (7)$$

where H_1 to H_n can refer to any separation of the Hamiltonian either in terms of force field parameters, residue–residue interactions or solvent–protein interactions. The flaw in this approach is that for any given perturbation the type of separation that is possible and the magnitudes of the calculated free energy components $\Delta F_1(X \rightarrow Y)$ to $\Delta F_n(X \rightarrow Y)$ will depend on the λ-dependence of the Hamiltonian. The λ-dependence of the Hamiltonian defines the pathway taken to go from the initial to the final state. The choice of the λ-dependence of the Hamiltonian or pathway is not unique and hence the calculated free energy components are not unique. Detailed analysis of free energy components based on such calculations is, therefore, meaningless (Shi *et al.*, 1993; Mark and van Gunsteren, 1994).

Summary

Central to any rational design process is the ability to predict the effect of a proposed modification on the properties of interest. In the case of drug design, the properties of interest depend directly on the associated changes in free energy. The basic methodology to predict changes in free energy based on molecular simulation techniques is well established and potentially highly accurate. Despite this, the quality of published free energy calculations varies greatly. This is because reliable estimates from such calculations can only be obtained if the basic assumptions in terms of equilibrium and sampling on which the methods are based, are met. The absolute requirements for a specific mutation are of course system dependent. The application of the simple rules outlined above should, nevertheless, assist in obtaining reliable free energy estimates.

References

Berendsen, H.J.C. (1991). *In* 'Proteins: Structure, Dynamics and Design' (V. Renugopalakrishnan, P.R. Carey, I.C.P. Smith, S.G. Huang and A.C. Storer, eds), pp. 384–392. ESCOM, Leiden.

Beutler, T.C., Mark, A.E., van Schaik, R.C., Gerber, P.R. and van Gunsteren, W.F. (1994). *Chem. Phys. Lett.* **222**, 529–539.

Beveridge, D.L. and DiCapua, F.M. (1989). *Annu. Rev. Biophys. Biophys. Chem.* **18**, 431–492.

Brooks, B.R., Bruccoleri, R.E., Olafson, B.D., States, D.J., Swaminathan, S. and Karplus, M. (1983). *J. Comput. Chem.* **4**, 187–217.

Dang, L.X. and Kollman, P.A. (1991). *In* 'Proteins: Structure, Dynamics and Design' (V. Renugopalakrishnan, P.R. Carey, I.C.P. Smith, S.G. Huang and A.C. Storer, eds), pp. 393–398. ESCOM, Leiden.

Dang, L.X., Merz, K.M. and Kollman, P.A. (1989). *J. Am. Chem. Soc.* **111**, 8505–8508.

Gao, J., Kuczera, K., Tidor, B. and Karplus, M. (1989). *Science* **244**, 1069–1072.

Kuczera, K., Gao, J., Tidor, B. and Karplus, M. (1990). *Proc. Natl Acad. Sci. USA* **87**, 8481–8485.
Mark, A.E. and van Gunsteren, W.F. (1994). *J. Mol. Biol.* **240**, 167–176.
Mark, A.E., van Gunsteren, W.F. and Berendsen, H.J.C. (1991). *J. Chem. Phys.* **94**, 3808–3816.
Mark, A.E., van Helden, S.P., Janssen, L.H.M., Smith, P.E. and van Gunsteren, W.F. (1994). *J. Am. Chem. Soc.* **116**, 6293–6320.
Miyamoto, S. and Kollman, P.A. (1993). *Proteins: Struct. Funct. Genet.* **16**, 226–245.
Pearlman, D.A. (1993). *J. Chem. Phys.* **98**, 8946–8957.
Pearlman, D.A. and Kollman, P.A. (1989). *J. Chem. Phys.* **90**, 2460–2470.
Prod'hom, B. and Karplus, M. (1993). *Protein Engng* **6**, 585–592.
Ryckaert, J.-P., Ciccotti, G. and Berendsen, H.J.C. (1977). *J. Comput. Phys.* **23**, 327–341.
Shi, Y.Y., Mark, A.E., Wang, C.X., Fuhua, H., Berendsen, H.J.C. and van Gunsteren, W.F. (1993). *Protein Engng* **3**, 289–295.
Simonson, T. and Brunger, A.T. (1992). *Biochemistry* **31**, 8661–8674.
Smith, P.E. and van Gunsteren, W.F. (1994). *J. Chem. Phys.* **100**, 577–585.
Straatsma, T.P., Zacharias, M. and McCammon, J.A. (1992). *Chem. Phys. Lett.* **196**, 297–302.
Tidor, B. and Karplus, M. (1991). *Biochemistry* **30**, 3217–3228.
van Gunsteren, W.F. and Berendsen, H.J.C. (1987). *Groningen Molecular Simulation (GROMOS) Library Manual.* Biomos, Nijenborgh 4, 9747 AG Groningen, The Netherlands.
van Gunsteren, W.F. and Mark, A.E. (1992). *Eur. J. Biochem.* **204**, 947–961.
van Gunsteren, W.F., Beutler, T.C., Fraternali, F., King, P.M., Mark, A.E. and Smith, P.E. (1993). *In*: 'Computer simulation of biomolecular systems, theoretical and experimental applications'. vol. 2, (W.F. van Gunsteren, P.K. Weiner, A.J. Wilkinson, eds.), pp. 315–348. ESCOM, Leiden.
Wood, R.H. (1991). *J. Phys. Chem.* **95**, 4838–4842.

Discussion

P.M. Dean

Thank you for clearly outlining where the future lies here. Important advances will have to include the development of new hardware. Is that the case? You gave a masterful demonstration of what should go on and how to do it, but your limitations, presumably, are still the power of the computer.

A.E. Mark

It is not just the computing time. In terms of computing, we are still 15 or 16 orders of magnitude slower than nature – we would like, of course, to be much quicker. However, while nature is limited to physical pathways, the simulations are not so limited. We can allow for a lot more rearrangements and better sampling by doing things, say, in four dimensions, using soft-core potentials or various other things, that give us major advances in the efficiency of our calculations. It is not just a question of waiting for more computer time – but any more always helps.

J. Goodman

Previous speakers have estimated relative binding by considering some form of internal energy and hoping that entropy effects cancel. How dangerous is this likely to be?

A.E. Mark

It depends – if there is an extremely tight binding constant, it is likely that the enthalpy terms dominate or a simple entropy correction for loss of solvation by water can be used. If it is considered to be a purely hydrophobic binding, and it is a nice simple molecule, an estimate of the range in free energy can be made based on the burial of surface area or something similar, and we may also get a reasonable estimate.

The problem is that such estimates can never be trusted. In some cases these methods will work well, whereas in others they will give a completely wrong answer. Unfortunately, this has just been illustrated in respect to DOCK: another configuration, binding in a completely different way, can be often found in the crystal structures, even though from a medicinal point of view we have hit exactly what we wanted, i.e. prediction of a compound that binds. The docking algorithm itself, unfortunately, only works on particular cases. This is really the message: any empirical method or any type of fitting procedure will work only on the particular cases for which it is paramaterized – they are not general.

E. Westhof

You mentioned that long simulations are needed to get convergence. What about equilibration of the system before starting the simulation from which the free energy changes will be extracted? How is the system equilibrated at the start, and for how long?

A.E. Mark

The equilibration time required depends on what property we wish to look at. Something like the potential energy equilibrates quickly in the simulation, whereas structural equilibration is very slow. To judge when we are in equilibrium in free energy calculations we look at the change in the derivative of the potential – the free energy component – and how this converges. Basically, for each individual system the convergence of the derivative is traced until it no longer changes, and then we consider that the system is equilibrated for the quantity that we wish to measure. Generally, we run for about 100 or 200 ps to allow the protein to stabilize.

E. Westhof
At what temperature is this done, and are cut-offs used?

A.E. Mark
This is done at 300 K – calculations have to be run at realistic temperatures. Taking higher temperatures to improve sampling is meaningless in free energy calculations. These are standard simulations, with all the problems of standard simulations. I use a short-range cut-off in protein simulations of about 8 Å and a long-range cut-off of perhaps 15 Å to allow for longer-range charge effects.

There are many improvements we would want to make in order more accurately to determine the derivatives. For example, no allowance is made for the very long-range electrostatic effects which, of course, if a charge is being created, are a huge problem in the system. In such cases we really need to include something like a reaction field correction.

E. Westhof
In simpler systems, depending on the equilibration, one can get different results.

A.E. Mark
(*interrupting*) Yes – but the other point to remember is that it may not be just equilibration. All the states that are sampled in the simulations are probably equilibrium states. This is something people often forget in free energy calculations. For example, I have performed some calculations trying to mutate *trans*-butane into *gauche*-butane. When we made the mutation we started from all *trans* (I started with 64 molecules of *trans*), and changed the potential so that the system wanted to become predominantly *gauche*. People think that at the halfway point all molecules will change over. This is not what we want: we want to start from 99% *trans* and, as the mutation is performed for the percentage of *trans*, to go 98%, 97%, 96%, 95% – right the way through the entire simulation. If, however, we start initially with, say two molecules of *gauche*-butane, both of which are valid equilibrium structures, we will get a different answer unless there has been very extensive sampling. The system may not be out of equilibrium, but is just starting from a different initial state. The two aspects are not quite the same. An ensemble is needed; it cannot be avoided.

A.R. Leach
Another major source of worry and potential error in all these kinds of calculations is the force field parameters. Have you done any similar studies investigating more the underlying theory to see how sensitive the results obtained are to the force field parameters being used? Where do you see that the major focus of our activity in this area should be directed?

A.E. Mark

The sort of method used to calculate free energy derivatives was initially proposed by C.F. Wong (Mount Sinai School of Medicine, New York) precisely to look at how to predict what changes need to be made to the force field in order to get the right free energies. In my talk I presented a number of calculations involving cyclodextrin that performed badly – it turned out that this was due to an incorrect water–carbon parameter inside the force field.

It is difficult to say which is the major error because it will be different in different cases. The advantage in free energy calculations is that we are making only a perturbation to the force field. The perturbation can often be made in the right direction even if in absolute terms the force field is incorrect. I do not know what sort of accuracy the GROMOS or any other empirical force field has in absolute terms. It is something that certainly has to be improved and is currently most likely not good.

R.F. Hirschmann

If you have a small molecule and a macromolecule, for both of which there is an X-ray structure, and when the small molecule binds to the macromolecule the X-ray structure of the complex shows that the conformation of one or both components is different from either component prior to binding, can it be assumed that the energy change for both molecules will not have been very large?

A.E. Mark

Not necessarily. All energy terms including conformational changes should be taken into account. It should, however, be realized that a protein can be deformed dramatically with an extremely tiny energy cost. It does not take much energy to shift parts of proteins around. The classic example is that when a protein unfolds it goes from a folded to an unfolded state with no energy cost at its unfolding temperature. Just because we see a rearrangement in a protein does not necessarily mean that it has cost any energy, or that it must have cost only a tiny amount of energy. However, in both cases it must of course be included.

11

Conformational Analysis in Site-Directed Molecular Design

A.R. LEACH

Department of Chemistry, University of Southampton, Southampton, Hampshire SO9 5NH, UK

Introduction

The interactions between small molecule ligands and biological macromolecules are crucial to the activity of many drugs. The design of small molecule ligands which cause a desired effect at a receptor has been, and will continue to be, a major focus of many drug discovery programmes. In an increasing number of cases, a detailed three-dimensional structure of the target macromolecule is available from X-ray crystallography, NMR or molecular modelling. These structures can provide vital information in the search for new molecules that will form strong intermolecular complexes with the biological targets* and act as lead compounds. Of course, not all tight-binding inhibitors are successful drugs; other properties such as transport, bioavailability, metabolism and toxicity are also important. Nevertheless, a good inhibitor is often the required starting point for a drug design programme.

Finding new lead compounds is a difficult task, but a number of promising theoretical approaches have been developed in recent years, some of which are discussed in this volume (see Chapters 4, 8 and 12). These methods fall into two broad categories (Lewis and Leach, 1994). The first category comprises those methods that attempt to identify leads from among a list of known molecules, usually by searching a database. This approach has the advantage that any molecules will be readily available for testing (or at least

* We will henceforth use the term 'receptor' to refer to all types of macromolecule with which we might wish to form an intermolecular complex.

New Perspectives in Drug Design
ISBN 0–12–208070–X

the synthesis should be known), but suffers from the disadvantage that the suggested compounds will not be 'novel'. Alternatively, one can attempt to find completely new compounds – *de novo* drug design. The obvious disadvantage here is that the suggestions may be difficult (if not impossible) to synthesize.

In this chapter we consider two problems in structure-based design. The first problem is concerned with identifying a representative set of conformations of a molecule. It is often desired to select a manageable number of conformations of a molecule to represent its accessible conformational space. Such a set could be obtained by performing a conformational search and then using cluster analysis. However, a significant proportion of molecules have a very large number of minimum energy structures – tens if not hundreds of thousands – which can take a long time to generate, let alone to cluster. We shall then consider a new method which can take the conformational space of the receptor into account during structure-based design. At present, the receptor is invariably maintained in a fixed conformation (the 'rigid receptor' approximation). What our algorithm provides is an efficient way to rigorously sample a significant proportion of the receptor's conformational degrees of freedom and to investigate the implications of the rigid receptor approximation.

Some Relevant Concepts

To tackle these two problems we use the concept of a directed search. Many problems encountered in molecular modelling have a large number of possible solutions. Finding the minimum energy conformations of a flexible molecule is a pertinent example. In such cases, it may be impractical – if not impossible – to try to identify all the solutions. This being so, it is obviously desirable that the solutions we can consider should be the most relevant ones. We therefore want to direct the search towards the most desirable solutions. For example, there are many ways to travel between Southampton and Turnberry, but for the purposes of attending this conference I am only interested in those which correspond to the shortest or quickest journey. A route that requires me to drive on minor roads all the way from Southampton to Turnberry is a 'solution' that I am happy to ignore. Giving 'direction' to a search in molecular modelling can be done in various ways. For example, experimental information about the distances between pairs of atoms (e.g. from NMR) is easily incorporated into the distance geometry or restrained molecular dynamics methods for exploring conformational space. In other cases where no experimental data are available it is necessary to discriminate between solutions using some measure of their 'quality'. For example, in a conformational search we are typically interested in the lowest energy conformations.

An appropriate function here would be the intramolecular energy, as might be calculated using molecular mechanics. Global optimization methods aim to identify the optimal solutions to a problem; simulated annealing and genetic algorithms are two particularly popular examples being applied in molecular modelling at present. Most global optimization methods are stochastic: they inherently rely upon a random exploration of the search space, albeit with sophisticated mechanisms for directing the search towards optimal solutions. However, random-based methods provide no *guarantee* to find the optimal solution, nor can they always locate all the solutions required (for example, the global minimum energy conformation of a molecule and all conformations within some energy cutoff of the global minimum). The traditional alternative to the stochastic methods is the systematic search. This is often believed to be impractical for problems larger than a modest size due to the combinatorial explosion in the number of possibilities. One of the aims of the work reported here is to show that it is possible to explore systematically the search space and to identify with no element of uncertainty not only the optimal solution but also *all* of the 'best' solutions.

The methods that we shall describe are most easily understood using a *search tree* representation of a problem. A search tree is an abstract entity comprising nodes that represent the states available to a problem (Fig. 11.1). The nodes are connected by *edges*. There may be a *cost* associated with each edge. The *root node* corresponds to the initial state of the problem. *Goal nodes* correspond to acceptable solutions to the problem. There may also be other *terminal nodes* which represent 'dead ends'. Nodes between the root node and the goal nodes represent partial solutions to the problem. Sometimes the objective is to find just a single acceptable solution; in other cases we

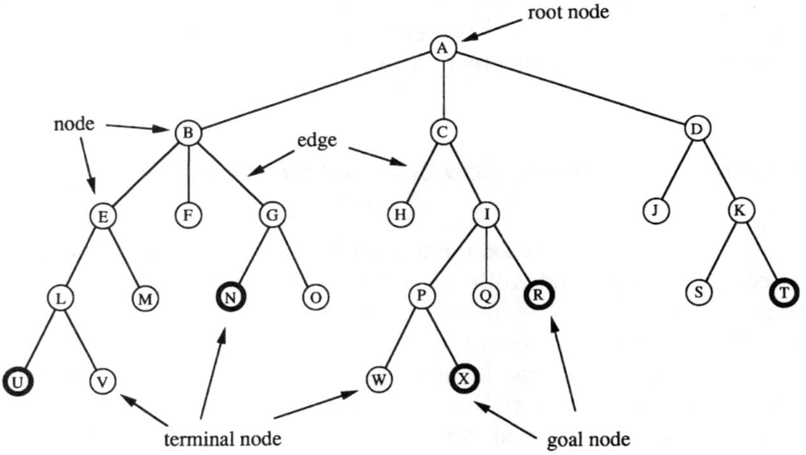

Fig. 11.1 A simple search tree that contains five goal nodes.

would like to find all possible solutions. In such situations, the well-known depth-first or breadth-first algorithms can be used to explore the search tree (Winston, 1992). However, for many problems the number of possible solutions is so large that it is not feasible to find them all. Moreover, a large proportion of the potential solutions may be of little or no interest because much 'better' solutions exist. To find the 'best' solutions (i.e. those with the lowest cost from root to goal node) alternative methods can be used to explore the search-space which do not require that all solutions are first generated. One of these alternative search methods is the A* algorithm (Hart *et al.*, 1968; Nilsson, 1982). The A* algorithm uses an evaluation function denoted f^*. There are two components of f^* for any node n; the cost of reaching the node from the start node (denoted g^*) and the estimated cost of reaching a goal node from $n(h^*)$. Thus:

$$f^* = g^* + h^* \tag{1}$$

where g^* is the cheapest path found so far for the node, and h^* carries heuristic information, defined in a way appropriate to the problem. However, h^* must never overestimate the cost of reaching a goal node. If it were to overestimate the actual path cost then we might ignore a path that would be cheaper than the one ultimately found. A list of nodes is maintained by the algorithm, ordered according to their values of f^*. At each stage, the node at the head of the list (the one with the smallest value of f^*) is expanded and new values of f^* calculated for its successor nodes. These successor nodes are added to the list in the appropriate position. The first goal node to reach the head of the list has the minimum cost path from the root node. By continuing to process the list, other solutions of increasing cost can be found. It should be noted that the A* algorithm can also be used to identify 'maximum cost' paths. Here, the list of nodes is ordered so that the node with the largest value of f^* is at its head and the h^* values should now be overestimates rather than underestimates.

Generating a Molecule's 'Most Different' Conformations

A variety of methods is now available for searching the conformational space of molecules (Howard and Kollman, 1988; Leach, 1991). In our approach to conformational analysis (Dolata *et al.*, 1987; Leach *et al.*, 1990a,b; Leach and Prout, 1990), low-energy conformations of a molecule are generated by breaking a molecule into small fragments (called units) as illustrated in Fig. 11.2 for 3-acetamido-3-deoxythymidine. Associated with each fragment are one or more three-dimensional 'templates' that give the conformations available to the unit. For example, the pyrimidine unit has just one template but the amide fragment has two (*cis* and *trans*). Conformations of the molecule are

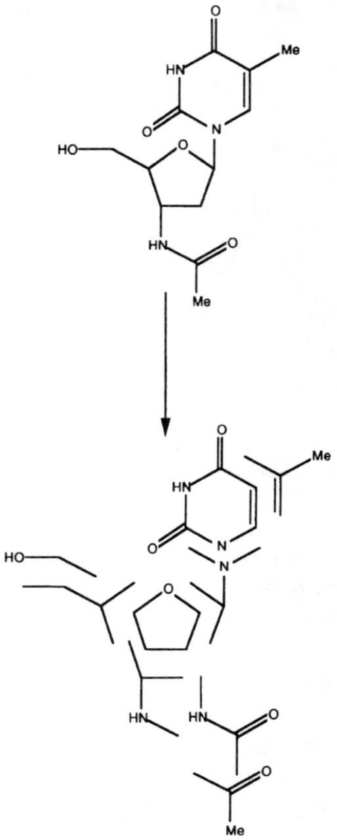

Fig. 11.2 3-Acetamido-3-deoxythymidine is constructed from the nine fragments (units) indicated.

constructed by joining the templates together, one template for each unit. Different combinations of templates give rise to different molecular conformations. The total number of possible conformations for the molecule equals the product of all fragment conformations. However, for many molecules a large proportion of these combinations are unsatisfactory due to steric overlaps or ill-fitting templates. The space explored by the method can be represented using a search tree. For example, the search tree appropriate to a simple molecule containing three units A, B and C such that unit A has three templates, unit B has two templates and unit C has two templates is shown in Fig. 11.3.

We have previously described how the A* algorithm can be used to identify the lowest energy conformations of a molecule (Leach and Prout, 1990) where the cost associated with each edge in the search tree is the intramolecular

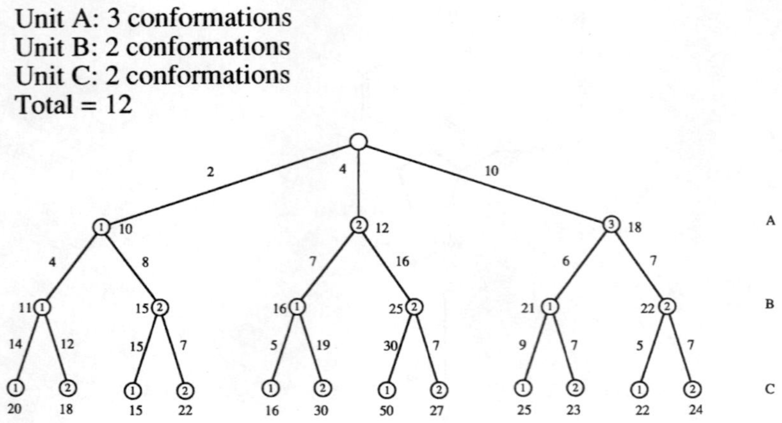

Fig. 11.3 A molecule with three fragments that has a total of 12 possible conformations.

energy. We have often found that the lowest energy conformations of a molecule are very similar, often differing by the rotation of just one or two bonds. However, the relative energies of the conformations of the isolated ligand often bear no relationship to the relative energies when bound to a receptor. Thus the global minimum energy conformation for the isolated molecule is rarely the conformation in the intermolecular complex. Consequently, if there is a restriction on the number of conformations that can be considered, it is sensible to consider structures that span the range of possible conformations. Cluster analysis can be used to find such a set of representative structures from a previously generated group of conformations. Cluster analysis requires a means to quantify the differences between two conformations. In this work we will use the following torsion-based expression:

$$d_{ij} = \sqrt{\frac{\sum_{k=1}^{N} (\tau_{ik} - \tau_{jk})^2}{N}} \tag{2}$$

Here, d_{ij} is the torsional 'distance' between the two conformations i and j, and $(\tau_{ik} - \tau_{jk})$ is the difference between the values of the torsion angle k in the two structures, taking into account the 2π periodicity of torsion angles. The index k runs over all bonds involving at least four heavy atoms in sequence. A wide variety of clustering algorithms have been devised (Hartigan, 1975); one that we found useful in our ligand docking studies (Leach and Kuntz, 1992) is the improved leader algorithm. As originally described, this algorithm first identifies a 'central' object; in our case this could for example be the conformation that is closest to the average structure. This central conformation defines the first 'leader'. The distance between the first leader and the other conformations is then calculated using the currently operable difference measure (e.g. expression (2)). The structure that is furthest from the first leader then becomes the second leader. The remaining conformations are then sorted into two clusters depending upon whichever of the first two leaders they are closest to. The conformation most dissimilar from its leader then becomes the third leader. In the next step the orientations are sorted into three clusters, and so on. After $N-1$ passes the orientations are thus divided into N clusters. This algorithm has the advantage of speed over other methods which require a similarity matrix of order N to be pre-computed, without some of the drawbacks associated with other quick-partition algorithms.

A major drawback of adopting this two-stage approach to the problem of finding a set of representative conformations is that the conformational search may generate an extremely large number of low-energy structures, which would then constitute a major clustering problem. We have devised a way to combine the conformational search and the cluster analysis that does not require all structures to be generated, an algorithm that we term a 'directed clustering conformational search'. In our algorithm, the energy-based A* search is used to find the global minimum energy conformation. We next require the structure that is 'most different' to this first conformation. To do so we use the A* algorithm, but now the cost associated with each edge is given by the value of the torsional distance function above, rather than the energy (Leach, 1994b). Moreover, as we now seek the structure that is 'most different' from the first conformation, we aim to find the conformation that maximizes the function (2). Having found the second conformation, the third conformation that we require is the one that would be the third leader according to the improved leader clustering algorithm. It may be necessary to amend some of the f^* values used by the A* algorithm as some of the nodes in the list (which represent partially constructed conformations of the molecule) may be closer to the second conformation than the first. A detailed illustration of the method is available elsewhere (Leach, 1994b).

As anticipated, the advantages of this algorithm are most significant for flexible molecules. For example, more than 100 000 structures are generated by a 'full' conformational search for arachidonic acid. The directed clustering search algorithm is able to locate the 'most different' structures much more quickly than the two-stage approach (4 min to find the five 'most different' conformations versus 102 min just to generate 100 000 structures for arachidonic acid). The method can also be used to generate a series of diverse conformations to store in a database. A recent paper (Ricketts *et al.*, 1993) has compared the ability of a variety of structure-building algorithms to generate conformations of molecules which are present in protein–ligand intermolecular complexes in the Protein Databank (Bernstein *et al.*, 1977). A total of 53 intermolecular complexes containing 48 unique ligands were considered (Table 11.1). The crystallographic coordinates of the ligands were extracted

Table 11.1
Protein Databank codes of the 53 protein–ligand complexes used to evaluate the clustering search algorithm

2aat	8atc	1cla	3cpp	3dfrm	4dfr	7dfr	2dhf	1fcb	1fx1
1gox	2gbp	8ldh	3ptb	8rsa	2trm	4xia	5xia	4cts	3drf
4erl	2est	3gap	7gch	3gpd	4pad	5pad	6pad	2r04	2r06
2r07	1r08	2rm2	1rnt	2rnt	2rr1	2rs1	2rs3	2rs5	9rsa
1sgc	1snc	2sns	5tln	7tln	1tlp	1tmn	4tmn	5tmn	6tmn
1tpp	3ts1	2yhx							

from the appropriate entries in the Protein Databank and converted into a format suitable for input to our conformational search program Cobra. The configuration of each ligand was taken to be that defined by the X-ray data. We used our directed clustering conformational search to find the 10 'most different' structures as described above, but with a slight modification: rather than first identifying the global minimum energy conformation, the depth-first search was used to generate a single structure which then acted as the first conformation for the clustering search. In a separate calculation, the default depth-first search method was used to generate systematically conformations of each ligand. No limit was imposed on the number of conformations that were generated by the depth-first search, but no conformational search was permitted to continue for more than 30 min. Each of the conformations generated by either approach was compared to the crystallographically determined structure of the ligand, using a variety of measures. These included the torsional measure above (2), together with one of the measures used by Ricketts *et al.*, who counted the number of acyclic torsion angles that were within $\pm$ 60° of their values in the intermolecular complexes.

We compared the actual conformations generated in each case against the crystallographically determined structure of the ligand. The results are presented graphically using the torsional measure of Ricketts *et al.* in Fig. 11.4. As we would expect, the likelihood of finding a conformation that is similar to the crystal structure is greater when all conformations are considered rather than the smaller number obtained from the clustering search. However, this result must be tempered by two facts. First, the time required to perform the search is much greater for the depth-first algorithm than for the clustering search (with the exception of relatively rigid molecules that can in any case be processed rapidly). The total time to generate the 10 'most different' conformations for the 53 ligands was 148 min with the search being terminated for just one molecule due to the time limit of 30 min being exceeded. By contrast, the total time for the 'total' search was 533 min with 14 molecules exceeding the time limit. Second, even if it were feasible to generate all the accessible conformations (for all molecules), it may not be possible to consider them all in the subsequent calculations. We would still be left with the problem of identifying the 'representative' conformations. For

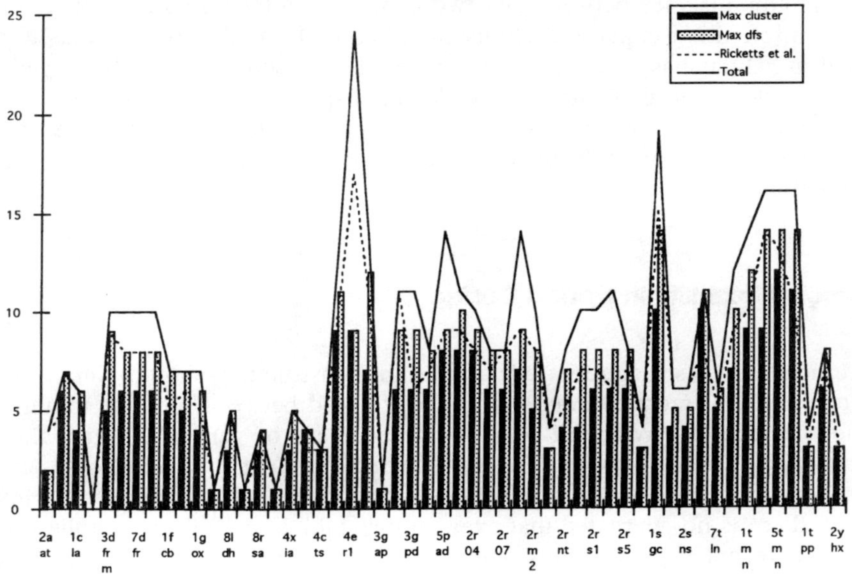

Fig. 11.4 A comparison of the results obtained by applying the directed clustering search and the depth-first search to 53 ligands from protein–ligand complexes in the Protein Databank (PDB). The comparison is made using the torsional measure of Ricketts *et al.* (1993) which counts the number of torsional angles in any one conformation within 60° of their values in the crystal structure. The solid column gives the results obtained from the 10 conformations produced by the clustering search and the dotted column gives the results from the depth-first search. The solid line is the number of dihedral angles in each molecule and the dotted line gives the best result obtained by Ricketts *et al.* (1993) using a variety of alternative structure-generation programs. The labels along the *x*-axis are the PDB codes of the protein–ligand complexes examined.

example, for a significant number of the molecules in the set considered here several tens of thousands of conformations were generated.

Visual examination revealed that the ligands tend to adopt extended structures in intermolecular complexes. This is not unexpected; only in an extended conformation will a ligand be able to maximize its interaction with the receptor (subject of course to the shape constraints of the binding site). In ligand design it might therefore be desirable to direct a search for ligand conformations towards a molecule's more extended conformations. Our investigations also suggest that alternative ways to measure the 'difference' between conformations might usefully be considered. For example, properties such as the molecular electrostatic potential might be more appropriate. Our directed search algorithm has potential applications in other areas. For example, we have used it to identify the conformations in which the interatomic distance between any two atoms is a minimum and a maximum. Such information is particularly useful when deriving distance screens to be used in 3D database searches (see Chapter 12). It could also be employed in *de novo* design to generate molecules which span a range of properties (e.g. dipole moment, molecular weight, partition coefficient, etc.) rather than generating a set of molecules that all have very similar values for these properties.

Protein Flexibility in Ligand Design

A crucial step in structure-based design is the construction of three-dimensional models of the intermolecular complexes formed between putative inhibitors and the receptor. We shall refer to the problem of generating such three-dimensional models as the 'ligand docking problem'. In some cases it is known how the substrate or a substrate analogue binds to a receptor. However, there is no guarantee that even similar inhibitors will bind in the same way, as recent experimental results have demonstrated (Mattos *et al.*, 1994). In addition, a significant number of X-ray structures are of the receptor alone and do not contain a bound substrate or ligand. The ligand docking problem is characterized by a large number of degrees of freedom: the three degrees of translational and three degrees of rotational freedom of one body relative to another, the conformational degrees of freedom of the ligand, and the conformational degrees of freedom of the receptor.

Current ligand docking algorithms can be usefully classified according to the degrees of freedom which they ignore. The earliest approaches to the problem (Kuntz *et al.*, 1982) (and indeed, many of the more recent approaches (Lawrence and Davis, 1992; Kasinos *et al.*, 1992)) treat both ligand and receptor as rigid bodies, only exploring the six degrees of translational and rotational freedom. The receptor is fixed in the experimentally determined conformation. The conformation of the ligand may be obtained from X-ray crystallography, or from a theoretical structure-generation program. An obvious limitation of methods that use a rigid ligand (leaving aside the approximations inherent in the use of a rigid receptor, to which we shall return later) is that the ligand conformation may not correspond to that adopted in the intermolecular complex. For this reason, methods have been developed that attempt to take account of the conformational degrees of freedom of the ligand (DesJarlais *et al.*, 1986; Ghose and Crippen, 1985; Goodsell and Olson, 1990; Hart and Read, 1992; Leach and Kuntz, 1992; Dixon, 1993).

But what of the degrees of freedom of the receptor? Evidence for the role of conformational flexibility in protein structure and function is available from both experiment and theory. In a number of protein X-ray structures multiple conformations have been reported, often manifested as alternative side-chain conformations. The 'real' number of structures which contain different side-chain conformations may in fact be much higher than would appear from an examination of the protein databank. In most cases refinement of X-ray data is terminated when the R factor is less than approximately 20% and there are no interpretable features in the difference Fourier maps (Wlodawer *et al.*, 1988). However, satisfactory refinement to lower R factors of high-resolution data can often require some residues to adopt more than one conformation. For example, the structure of ribonuclease A when refined at 1.26 Å resolution to a final R factor of 0.15 contains 13 side-chains with two alternative conformations (Wlodawer *et al.*, 1988). Data from NMR experiments can also in some cases be interpreted only by assuming the existence of multiple conformations (Mierke *et al.*, 1994). Theoretical methods have also provided detailed information about the dynamics of biological macromolecules. Since the first molecular dynamics simulation of a protein was reported, an increasing number of papers have been published describing the application of this technique to biological macromolecules. A wealth of information can be produced by such simulations. For example, molecular dynamics simulations, used in conjunction with energy minimization, have suggested that many minima lie on the energy surface (Elber and Karplus, 1987). However, molecular dynamics simulations require the expenditure of a considerable amount of computer time and tend to explore the conformational space in the vicinity of the starting structure (indeed, it is often regarded as an indication of a stable simulation if the structure remains close to the initial X-ray conformation!). The time scales over which such simulations can be performed (simulations of a few hundreds of picoseconds are still the exception rather than the rule) are much smaller than many molecular processes of interest. The nature of ligand design is such that a large number of candidates must be considered, and consequently requires a compromise between speed and the level of approximation.

As a first step towards incorporating protein flexibility in ligand design, we have made the following two approximations. First, that the protein backbone is fixed. Second, the side chains are restricted to discrete conformations or rotamers. The problem then is to find a suitable combination of side-chain rotamers for the backbone structure. This is a difficult problem given the large number of possible combinations of side-chain rotamers. A variety of algorithms have been described to tackle this problem, all of which aim to identify a 'low-energy' structure. A variety of algorithms are used to explore the conformational space, including systematic search (Bruccoleri and Karplus, 1985, 1987), Monte Carlo/simulated annealing methods (Lee and Subbiah, 1991; Holm and Sander, 1992) and genetic algorithms (Tuffery *et al.*, 1991). These methods are able to identify low-energy structures, but they cannot guarantee to locate the very lowest energy structure, nor can they determine exactly how many structures are within some energy cut-off of the energy minimum.

An algorithm that is (in principle) able to locate the global energy minimum conformation has been described recently by Desmet and colleagues (Desmet *et al.*, 1992; Lasters and Desmet, 1993). Their procedure is called 'Dead-end elimination' (DEE). The DEE algorithm identifies those side-chain conformations that are incompatible with the global minimum energy combination (GMEC). The energy of a combination of side-chain rotamers is given by:

$$E_{\text{total}} = E_{\text{template}} + \sum_{i=1}^{nres} E_{i_r,template} + \sum_{i=1}^{nres-1} \sum_{j>i}^{nres} \varepsilon_{i_r,j_s} \quad (3)$$

where E_{template} is the internal energy of the backbone and conformationally inflexible residues (the template), $E_{i_r,template}$ is the energy of interaction between residue i in rotamer r and the template, and ε_{i_r,j_s} is the interaction energy between rotamer r of residue i and rotamer s of residue j. A rotamer i_r is incompatible with the global energy minimum structure if it satisfies the following inequality:

$$E_{i_r,\text{template}} + \sum_j \min_s \varepsilon_{i_r,j_s} > E_{i_t,\text{template}} + \sum_j \max_s \varepsilon_{i_t,j_s} \quad (4)$$

In this expression, $\min_s \varepsilon_{i_r,j_s}$ is calculated by taking the rotamer i_r, examining its interaction energy with all currently permitted rotamers s of residue j and finding the minimum value. The value of $\max_s \varepsilon_{i_t,j_s}$ is found similarly. To implement the DEE algorithm, the values of $\sum_j \min_s \varepsilon_{i_r}$, and $\sum_j \max_s \varepsilon_{i_r}$, are determined for each rotamer. Pairs of rotamers are then examined, and rotamers which satisfy the inequality (4) are flagged as being incompatible with the GMEC. This procedure is repeated for all residues in the protein. The process is then repeated, ignoring those rotamers that have just been flagged, until no more rotamers can be eliminated.

The DEE inequality can be generalized to any number of rotamers. Thus, it is possible to derive an expression that permits pairs of rotamers that are incompatible with the global energy minimum to be identified. This information can then be used in the single-rotamer DEE algorithm in two ways. First, if all rotamers of a residue j are deemed incompatible with a rotamer r of residue i, then rotamer r can be eliminated from further consideration. Second, incompatible pairs can be discarded from the calculation of $\min_s \varepsilon_{i_r,j_s}$. It is therefore possible to repeatedly apply the one- and two-rotamer versions of the DEE algorithm, until eventually no further rotamers can be discarded. At this point, Desmet *et al.* found that the number of possible combinations remaining was sufficiently low to enable them to use the generalized DEE method as applied to three, four, etc. rotamers in a combinatorial fashion, until the GMEC was found.

The DEE method as originally described thus guarantees to identify the global minimum energy combination of side-chain rotamers. However, our own implementation showed that the algorithm did not always give the dramatic decrease in the number of combinations observed by Desmet *et al.* We anticipate that this is partly due to the fact that we used a different energy model (based on the AMBER force field (Weiner *et al.*, 1984, 1986)) but also that there may have been an error in the original paper (Lasters and Desmet, 1993). Moreover, uncertainties in the force field and the fact that some contributions (e.g. solvation) may not be included in the energy model means that the true free energy global minimum may not correspond to that of the energy function. Other structures may contribute to the partition function. For these reasons we strongly believe that a method which can locate all accessible structures is far superior to an approach that only provides a single structure, even if that structure is at the global minimum of the potential energy function. Our objective was thus to develop an algorithm that would be able to directly locate the global energy minimum and also provide all structures within some specified energy of the lowest energy structure. The conformations obtained would then provide a more complete picture of the accessible conformational space. In our approach to the problem a modified DEE expression is used to eliminate amino acid rotamers which are incompatible with a structure of the intermolecular complex within a given energy of the global energy minimum. This is done using the following trivial modification of equation (4) which identifies rotamers i_r that cannot be in a structure within E_{cut} of the global energy minimum:

$$E_{i_r,\text{template}} + \sum_j \min_s \varepsilon_{i_r,j_s} > E_{i_t,\text{template}} + \sum_j \max_s \varepsilon_{i_t,j_s} + E_{\text{cut}} \quad (5)$$

This first stage usually eliminates a significant number of amino acid rotamers from further consideration. However, the number of possible combinations of rotamers may still be extremely large (10^{10}–10^{20} is quite common). This search space is then explored using the A* algorithm, to identify first the global minimum energy combination of side chains, and then other structures of increasing energy. In order to achieve this objective we use the A* algorithm. Each node in the search tree represents a partially constructed model in which some of the amino acids have been assigned a rotameric state. The energy of this partial conformation, g^* is calculated using the expression above. An estimate of the minimum energy required to complete the model, h^*, can be obtained from the precalculated values of $E_{i_r,\text{template}}$ and ε_{i_r,j_s}. The secret to success lies in obtaining the best possible estimates of the energies and in processing the residues in the correct order, else the algorithm can become bogged down in the immense space of possible solutions. The first goal node to reach the head of the list is the global energy minimum; the list of nodes can then be processed further in exactly the same fashion to generate a succession of conformations of increasing energy.

Our algorithm can obviously be used to examine the conformational space of isolated proteins. For example, we can determine which residues adopt alternative side-chain conformations and which residues remain fixed, as structures of higher energy are considered. Similarly, we can investigate whether side chains act independently to give rise to higher energy conformations or whether concerted changes dominate. Our initial investigations with small proteins such as BPTI and insulin indicate that little concerted change occurs; this is not surprising as most of the changes are to surface residues which would be expected to have a greater range of conformational freedom. Current work is directed towards an examination of protein cores.

Our approach generates all combinations of side-chain conformations within a specified energy of the global energy minimum, and as such it provides a unique picture of the range of accessible conformational states. We have investigated the effects of ligand binding on the range of conformational states available by determining the number of combinations of side-chain rotamers within 5 kcal/mol of the global energy minimum both for the isolated protein and for the intermolecular complex with the ligand present in its crystallographically determined position. Only residues within 10 Å of the ligand in the crystal structures were allowed to vary. An interesting and somewhat surprising result was that in some cases more conformational states were predicted to be available to the protein in the intermolecular complex than in the isolated molecule. This is due to a modification of the protein's energy surface by the ligand which makes more combinations accessible. For example, for benzamidine/trypsin, 3144 combinations of side-chain rotamers were found for the isolated protein and 3355 for the ligand–protein system. For phosphocholine/McPC 603 the values are 42 and 79 respectively. The conformational entropy may thus increase on formation of the intermolecular complex, rather than decrease as might intuitively be imagined. We do stress, however, that counter examples can be found: for ribonuclease A/sulphate, 65 combinations were found for the protein and 57 for the protein–ligand complex.

The potential importance of receptor flexibility in computer-aided ligand design has long been recognized. However, as noted above, this problem has been largely ignored in theoretical approaches to ligand docking, the receptor being treated as a rigid molecule fixed in the conformation determined by the X-ray experiment. Our method can be applied to problems in ligand design. For example, we can perform ligand docking with both ligand and receptor flexibility. Part of the ligand (the 'anchor region') is positioned at all points on a regular grid which covers the binding site. At each grid point, the rotational degrees of freedom are also explored systematically. For each position of the anchor region all possible conformations of the ligand (previously calculated) are generated and tested for unfavourable interactions with the backbone. The remaining ligand conformations define a family of ligand rotamers which are then added to the amino acid rotamers and the lowest energy structures of the intermolecular complex are determined. Applications of this docking method to benzamidine/trypsin and phosphocholine/McPC 603 have been described (Leach, 1994a).

A related application of our algorithm is in finding favourable regions for binding functional groups, and the consequent generation of potential energy grid maps which take account of receptor flexibility. A popular approach to *de novo* ligand design is first to identify regions in the site where strong binding to specific functional groups would be expected. Goodford's GRID method (Goodford, 1985) is widely used to identify such locations, but suffers from the possible limitations of a rigid receptor, insofar as the movement of a few side chains may change the nature of the binding site. The MCSS approach developed by Karplus and co-workers is, in principle, able to deal with protein flexibility using molecular dynamics, but all of the reported applications of this approach have been based on a rigid receptor (Miranker and Karplus, 1991). Our DEE/A* search can be used to generate 'flexible receptor' potential energy maps. The probe group is positioned at all points on a regular grid. The interaction energies between the probe and the amino acid side chains and between the probe and the protein backbone are calculated at each point and the DEE/A* search is then used to find the lowest energy combination of side-chain rotamers.

To illustrate the procedure, we have generated potential energy maps in the active site of ribonuclease A, using a rigid protein model (corresponding to that determined by X-ray crystallography (Howlin *et al.*, 1989)). We have also repeated the calculation using a flexible protein model, in which the side chains are free to move within the confines of our search algorithm. We illustrate the approach here using a sulphate anion as probe. A 21 × 21 × 21 grid (1 Å separation) was positioned in the active site. Grid points further than 10 Å from the position of the sulphate anion in the crystal structure were ignored, leaving a total of 4170 grid points.

For a significant proportion of the grid points a high-energy position with the rigid receptor was replaced by a low-energy structure with the flexible receptor. Thus, 72 grid points were within 40 kcal/mol of the very lowest energy position with the rigid receptor but 137 points satisfied this criterion with the flexible receptor. In Fig. 11.5 we show an example in which the probe has a severe interaction with the crystallographically determined orientation of the side chain of Gln11. With a flexible receptor, however, an alternative arrangement of side-chain conformations can be found to give a low-energy structure, as illustrated. It should be noted, however, that for ribonuclease A/sulphate, no dramatically different binding pockets were revealed by the use of a flexible receptor; this reflects the nature of the active site of ribonuclease

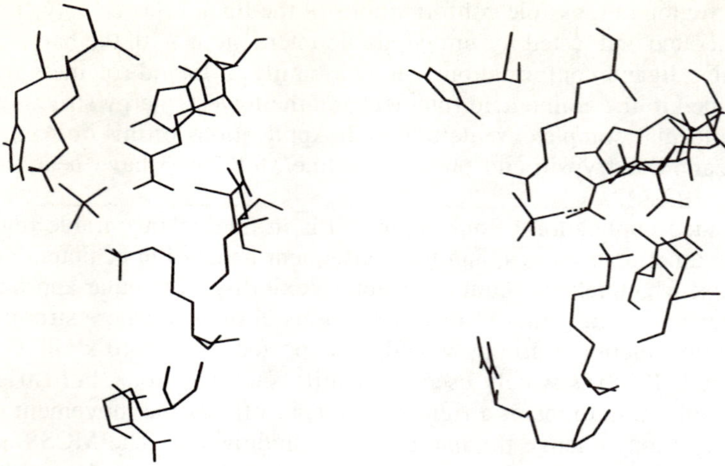

Fig. 11.5 On the right is shown an orientation of a sulphate anion probe in the active site of ribonuclease A which has a high-energy interaction with the crystallographically determined orientation of the side chain of Gln11. When the flexible receptor model is used, however, an alternative arrangement of side chains is possible (left) giving rise to a low-energy structure.

A with its preponderance of positively charged side chains. We do nevertheless anticipate that this may be the case for other systems which are under investigation.

Our combined DEE/A* algorithm offers a unique way to explore the side-chain conformational space of a protein, a particular advantage being that it guarantees to find, in order, all of the lowest-energy combinations of side-chain rotamers. It is important to recognize the approximations inherent in the approach. There are three major approximations:

1) The backbone is rigid.
2) The side chains are restricted to discrete conformations.
3) The energy function may not provide an accurate representation of the interactions.

Our present implementation uses the AMBER force field (Weiner *et al.*, 1984, 1986). Different variants of this force field are possible and in this section we report a comparison of united atom/all atom models, constant and distance-dependent dielectrics and employing different non-bonded cut-offs. In addition, we have investigated the effects of using two different rotamer libraries: one due to Desmet *et al.* (1992) that is closely based on that of Ponder and Richards (1987) and the other from Lavery's group (Tuffery *et al.*, 1991). We have used the 13-residue sequence Lys–Glu–Thr–Ala–Ala–Ala–Lys–Phe–

Table 11.2
A comparison of the numbers of conformations within energies of 1, 2, 5, 10, 15 and 20 kcal/mol of the global minimum energy conformations using various force field models and rotamer libraries. 'Lavery' refers to the rotamer library of Tuffery *et al.* (1991); 'Desmet' to the rotamer library of Desmet *et al.* (1992) (based on the Ponder and Richards, 1987, library). The models comprise united and all atom descriptions with varying non-bonded cut-offs and dielectric model (constant dielectric of 1 or distance-dependent dielectric, $\varepsilon = r$)

Energy (kcal)	6 Å; $\varepsilon \propto$ r	8 Å; $\varepsilon \propto$ r	12 Å; $\varepsilon \propto$ r	8 Å; ε = 1
Lavery: united atom				
1	9	10	9	2
2	25	35	25	5
5	91	103	95	14
10	660	723	901	60
15	2482	2609	2509	183
20	7485	7841	7510	511
Lavery: all atom				
1	2	3	2	5
2	7	8	6	7
5	74	84	71	22
10	849	894	821	111
15	3753	3911	3713	359
20	>10 000	>10 000	>10 000	964
Desmet: united atom				
1		2		
2		4		
5		54		
10		962		
15		>10 000		
20		>10 000		

Glu–Arg–Gln–His–Met (the C-peptide) which constitutes the N-terminus of ribonuclease A for these investigations. This peptide has been widely studied due to its ability to form an isolated α-helix in solution. Our first experiments were performed with the backbone in an ideal α-helical conformation. We then compared the results with those obtained using the backbone conformation from the X-ray structure of ribonuclease A. For each set of parameters the global minimum energy combination of side chains was identified, together with all other combinations within 20 kcal/mol. Table 11.2 gives the number of conformations within a given energy of the global energy minimum for each parameter set.

A visual comparison of the global minimum energy combinations obtained in each case revealed that, for the C-peptide, there was little difference between the united and all atom models. The effect of varying the electrostatic term in the potential energy function did, however, have a significant impact: with a constant dielectric of 1 the global minimum energy structure has a strong electrostatic interaction between Lys7 and Gln11. With a distance-dependent dielectric, this interaction is reduced and an alternative arrangement of side-chain rotamers is suggested. In addition, whilst there is relatively little difference in the numbers of conformations within a given energy cut-off of the global energy minimum as the non-bonded cut-off is varied, the results are significantly different when the dielectric model is changed, with far fewer structures being obtained for $\varepsilon = 1$ than for $\varepsilon = r$. This is again due to the greater magnitude of the electrostatic interactions with the constant dielectric.

Significant differences were observed in the results obtained using the two alternative backbone conformations for the C-peptide. Only residues 3–13 of the sequence were considered as the first two residues in the crystal structure adopt a random structure. The RMS fit (backbone atoms) between the ideal α-helical structure and the experimentally determined structure was 0.9 Å. When subject to the side chain placement algorithm, the structures obtained show significant differences; for example, some residues adopted a side chain conformation in the global minimum energy conformation that was not present in any of the conformations generated using the alternative backbone structure. This result can be attributed both to the use of a discrete rotamer model but particularly to the sensitivity of the energy model to relatively small changes in orientation when the different backbone conformation is employed. Ligand design is – at present at least – a discipline that is subject to many approximations, and it is important that no part of the procedure uses a more accurate representation than is justified (van Gunsteren and Mark, 1992).

The sensitivity of the results to the force field model is further illustrated by examining some of the results obtained for the ribonuclease A/sulphate intermolecular complex. The crystal structure of this particular system contains two alternative conformations for His119 (Howlin *et al*., 1989), though other authors have failed to find evidence for two conformations, albeit for structures obtained in the absence of sulphate (Wlodawer *et al*., 1988). Using the AMBER united-atom force field model, rotamers corresponding to both conformations of this histidine are observed. However, with the all-atom model, high-energy steric interactions with the hydrogen atoms on the side chain of Val118 result in one of the two histidine rotamers being rejected (although the rejected rotamer does correspond to the 'disputed' histidine conformation).

Conclusions

Algorithms which find optimal solutions are very important in molecular modelling and computational chemistry and the development and application of new methods continues to be an area of significant activity. The methods can be divided into two broad categories: those that use a stochastic method to explore for solutions, and those that involve a systematic exploration of the problem space. Stochastic methods in general have the advantage that they are able to provide 'good' answers relatively quickly; however, by their very nature they are unable to guarantee to locate globally optimal solutions. In addition, only by repeated sampling can we obtain an accurate picture of the energy surface. Systematic search methods are traditionally subject to the effects of combinatorial explosion. However, new search techniques may provide the way to directly and efficiently identify all solutions of interest. The systematic search is not dead!

Acknowledgement

The author is supported by the SERC under the Advanced Fellowship Scheme.

References

Bernstein, F.C., Koetzle, T.F., Williams, G.J.B., Meyer, E., Bryce, M.D., Rogers, J.R., Kennard, O., Shikanouchi, T. and Tasumi, M. (1977). *J. Mol. Biol.* **112**, 535–542.

Bruccoleri, R.E. and Karplus, M. (1985). *Macromolecules* **18**, 2767–2773.

Bruccoleri, R.E. and Karplus, M. (1987). *Biopolymers* **26**, 137–168.

DesJarlais, R.L., Sheridan, R.P., Dixon, J.S., Kuntz, I.D. and Venkatarghavan, R. (1986). *J. Med. Chem.* **29**, 2149–2153.

Desmet, J., DeMaeyer, M., Hazes, B. and Lasters, I. (1992). *Nature* **356**, 539–542.

Dixon, J.S. (1993). *In* 'Trends in QSAR and Molecular Modelling' (C.G. Wermuth, ed.), pp. 412–413. ESCOM, Leiden.

Dolata, D.P., Leach, A.R. and Prout, K. (1987). *J. Comput.-Aided Mol. Des.* **1**, 73–85.

Elber, R. and Karplus, M. (1987). *Science* **235**, 318–321.

Ghose, A.K. and Crippen, G.M. (1985). *J. Comput. Chem.* **6**, 350–359.

Goodford, P.J. (1985). *J. Med. Chem.* **28**, 849–857.

Goodsell, D.S. and Olson, A.J. (1990). *Proteins* **8**, 195–202.

Hart, P.E., Nilsson, N.J. and Raphael, B. (1968). *IEEE Trans on SSC* **4**, 100–114.

Hart, T.N. and Read, R.J. (1992). *Proteins – Struct. Funct. Genetics* **13**, 206–222.

Hartigan, J.A. (1975). *In* 'Clustering Algorithms'. John Wiley, New York.

Holm, L. and Sander, C. (1992). *Proteins – Struct. Funct. Genetics* **14**, 213–223.

Howard, A.E. and Kollman, P.A. (1988). *J. Med. Chem.* **31**, 1669–1675.

Howlin, B., Moss, D.S. and Harris, G.W. (1989). *Acta Crystallogr.* **A45**, 851–861.

Kasinos, N., Lilley, G.A., Subbarao, N. and Haneef, I. (1992). *Protein Engng.* **5**, 69–75.

Kuntz, I.D., Blaney, J.M., Oatley, S.J., Langridge, R. and Ferrin, T.E. (1982). *J. Mol. Biol.* **161**, 269–288.

Lasters, I. and Desmet, J. (1993). *Protein Engng.* **6**, 717–722.

Lawrence, M.C. and Davis, P.C. (1992). *Proteins – Struct. Funct. Genetics* **12**, 31–41.
Leach, A.R. (1991). *In* 'Reviews in Computational Chemistry, vol. II'; (K.B. Lipkowitz and D.B. Boyd, eds), pp. 1–55. VCH, New York.
Leach, A.R. (1994a). *J. Mol. Biol.* **235**, 345–356.
Leach, A.R. (1994b). *J. Chem. Inf. Comput. Sci.* **34**, 661–670.
Leach, A.R. and Prout, K. (1990). *J. Comput. Chem.* **11**, 1193–1205.
Leach, A.R. and Kuntz, I.D. (1992). *J. Comput. Chem.* **13**, 730–748.
Leach, A.R., Dolata, D.P. and Prout, K. (1990a). *J. Chem. Inf. Comput. Sc.* **30**, 316–324.
Leach, A.R., Prout, K. and Dolata, D.P. (1990b). *J. Comput. Chem.* **11**, 680–693.
Lee, C. and Subbiah, S. (1991). *Nature* **253**, 448–451.
Lewis, R.A. and Leach, A.R. (1994). *J. Comput.-Aided Mol. Design* **8**, 467–475.
Mattos, C., Rasmussen, B., Ding, X., Petsko, G.A. and Ringe, D. (1994). *Nature Struct. Biol.* **1**, 55–58.
Mierke, D.F., Kurz, M. and Kessler, H. (1994). *J. Am. Chem. Soc.* **116**, 1042–1049.
Miranker and Karplus, M. (1991). *Proteins – Struct. Funct. Genetics* **11**, 29–34.
Nilsson, N.J. (1982). *In* 'Principles of Artificial Intelligence', pp. 74–88. Springer-Verlag, Berlin.
Ponder, J.W. and Richards, F.M. (1987). *J. Mol. Biol.* **193**, 775–791.
Ricketts, E.M., Bradshaw, J., Hann, M., Hayes, F., Tanna, N. and Ricketts, D.M. (1993). *J. Chem. Inf. Comput. Sci.* **33**, 905–925.
Tuffery, P., Etchebest, C., Hazout, S. and Lavery, R. (1991). *J. Biomol. Struct. Dyn.* **8**, 1267–1289.
Van Gunsteren, W.F. and Mark, A.E. (1992). *J. Mol. Biol.* **227**, 389–395.
Weiner, S.J., Kollman, P.A., Case, D.A., Singh, U.C., Ghio, C., Alagona, G., Profeta, S. and Weiner, P. (1984). *J. Am. Chem. Soc.* **106**, 765–784.
Weiner, S.J., Kollman, P.A., Nguyen, D.T. and Case, D.A. (1986). *J. Comput. Chem.* **7**, 230–252.
Winston, P.H. (1992). *In* 'Artificial Intelligence', 3rd ed, pp. 63–100. Addison-Wesley, Reading Massachusetts.
Wlodawer, A., Svensson, L.A., Sjölin, L. and Gilliland, G.L. (1988). *Biochemistry* **27**, 2705–2717.

Discussion

I.D. Kuntz
First, you did not give a time estimate in the case of flexible docking for the A* dead-end combination. Roughly what do you expect there?

A.R. Leach
It certainly takes longer than docking a rigid crystal structure, as would be expected. In one of the cases to which I alluded, the phosphocholine example, the whole of the binding site (which is quite large) can be searched overnight. By comparison, a rigid search would take perhaps 20% of that time. Perhaps the most significant point is that the energy calculations in those docking studies take about 75% of the total cpu time, which is one reason for stressing that these methods are too slow and that some sort of grid-based approach would perhaps be more appropriate.

I.D. Kuntz

Second, how complicated is it to get that estimate function (h^*) in the A* algorithm? This is an area that I do not know much about, and it seems to be the tricky part.

A.R. Leach

I did not go into detail on that because of the difficulties of trying to explain exactly how the estimates are obtained. The estimate must be lower than the actual cost required. I think intuitively this is correct. What is required is to work through the mathematics to find an expression that is guaranteed to be lower than the actual cost, and then see how it works.

In the case of the side chains, it is also important to consider them in the most appropriate order, rather than just taking 1, 2, 3, 4, 5 and so on which can be an inefficient order of considering the residues. I have not yet come up with a universally held equation that will always guarantee to consider the rotamers in the correct order, but there are methods that we have looked at that provide an indication of which should be looked at first. They certainly perform better than an arbitrary sequence.

S. Pickett

The water around in the system in real life will bind to those side chains, again changing the energy – how can this be incorporated into the calculations?

A.R. Leach

That is certainly true. It would be anticipated that incorporating some sort of solvation model might take account of that. I hesitate slightly because again, as was illustrated earlier, there are differences between bound waters and the general water of solvation. It needs investigating whether one of these simple solvation models is able correctly to distinguish between them.

S. Pickett

The number of conformations of side chains with a ligand bound is dependent on the energy cut-off used. As you say, if a particular sidechain is no longer bound to the surface, the energy cut-off used may influence whether that is good or bad.

A.R. Leach

It certainly does matter. Based upon the work with the C-peptide from ribonuclease A, investigating the effect of varying these different parameters, in this case it was a dielectric model that gave vastly different results. Going from, say, a distance-dependent dielectric to a constant dielectric (there are obvious reasons why this holds) is much more significant than the non-bonded cut-off that is used.

S. Pickett
I was not thinking so much in that case of the non-bonded cut-off, but rather the cut-off being taken to determine whether or not conformation was accepted.

A.R. Leach
Yes, that is true. I hesitate to say it is an arbitrary energy scale because AMBER has been well parameterized against certain model systems. It is, however, an arbitrary cut-off in the context of these discrete conformations – fairly arbitrary, anyway – which are chosen as a compromise between a number that is far too small and a number that is far too large. It we were to go back and do energy minimization on all the results obtained there might be considerably different results – which, again, I think points to the need for alternative energy models in these sorts of problems.

G.A. Petsko
How do you know what the right answer is when you find it? The sense that I have about protein structures is that if just one property is considered, say, side-chain rotamers, they are not at a global minimum: Peter has been robbed in one or two places to pay Paul somewhere else. Quite properly, you seem to be trying to take this into account by allowing some deviation from the global minimum in your search, but if that gives, say, 20 different structures, how do you know which is the one you really want?

A.R. Leach
I do not know. I have to ask someone like yourself to solve the crystal structure. There are two ways of approaching this: first, as an interesting intellectual problem. Perhaps we can think of using methods such as these in smaller systems, going back to statistical mechanics and putting them into models of that sort to say something more about, for example, protein folding. The problem is that these methods have to be restricted to very small systems because of the computer time. I know that work has been done using Monte Carlo simulations on very short peptides. Models such as these might allow us to look at larger systems, though still of the peptide type rather than proteins.

The alternative point I would make is that in some ways the results obtained from crystallography – particularly with the high-resolution work – are the sort that should be incorporated into all these energy models that I have discussed in order to try to establish the correlation between what a theoretical approach can produce and what is observed experimentally.

G.A. Petsko
That is rather what I was driving at. One of the things we do not know, that we need to be able to tell someone like you, is why the structure has chosen to rob Peter in *this* way to pay Paul in *that* way, among what seem to be a set of

equally likely alternative possibilities. Clearly, they must not be equally likely in some fashion, and we need to try to understand what it is that has led to the choice of a few bad rotamers here as opposed to a few bad rotamers somewhere else.

A.R. Leach
I think this comes back to the synergy between experiment and theory. Again, as you said earlier, it is only now, as an increasing number of protein structures are obtained at the sorts of resolutions compatible with what theoreticians claim to be able to do, that we can start to think about getting a closer correlation between the two and refining the energy models more precisely.

I.D. Kuntz
We also have to be careful how these questions and answers are phrased. As we look at things in more detail, both experimentally and theoretically, as Dr Mark said earlier, for example, we should think about thermodynamic states and not about individual snapshot conformations or configurations. As Professor Petsko knows well, we cannot say what is the right conformation of one of these systems because it is sampling many at room temperature in a crystal; and even more in solution. It has to be kept in mind that the numbers reported in experiments are averages over a large number of different geometries, even in the best binding systems.

A.R. Leach
I think this ties in with what I said about deriving statistical mechanical models: because these methods are able to provide a range of solutions, it might be possible to compare them with these average results that are obtained.

12

Applications of Computer-Aided Drug Design Techniques to Lead Generation

J.S. MASON[†], I.M. McLAY[†] and R.A. LEWIS*

[†]*Rhône-Poulenc Rorer Central Research, 500 Arcola Road, PO Box 1200, Collegeville, PA 19426–0107, USA and*
**Dagenham Research Centre, Rainham Road South, Dagenham, Essex RM10 7XS, UK*

Introduction

The generation of new chemical leads for biological targets is one of the most challenging tasks faced in the drug design process. Recent advances in computer-aided drug design (CADD), particularly in the areas of conformationally flexible three-dimensional (3D) database searching and *de novo* design, have allowed CADD to play an ever increasing role in lead generation. Important advances have also been made in lead optimization methods, such as 3D-QSAR (quantitative structure–activity relationship) analysis using molecular fields. The development of these new tools has enabled CADD to make a greater impact on the drug design process, to pass beyond explanatory models restricted to closely related compounds and on to the analysis of complex data for sets of diverse structures, and thus to the design and evaluation of novel structures.

A schematic division of CADD lead generation methods is shown in Fig. 12.1; passing from left to right, we move from methods which need little or no information about either the target or ligands, to methods in which a 3D model of the target enzyme or receptor is needed. This latter situation is relatively rare at present, although advances in protein structure determination by X-ray

New Perspectives in Drug Design
ISBN 0–12–208070–X

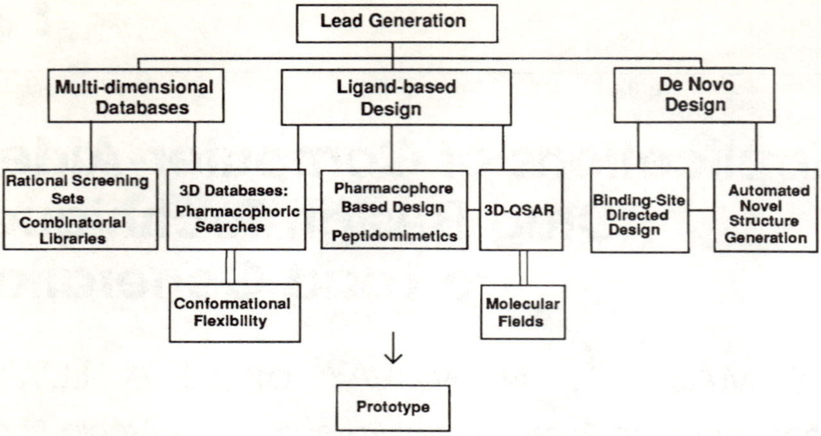

Fig. 12.1 A strategy for drug design.

crystallography, NMR spectroscopy and homology modelling mean this type of design will become increasingly common. However, for the present, the problem of determination of high-resolution structures for many proteins, particularly membrane-bound receptors, still remains to be solved. Fortunately, automated structure generation is now possible not only for both binding-site directed tasks, but also for envelope-directed tasks; in this latter mode a mould with complementary shape and electrostatic properties is generated from one or more active ligand(s) in their proposed bioactive conformation(s).

A common situation is one in which the structures of molecules that interact with the desired biological target are known; from this information, pharmacophoric models can often be proposed. A pharmacophore model is a spatial model defined from those features of a molecule hypothesized to be essential for biological activity, often defined in terms of generic features such as hydrogen bonding groups or aromatic ring centres, and in terms of the distances separating the features. From these models, 3D requirements for bioactivity can be proposed. Three-dimensional database searching enables the identification of compounds that match the pharmacophore model; compounds found from searches of company registries should rapidly be available for screening. It may be noted that the identification of a pharmacophore model is key to this approach. Three-dimensional searches can also be used to generate ideas or scaffolds for the design of novel compounds.

Where the structure of the target enzyme or receptor is known, e.g. from X-ray or NMR studies, then *de novo* structure-based design is also feasible. In this case, lead generation is possible both through the application of 3D searches to identify existing compounds, and by the *de novo* design of novel structures, including automated structure generation. The 3D searches can be either complementarity-based, using all the information of the binding site to identify structures with shape and electrostatic complementarity, or pharmacophore-based, using models derived from an energy-based survey of the site (Goodford, 1985) and/or from the interactions of a bound ligand.

Rational screening sets may be used in any lead generation situation, but are particularly important where no, or very limited, structural information is known about the receptor or suitable ligands. These sets are a development of the quasi-random method that has had a role in drug discovery for many years. One approach is to select small sets of compounds, in which maximal diversity is represented, from large databases. A new method based on diversity of molecular properties has been implemented for our corporate databases.

This paper describes our experiences with the design and development of suitable methods and the practical use of these different approaches for lead generation, all within the context of pharmaceutical discovery.

Three-dimensional Database Searching

Three-dimensional database searching can greatly enhance the speed of the lead generation step within the drug design process, enabling structures to be selectively extracted from large databases of 3D structures based on some type of molecular similarity, complementarity or topology. The use of 3D databases in drug design is a subject of much current interest, with several new commercial software packages for 3D database searching now being available. Recent reviews on this subject are available (Martin, 1992), and also on the generation and use of 3D molecular structures in 3D searching (Pearlman, 1993); software for general molecular modelling, often needed for defining the search criteria or analysing the results, has also recently been reviewed (Boyd, 1994).

Large databases of compounds from any source (company registries, external databases, active ligands or hypothetical structures) can now be searched in 3D, taking into account the full conformational flexibility of the structures. Three-dimensional database searches can play an important role in the lead generation and optimization steps in the drug design process. Small screening sets tailored to a specific biological target can be generated from large company databases; the idea-based design process can be optimized; *de novo* ligand design is possible through the identification of complementary fragments and new molecular scaffolds; automated pharmacophore identification is possible from a set of compounds of known activity. A schematic diagram of some of our applications of 3D database searching is shown in Fig. 12.2.

Two main approaches for using 3D database searching in drug design can

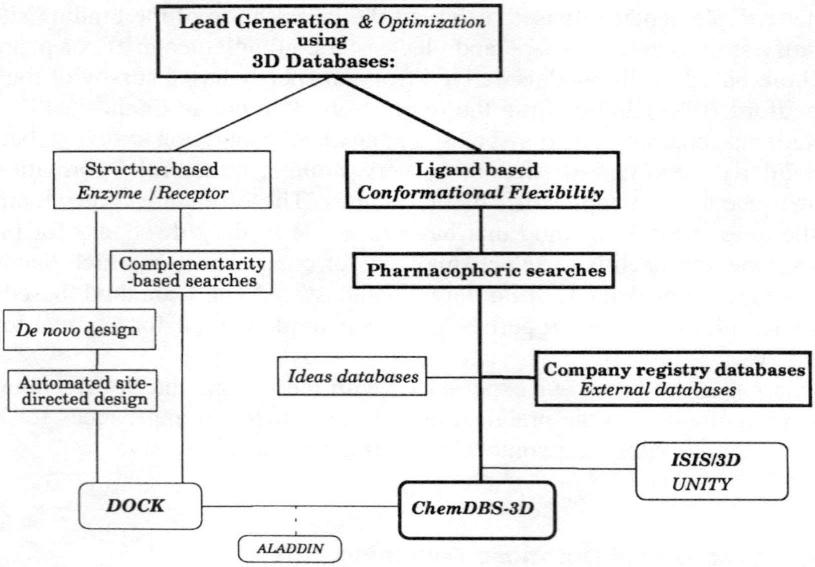

Fig. 12.2 In-house use of different 3D databases for lead generation.

be distinguished, based on either pharmacophoric distances or shape and electrostatic complementarity. The pharmacophore-based method uses only those features of a molecule hypothesized to be essential for biological activity, often defined in terms of generic features such as hydrogen bond acceptors and donors, aromatic ring/hydrophobe centres, positive charge centres and acidic and basic centres. Conformational flexibility can now be handled in most pharmacophore-based systems (see below for ChemDBS-3D, ISIS/3D, and UNITY); ALADDIN (Martin *et al.*, 1993; Van Drie *et al.*, 1989) only searches explicitly stored conformations, but can automatically modify and re-evaluate hit structures. The second method involves the identification of molecules whose overall shape and electrostatic properties are complementary to a defined binding site. This method is ideally used when the 3D structure of an enzyme or receptor is known, although a site can be defined from a ligand, projecting complementary properties. The method has been developed as the DOCK program (DesJarlais *et al.*, 1988; Kuntz *et al.*, 1982); published drug design applications of this type of 3D search include the structure-based design of inhibitors of thymidylate synthase (Shoichet *et al.*, 1993). Conformational flexibility is, however, much less readily handled in this approach and is currently generally approached by storing multiple conformations; a method that can be applied to achieve this more efficiently is discussed below (Complementarity-based 3D Database Searching).

Another use of 3D database searching in drug design is the identification of molecular scaffolds; this can be achieved using the distance or shape-based 3D searching programs already described, or using specialist programs such as CAVEAT (Lauri and Bartlett, 1994) which focuses on the orientation of bonds rather than the location of atoms in the 3D searching. Using this approach, structures can be identified that match the position and direction of bonds. A major application of these types of 3D searches is in the design of peptidomimetics; potential replacements for secondary structures such as β-turns can be identified from both corporate and public databases, now including massive resources such as the Chemical Abstracts (CAS) database. The identification of suitable 3D scaffolds or linking groups is of general application in small molecule design and combinatorial screening library design, and is discussed further in Chapter 13.

Pharmacophore Identification

A pharmacophoric model can be proposed from the analysis of a set of biologically active ligands or from the analysis of a receptor or enzyme active site structure, preferably determined with a bound ligand. New methods that can analyse automatically sets of active ligands to produce hypothetical pharmacophoric models, are becoming available; here a model of 3D molecular similarity is being defined based on interpoint distance comparisons. Enzyme and receptor structures can be surveyed energetically by a program such as GRID (Goodford, 1985) to identify favourable interaction sites for a large variety of different functional group probes, such as a carbonyl group, an amine NH and an aromatic CH. Those regions having favourable interactions can then be used to define sets of pharmacophoric queries for 3D searches based on different combinations of inter-region distances.

The more common situation is where only the structures of several active but flexible ligands are known. Several automated methods that try to identify potential pharmacophores are now available. The most common approach is to analyse a predefined set of conformations for each ligand to suggest possible common features having similar inter-feature 3D distances, such as in DISCO (Martin *et al.*, 1993; Bures *et al.*, 1994), APEX (Golender and Vorpagel, 1993) and CATALYST (Sprague, 1991). An alternative approach is to analyse distance keys derived from a full conformational analysis of the active ligands to generate rapidly potential models. These distance keys are calculated in ChemDBS-3D/Chem-X (Chemical Design, 1990) from all the observed distances between all the pharmacophore centres (normally hydrogen bond donors, hydrogen bond acceptors, positive charge centres and aromatic ring centroids) in the molecule; the composite result for all conformations generated is stored (Murrall and Davies, 1990, 1993). The models proposed by these programs should be validated by using them as queries for a 3D search on the database of active ligands; many, if not all, ligands should be retrieved, before the model can be considered valid. This method is implemented in Chem-X/ChemDBS-3D, with clustering and similarity methods also available to aid the selection of a suitable structure set for analysis.

Pharmacophore-Based 3D Database Searching

The most common approach in 3D database searching is to search large databases of structures to identify those which can present a particular pharmacophore. Here the idea of the search is to identify structures in a database with similar 3D geometric relationships between essential features. The criteria for similarity can be quite wide, and as the connectivity between the centres defining the 3D query is not considered, structures that are quite dissimilar in a two-dimensional chemical structural sense, can all match the same 3D query and be identified. The pharmacophore is often described only by a set of distance constraints between atom centres or centroids of a defined environment (e.g. acidic, basic, hydrogen bond acceptor/donor, aromatic ring centroid and/or other hydrophobe centre). The query can also contain other geometric constraints such as angles and other features including exclusion volumes, substructures and geometric objects (e.g. planes, lines, points and vectors). An important recent advance has been the ability to allow for the conformational flexibility of structures in the database during the 3D searches, as discussed here below; some experiences and applications have already been published (Haraki *et al.*, 1990; Mason, 1992, 1993).

Another use of conformationally flexible 3D database searching is to classify and optimize a set of 'idea' structures for a particular target. Given a potential pharmacophoric model, thorough systematic analysis (including all conformational and substructural possibilities) of a 3D database of designed structures enables the rapid selection of a small set of the most favourable compounds for synthesis. The automation achievable in both the construction of the 3D structures and in their evaluation in different pharmacophoric models, means that all substitution and isomeric possibilities can be easily evaluated, an otherwise time-consuming effort. The idea structures can be readily coded into SMILES line notation (Weininger, 1989) for 2D structure representation. Simple modification of these SMILES codes (single line per structure), before 3D structure generation with CONCORD (Pearlman, 1987; Pearlman *et al.*, 1988), enables the thorough investigation of structural variations for the idea structures; different chain length, substitution and isomeric possibilities can thus be evaluated in a systematic and automated way. From the 3D searches, with full conformer regeneration, superimposed best-fit conformations for each structure can be obtained; this facilitates the fine-tuning of the idea and the incorporation of other features not readily defined in the 3D query. The need to be able to view more than just the first conformation or substructure mapping found during the search became apparent during this type of project, when it was observed that the conformer regeneration could identify many quite different and interesting matches. The easy and rapid visualization of these multiple matches (different conformations and substructure mappings) for each structure fitted onto the query is a key feature of this method, from which new ideas are suggested and easily evaluated.

Conformational flexibility in 3D database searching

Three dimensional searching of a single low-energy conformation does not generally give a realistic appraisal of the ability of a flexible molecule to fit a particular pharmacophore geometry. An alternative low-energy conformation may match the query, as has been demonstrated recently (Haraki *et al.*, 1990; Mason 1992, 1993). Indeed, the bound conformation may not be a low-energy conformation, and receptor interactions may involve higher energy activated structures (Jorgenson, 1991). Conformational flexibility can now be readily taken into account for distance-based searches, requiring the storage of only a single conformation for each structure in the database. The flexibility is taken into account at search time by either generating new conformations, for example by systematic rule-based conformational analysis or random conformer generation, or by torsional fitting ('tweaking') where a minimization in torsional space occurs, using the query as constraints; this is discussed further below. The inclusion of conformational flexibility into 3D searching has been found to be the key for many of our lead generation applications, some examples of which are described below.

Lead generation from 3D database pharmacophoric searches

Pharmacophoric searches on the company databases have given very encouraging and interesting results. Many of the most interesting hits found have been in conformations other than the nominal low-energy conformation stored in the database, highlighting the extra capability of 3D searching with conformational flexibility. Two examples of lead generation are described below which illustrate the power of the method.

In the first, we were looking for new leads in an LDL (low density lipoprotein) receptor upregulator screen. This screen, part of our cardiovascular programme, was designed to identify compounds which may reduce blood LDL concentrations by this novel mechanism. Low-activity (IC_{50}: 1.7 μM) compounds based on the dibenzamide structure shown in Fig. 12.3 were known. A three-point pharmacophore model was derived from this compound, illustrated in Fig. 12.3. Three-dimensional searches of the corporate databases using this query in ChemDBS-3D yielded two new potent lead series. Figure 12.4 illustrates the 3D query together with one new active lead: a diaminoquinazoline (EC_{50}: 0.8 μM) which was identified following a 3D search of the stored CONCORD-generated conformation (a single conformation search). Figure 12.5 illustrates a second, more potent diaminopyrimidine series which was initially discovered using conformationally flexible 3D searching in ChemDBS-3D. This series provided compounds, from our

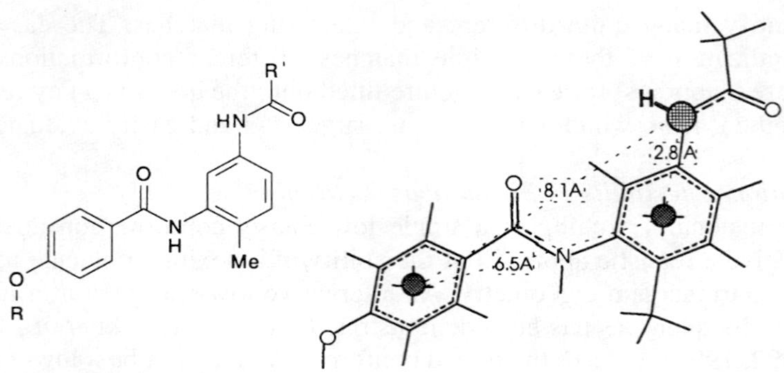

Fig. 12.3 Pharmacophore model used for LDL receptor upregulation 3D searches.

existing corporate registry, with activities as low as 5 nM. Interestingly, screening of the property-derived screening sets also identified a hit compound from this series: Fig. 12.5 illustrates related hit structures from the 3D search (**1a**, EC_{50}: 400 nM) and property-derived (**1b**, EC_{50}: 200 nM) sets. These compounds can fit the query in several quite different ways, as illustrated in Figs. 12.5 and 12.6 for compound **2** (EC_{50}: 6 nM); both substructure mappings of the amino groups are found when the second aromatic ring distance constraint is relaxed or modified based on the diaminoquinazoline lead. It is clear that the extended CONCORD conformation would not fit the query, showing the importance of allowing for conformational flexibility in the 3D searches.

A second example of the power of 3D pharmacophoric searches for the discovery of new leads comes from our endothelin receptor binding assay. Within our general new leads screening programme approximately 4000 compounds had been screened in this assay as part of routine screening,

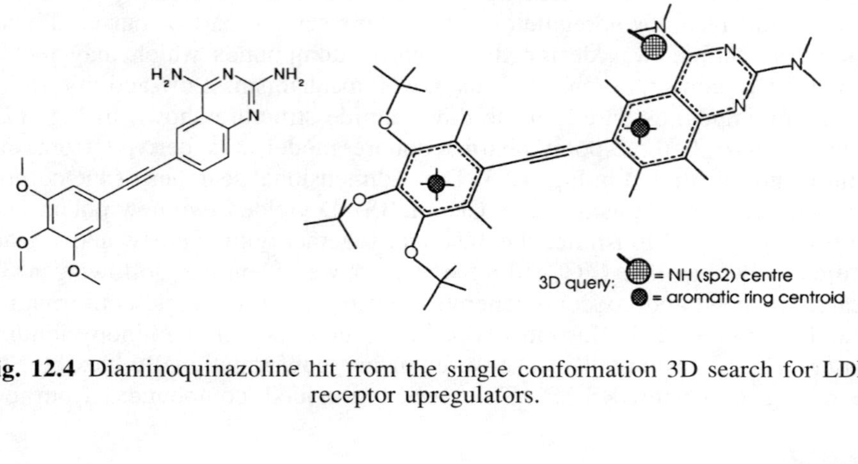

Fig. 12.4 Diaminoquinazoline hit from the single conformation 3D search for LDL receptor upregulators.

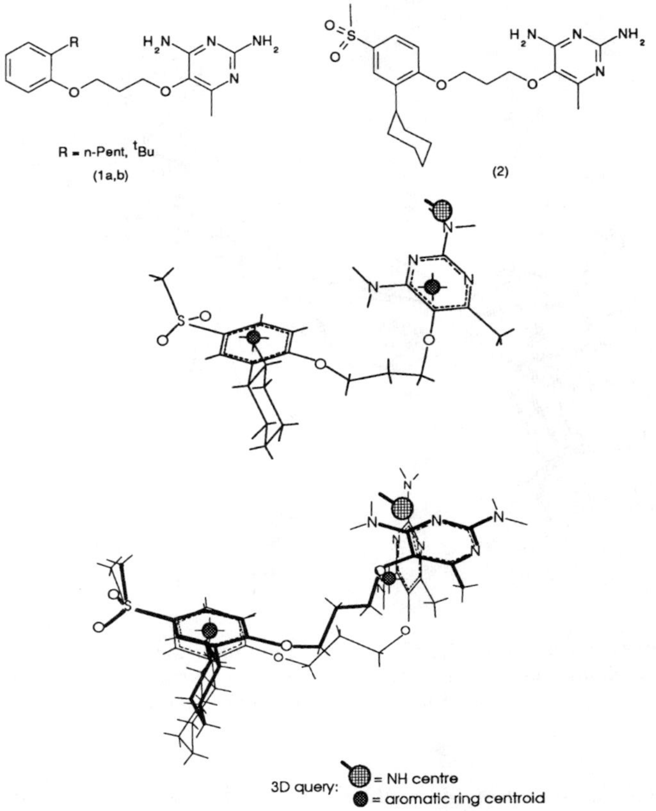

Fig. 12.5 Conformationally flexible hits for LDL receptor upregulation showing different conformations and substructure mappings for structure **2**.

and no leads of less than 10 μM had been found. Using a pharmacophoric model derived from molecular modelling studies on a cyclic pentapeptide structure and another active compound, 3D searches were performed on the corporate databases to identify 700 compounds of potential interest. Screening of this directed set of compounds identified ten new leads at less than 10 μM. The most potent compound (~ 500 nM) was only identified in the conformationally flexible 3D search; interestingly, screening of a further 400 compounds 2D-related to the 3D hits did not yield any further hits, indicating that the activity was indeed due to the correct 3D disposition of key groups, rather than the chemical family itself.

Three-dimensional database construction

The creation of a 3D database normally involves the generation of a reasonable 3D structure and the registration of this single conformation into the

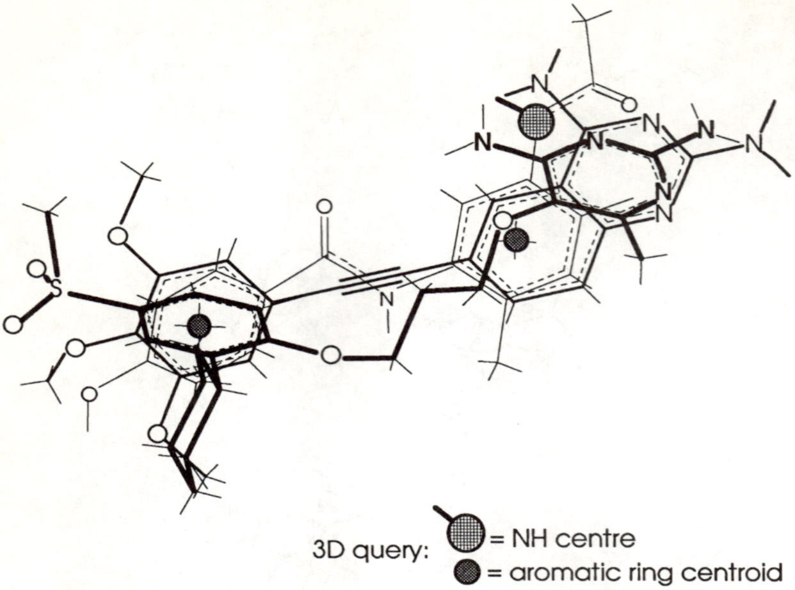

Fig. 12.6 Superimposition of the dibenzamide defining the 3D query (light) and the two hit series: diaminoquinazoline (normal); diaminopyrimidine (bold) from the 3D searches for LDL receptor upregulators.

database. The conversion of a 2D database of chemical structures to 3D structures involves the creation of a suitable '2D' connectivity table (CT) file with atom and bonding descriptions for each structure, which is used as input for an automated 3D structure generation program. The most compact and easily handled 2D structure representation is the SMILES line notation, which can be made unique for a given structure; extensions to the code have been developed to allow stereochemistry to be defined using both relative and absolute indicators. Several different methods for 3D structure generation are available, the most popular and rapid being bond- or fragment-based. Distance geometry-based methods are becoming more widely available, and although slower, are particularly powerful with fused ring systems and macrocycles. Methods for 3D structure generation were recently reviewed by Pearlman (1994).

The most robust and universally used program for 3D structure generation is CONCORD (Pearlman, 1987; Pearlman *et al.*, 1988). This program uses SMILES or SDfile (Dalby *et al.*, 1992) CT files as input, and produces reasonable low-energy conformations for most small organic structures; large (> 12) rings and peptides are not well handled, and most organometallic compounds cannot be converted. The program is rapid and gives useful structure quality information, including a close-contact ratio; this method was used to convert one of our company registry databases to 3D structures (~150 000 compounds).

The 3D database is created by reading a file of 3D structures; depending on the database system different actions occur at this stage. If atom types are used, then a parameterization database of special fragments is used to assign the desired atom types, ring centroids, and hydrophobe centres to each structure (this is the method used in ChemDBS-3D/Chem-X). The process is user-definable, allowing extensive tailoring to suit particular needs or structures. The ability to differentiate and link different atom types and environments can greatly affect the ease of use and efficiency of 3D searching. In many pharmacophoric searches used for lead generation, it has been found that it is very important to be able to search for centres that have a particular property but that are not limited to a single group; common examples are a basic nitrogen (both N sp^3 aliphatic amines and N sp^2 amidines and guanidines, but no other nitrogens), an acidic centre (both oxygens of a carboxylic acid and all nitrogens of a tetrazole) and aromatic ring centroids and/or hydrophobes (both 5- and 6-membered aromatic rings, optionally with other hydrophobic groups such as isopropyl and butyl groups).

Various element, substructure or distance range keys are used in 3D searching to screen out rapidly unsuitable structures. These may be set during or after the registration of structures in the database, or generated at search time. A relatively rapid distance key calculation based on a maximum and minimum distance defined by the connectivity is generally used, which is suitable for torsional fitting. An alternative method is the use of conformationally coded 3D keys; this option is available in ChemDBS-3D. Composite 3D distance keys, as described above, are calculated during a conformational analysis (normally rule-based systematic) applied to each suitable database structure; the conformations themselves are discarded. These keys define which distance ranges are accessible for each combination of the four 'pharmacophore' centre types, and are used as a very fast filter at the start of a search to eliminate all structures that could not possibly fit the query; the conformational analysis is then repeated to try to identify the conformations that simultaneously satisfy all the query requirements. An extra use of these distance keys, which represent accessible conformational space, was described above for the generation of potential pharmacophore models.

Identification of matching structures: search strategies

Key to the successful use of 3D searching for many drug design applications is the ability to deal with the conformational flexibility present in most drug molecules. For example, in one of our company databases (62 000 compounds registered for biological screening), only 5% had structures where flexibility would not normally play a role in defining potential pharmacophores. This was determined by finding out whether there were any rotatable bonds between atoms of any of the four 'pharmacophore' centres types used in ChemDBS-3D (hydrogen bond donor and acceptor centres, aromatic ring centroids and positively charged centres).

In ChemDBS-3D, the strategy is to store a single conformation and a set of distance keys as described above, and to generate conformational flexibility during the search process, normally using a rule-based approach. This strategy can be a systematic (or a random) conformational analysis, or a torsional energy minimization ('flexifit'). This principle of needing to store only one conformation is also used in the newly developed CFS module for the ISIS/3D (Moock, 1993) and MACCS-3D (Christie *et al.*, 1990) systems and the new UNITY (Hurst, 1994) system, but the handling of conformational flexibility is restricted to a torsional minimization technique ('directed-tweak' (Hurst, 1994) and 'CFS' (Moock, 1994) methods), which is query-directed rather than systematic.

Our experiences with ChemDBS-3D, UNITY and ISIS/3D find the fastest method to be torsional minimization, which can rapidly and thoroughly determine if a structure can fit a given set of distance constraints. The method readily handles very flexible molecules, and small tolerances on the distances, but is limited in that it is not systematic and can identify only a very limited number of possible conformational solutions; some implementations are even more restrictive in returning only one substructure mapping. This limitation is not important where the goal of a search is to identify all compounds in a database that can fit a particular pharmacophore, but can be restrictive for applications such as pharmacophore identification and idea evaluation. In a recent paper by Clark *et al.* (1994), the directed-tweak and genetic-algorithm methods were found to be most effective from a comparison of the efficiency and the effectiveness of the distance geometry, systematic search, random search, genetic-algorithm, and directed-tweak methods. In addition to handling conformational flexibility, we have also found it to be very important to differentiate different atom environments (e.g. a basic nitrogen, an acidic centre) and hydrophobe centres.

The fast rule-based systematic conformational analysis that can be used in ChemDBS-3D system is not suitable for very flexible molecules (e.g. > 14 rotatable bonds, ~ 5% in one of our libraries containing 62 000 compounds) or for use with small tolerance distances (a minimum of 0.5 Å or 20% of the distance is recommended). It does have, however, the advantage of allowing the systematic evaluation of all conformational and substructure mappings of a molecule to a particular 3D query, within a reasonable time scale for many structures. A full energy calculation is not yet feasible, but the use of the rules or a fast steric bump check is usually adequate. An alternative to torsional minimization for more flexible molecules is random conformational analysis, which allows the identification of multiple matches for a hit compound.

Each method of conformational regeneration has distinct advantages and disadvantages, depending on the application. A comparative study was made

Table 12.1
Comparison of 3D database search results

	Hits using initial CONCORD conformation only	Hits obtained when conformational flexibility was included	Hits obtained with VDW bump checking
Pharmacophoric distance search no. 1: Aromatic nitrogen to oxygen of carboxylic acid: N ↔ O 9.25 ± 0.75 Å			
ChemDBS-3D:	695	919	Rules implicitly exclude high energy conformations
ISIS/3D	594	961	954
UNITY	641	1016 (with ring flexibility) 1009 (with no ring flexibility)	990
Pharmacophoric distance search no. 2: Nitrogen to oxygen of carboxylic acid to aromatic ring (6-membered): N ↔ O 14 ± 0.5 Å; N ↔ AR6 14 ± 0.5 Å; O ↔ AR6 7 ± 0.5 Å			
ISIS/3D	1	152	
UNITY	1	151 (with no ring flexibility) 160 (with ring flexibility) 122 (with N = basic nitrogen)	
ChemDBS-3D: Systematic rule-based analysis	1	118 of the 122 hits from UNITY were too flexible (> 14 rotatable bonds) for this type of analysis	
ChemDBS-3D: Random conformational analysis		60/122 (tol = ± 0.5 Å) 90/122 (tol = ± 1.0 Å)	
ChemDBS-3D: Flexifit (torsional minimization)		122/122 (tol = ± 0.5 Å)	

ChemDBS-3D = rule-based systematic conf. analysis (single = 3, alpha = 4, double/conjugated = 2 points) or random rule-based (max. time = 2 mins), or flexifit (no VDW bump check); ISIS/3D & UNITY = torsional minimization (CFS and directed tweak).

using 58 000 compounds from one of our company libraries. Three-dimensional structures generated by CONCORD were built into 3D databases for ChemDBS-3D, ISIS/3D, and UNITY. The comparative results of some simple 3D pharmacophoric distance searches are given in Table 12.1.

The different number of hits for the initial CONCORD conformation in the three types of searches may be due to the way an aromatic nitrogen is interpreted (e.g. from Kekulé structures in ISIS database). It was clear from these studies that for very flexible molecules, torsional minimization techniques are the most effective, and that tolerance values need to be adjusted according to the method of conformational exploration used. The further effect of allowing for ring flexibility can be seen with the UNITY results. Considerations such as atom types vs. element types, or speed of search vs. thoroughness of conformational and substructure mapping search have an influence on the efficiency of any particular implementation or algorithm; the ability to evaluate instantly the hit compounds in 3D superimposed on the original query centres (as implemented in ChemDBS-3D) was found to be very useful.

We have found that structures with up to 14 rotatable bonds are readily handled using the rule-based conformational analysis; 2 (conjugated and double bonds), 3 (single bonds) and 4 (sp^2–sp^3 bonds) rotamers per bond were calculated in our databases for such structures. The default for 'alpha' (sp^2–sp^3) bonds is a 6-point analysis, but 4 points can offer a large gain in time without necessarily a reduction in yield. For a database of 62 000 company compounds, a total of 29 million conformations were accepted by the rules from a total of 912 million considered (on average, there were ~500 conformations accepted per compound, and about 3 s cpu for the calculation on a Silicon Graphics workstation; a maximum time of 60 s cpu was allowed). About 6000 compounds had no suitable bonds for rotation, and 1600 were too flexible (> 14 bonds for rotation); for the latter class of compounds, other analysis strategies such as torsional fitting or random conformation generation as discussed above are more effective.

Complementarity-based 3D Database Searching

Where the 3D structure of an enzyme or receptor is known, complementarity-based 3D searching can be applied; this is also possible where a site model can be defined from ligand(s), with projection of complementary properties. The major method used for this is DOCK (see Chapter 8). A structure-based design of inhibitors of thymidylate synthase (Shoichet *et al.*, 1993) illustrates its use in identifying new complementary structures, dissimilar to the enzyme substrate. The method is based on first identifying shape complementarity, using a negative image of the site, and, in DOCK version 3, by additionally scoring for electrostatic complementarity. Conformational flexibility is handled by searching multiple, pre-generated conformations of a molecule stored in a database. New methods to deal with conformational flexibility are being developed. One such method we are developing is to generate suitable subsets of conformations for searching. Key pharmacophoric points in the site are first identified, and these are used to perform a 3D pharmacophoric type search using rule-based conformational analysis and the retention of multiple conformational hits. The resulting 3D database of structures can then be used as input for a DOCK search, to identify those structures and conformers that fit the active site of the receptor. The structures are superposed on to the active site, making the evaluation of the results much simpler. The hit structures may also be used to provide seed ideas for *de novo* design. The advantage of using ChemDBS-3D to generate the conformers is that alternate conformers of equal or higher energy that match the query are generated. The advantage of DOCK is that structures that cannot fit into the site (due to bulky substituents) but still fit the query are eliminated rapidly. Each hit also receives a score, including electrostatic complementarity, allowing screening lists to be prioritized. Thus by linking ChemDBS-3D to DOCK, a set of conformations for DOCK analysis can be generated where at least one key interaction distance is fulfilled.

Three-dimensional QSAR

The aim of a QSAR analysis is to identify a statistical model which describes the biological activity as a function of numerical structural descriptors (variables). Ideally this model, which is derived using a training set of structures, may be used not only for activity prediction but also in the design of new, more potent molecules. Multiple linear regression (MLR) techniques have for many years been the mainstay of classical QSAR analysis (Martin, 1978); the parameters are usually either 1D (i.e. whole molecule parameters: cLogP, etc.), or 2D (i.e. substituent constants: π, σ, etc.) or pseudo-3D properties (i.e. STERIMOL parameters which attempt to describe the 3D shape of a substituent). However, 3D molecular structures may be described by their computed molecular potential fields; statistical analysis of these 3D fields is the principle of the CoMFA (comparative molecular field analysis) QSAR method introduced by Cramer *et al.* (1988). The molecular fields are created by a systematic energetic probing of the 3D space around a structure, simulating potential receptor interactions; the probes can be a single atom or an entire functional group.

The very large data sets involved in this type of analysis are handled in CoMFA by the PLS (partial least-squares projection to latent structures) technique. The ability to incorporate such large amounts of 3D data into QSARs represented an important advance over 'classical' MLR QSAR. Furthermore, visualization of the results, in terms of favourable and disfavourable 3D regions around the molecules, facilitates greatly the design of new structures; indeed the CoMFA fields can be used to direct novel structure generation (e.g. LEAPFROG, Tripos Associates). An alternative method for deriving QSARs from 3D fields was introduced by Good *et al.* (1993). This technique applies PLS techniques not to the analysis of the 3D fields themselves, but to the analysis of similarity indices generated from comparisons of 3D molecular fields using the Automated Similarity Package, ASP (Oxford Molecular Ltd.). The current problem with the use of orientation-specific 3D properties is that a method or rule for superposition must first be determined.

A Comparison of the MLR and PLS Techniques for QSAR Analysis and Design

To investigate the relative merits of the MLR and PLS techniques and the importance of 3D parameters, it was decided to explore the QSAR of a series of acyl-CoA:cholesterol *O*-acyltransferase (ACAT) inhibitors (see Fig. 12.7) which were under development as part of our cardiovascular program (Ashton *et al.*, 1992). Our object was to develop a QSAR which would deal with a diverse set of structures, be predictive for compounds not included in the training set, and be of direct use in the design of novel structures.

A training set of 20 compounds, believed to bind at the same site, was used in the analysis. These molecules have two parts, an invariant diphenyl

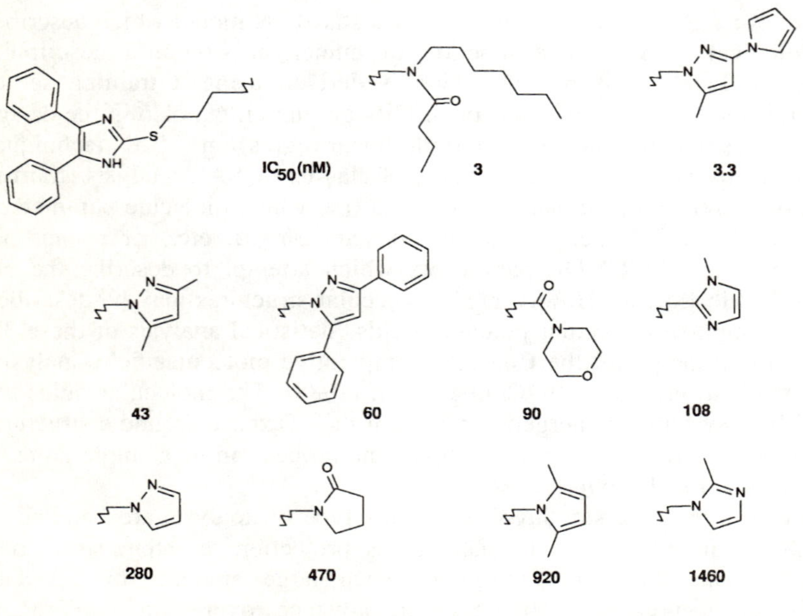

Fig. 12.7 Training set of ACAT inhibitors.

imidazole group, essential for activity, linked by an aliphatic chain to a highly variable group which is capable of modulating the activity over a wide range (IC_{50}: 3–1500 nM). Only the variant group, covering diverse structures such as heterocycle derivatives, alicycles and alkanes, was considered in the analysis. This was defined replacement of the variant portion, with a methyl group used to represent the point of attachment. A set of five compounds, with activities spanning the full range, was selected as a test set.

MLR analysis of ACAT inhibitors

Approximately 30 molecular parameters representing steric, electronic and hydrophobic properties were considered in the analysis. These included the calculated octanol–water partition coefficient (clog*P*,clogP^2), calculated molar refractivity (CMR), molar volume, HOMO and LUMO energies, dipole moment (μ, μ^2) and the STERIMOL parameters (B1, B2, B3, B4, B5, L). A statistical model could not be found until a '3D' parameter, a directional parameter of the coefficient of the group dipole in a specific direction, was included. A very predictive model was then obtained, as shown below and in Fig. 12.8. The requirement for such a parameter is evident when one considers the two *N*-substituted imidazoles (activities 108 and 1460 in Fig. 12.7) which are nearly identical in all their calculated molecule properties (there are small

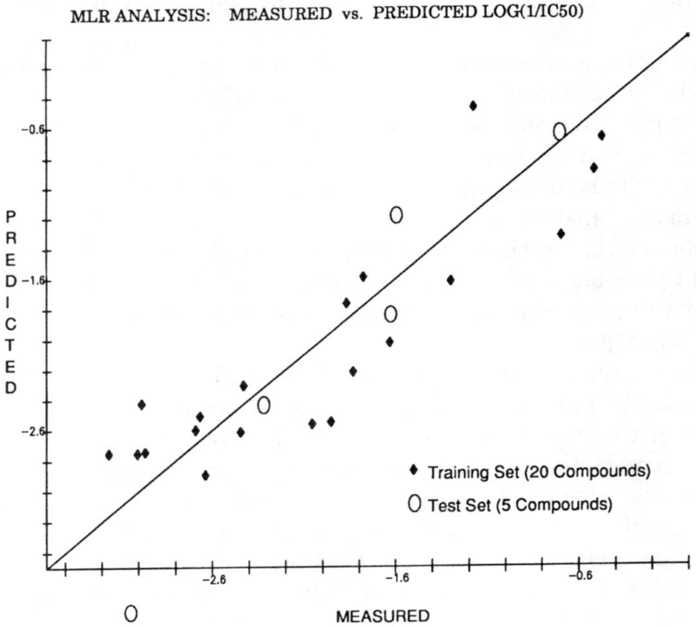

Fig. 12.8 MLR QSAR analysis of ACAT inhibitors.

differences in the STERIMOL parameters), but have widely differing activities. However, because these groups differ in their points of attachment, the directions of their dipoles differ greatly.

$$\log(1/IC_{50}) = 0.59(\pm 0.15)CMR + 0.38(\pm 0.15)\mu\cos(\theta_1 - 90) - 0.16(\pm 0.07)\mathrm{clog}P^2 - 10.05$$

$$SD = 0.4 \; F = 22 \; R^2 = 0.81 \; LOO \; Q^2 = 0.55$$

where θ_1 is the angle of the group dipole to the bond linking the variant group to the invariant.

Although a good predictive model was obtained, the discovery of the correct MLR parameters was time-consuming; furthermore, if new compounds, exploring new property space, are added to the training set then it is almost certain that this lengthy process would have to be repeated to derive additional parameters.

PLS analysis of ACAT inhibitors using CoMFA and similarity indices

As mentioned earlier, this type of analysis of molecular fields requires that structures be first superimposed. For these ACAT inhibitors this was achieved by an initial superimposition of the common linking bonds, with the remainder of the molecule being oriented to lie in the same plane, placing electronegative groups together. The similarity package ASP was used to effect a fit based on the electrostatic potentials when the choice of orientation was unclear.

Molecular fields were calculated using the SYBYL (Tripos Associates) Csp^{3+} probe (steric and electrostatic potentials), HINT (Kellogg *et al.*, 1991) for a hydrophobic potential, and GRID (Goodford, 1985, Molecular Discovery Ltd.) with CH_3, NH_3^+ and O^- probes. A map grid interval of 2 Å was used, with a 4 Å margin to the bounding box, to give 1820 points. These fields were used alone, and in combination, for PLS analysis in the SYBYL-QSAR module and in GOLPE (Baroni *et al.*, 1993), where data reduction techniques were applied. ASP was used to generate a full similarity matrix based either on electrostatic or shape similarity, the statistical analysis was then carried out using TSAR (Oxford Molecular Ltd.).

Some of the results are shown in Table 12.2. The ideal model should have a cross-validated Q^2 as close to 1 as possible, and a small standard error for the compounds in the training set SE(Tr) and for those in the test set SE(Te). Using these criteria, it can be seen that the SYBYL Csp^{3+} probe, with both steric and electrostatic potentials, gave the best overall relationship (a cut-off of 5 kcal/mol for the steric interaction was found to give best results with this probe). The GRID probes only gave a good predictive relationship after data reduction with GOLPE. The effect of including too many components (over-expressing the model) can also be seen, where an increase from two to five components improves the Q^2 for the model, but reduces the predictivity for the test set. GOLPE not only reduced GRID data dramatically, but gave the best

Table 12.2
PLS 3D-QSAR results for the ACAT inhibitors

	Method	Min σ	NC	Q^2	S.E.(Tr)	S.E.(Te)
SYBYL-CoMFA with SYBYL Csp^{3+} probe/HINT:	SYB_El	0.5	3	0.44	0.22	0.39
	SYB_St	0.5	2	0.59	0.28	0.49
	SYB_El_St	0.5	3	0.61	0.14	0.33
	HINT	0.5	1	0.36	*	*
	SYB_El_St+HINT	0.5	2	0.54	0.32	0.35
SYBYL-CoMFA with GRID probes:	GRID_CH_3	0.5	2	0.52	0.19	0.53
	GRID_O^-	0.5	1	0.56	0.40	0.42
	GRID_NH_3+	0.5	2	0.55	0.28	0.49
	GRID_3_Probes	0.5	5	0.64	0.10	0.56
	GRID_3_Probes	0.5	2	0.54	0.27	0.43
GOLPE with GRID probes:	GRID_3_Probes	0.001	2	0.92	0.11	0.35
ASP/TSAR similarity indices:	SHAPE	0.5	2	0.63	0.37	0.45
	ESP	0.5	1	0.14		
	SHAPE+ESP	0.5	4	0.59	0.25	0.42

Min σ = Minimum standard deviation for a variable to enter the analysis.
NC = Number of components.
El = Electrostatic field; St = Steric field.
Q^2 = Cross-validated predictive R^2.
S.E.(Tr) = Standard error for the TRaining set.
S.E.(Te) = Standard error for the TEst set.
SHAPE = Similarity based on molecular shape.
ESP = Similarity based on electrostatic potential.
*The Q^2 for this model was too low to be considered predictive, Standard errors were not calculated.

model as judged by Q^2 while maintaining the predictivity for the test set (in our hands we have found that with some data sets, not discussed here, GOLPE variable selection is essential to obtain a predictive model). For this series HINT, either alone or in combination with other probes, was not found to improve the models. The PLS analysis of similarity data provided a reasonable model based on SHAPE similarity alone with a slight improvement when electrostatic potential (ESP) similarity was included. The measured vs. predicted log(1/IC_{50}) values are shown in Fig. 12.9 for the SYB_El_St model.

Predictions from MLR and PLS for the ACAT inhibitors
The predictions for the test set of five compounds in the various MLR and PLS QSAR models are shown in Table 12.3. Based on these predictions it can be seen that PLS-CoMFA did not find a better predictive relationship than MLR, but it can be rapidly derived and used directly in the design of novel

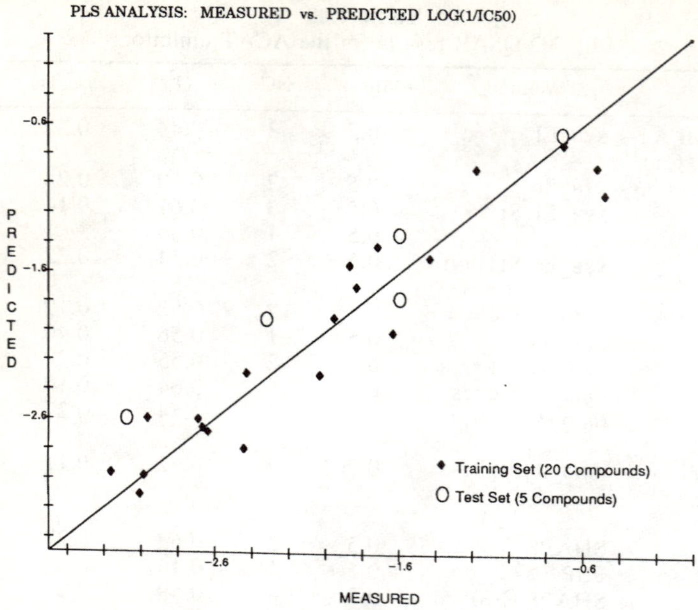

Fig. 12.9 CoMFA PLS analysis of ACAT inhibitors.

structures, with a relative ease of incorporation of new compounds; superposition of the structures can however be a problem. MLR can provide a very predictive model, but discovering the correct parameters can be time-consuming, and there are limited design and expansion possibilities. The PLS similarity matrices gave a predictive relationship (inferior to CoMFA and MLR) with simple and quick calculations, but the results are difficult to interpret for drug design.

De Novo Design

Structure-based lead generation is possible using the 3D structure of an enzyme or receptor for either direct *de novo* design or to direct 3D database searches of compound databases. The former technique leads to novel designed compounds which need to be synthesized, whereas the latter tries to identify existing compounds to create directed screening sets, using either pharmacophore-based or complementarity-based 3D searching, as discussed previously. Favourable binding sites in protein structures can be identified by programs such as GRID or from studies of a ligand complex, either experimental or from DOCK; these can be used to define 3D pharmacophoric queries.

Table 12.3
Predictions from the MLR and PLS 3D-QSAR analyses

Compound	Measured IC_{50} (nM)	MLR-predicted IC_{50} (nM)	GOLPE-predicted IC_{50} (nM)	SYBYL-predicted IC_{50} (nM)	TSAR-predicted IC_{50} (nM)
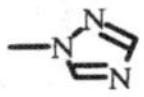	1140	4786	400	398	501
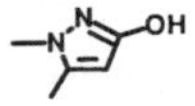	215	275	102	78	76
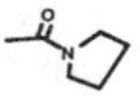	42	66	100	93	141
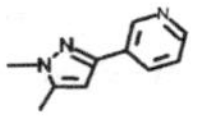	40	14	16	26	10
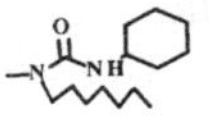	5	4	9	4	9

An important development in *de novo* design, applicable both to site-directed drug design using protein structures and envelope-directed drug design using ligand derived models, is automated structure generation (see Chapter 9). This may use 3D database searches to identify favourably binding fragments, or grow structures directly in this site. We have used this to generate putative skeletons within an active site, which were refined to give structures suitable for synthesis. Common to all methods is the problem of ease of synthesis of automatically generated structures. Further, the use of a rigid model of the protein binding site for initial structure generation necessitates many stages of validation and modification.

Rational Screening Sets

The use of quasi-random biological screening has played an important role in drug discovery for many years; this strategy is particularly applicable where little or no information is known about either the structure of the biological target or ligands which interact with it. Corporate databases of chemical compounds contain a wealth of information, and provide a very rich source of compounds for screening, but their very large size can preclude the systematic screening of all compounds. The brute-force method of screening is also time-consuming and wasteful of resources; the time taken to find a new lead is a critical step in any project. It is thus useful to abstract a small subset of a database that represents as many as possible of the key features of that database. One approach is to classify molecules by substructural features, such as the functional groups they contain, but a receptor or enzyme does not recognize particular atoms or groups, it interacts with the properties in space projected by these atoms. Subjectivity in the classification and selection stages of any method can also limit the true diversity of the final screening set.

An approach to try to rationalize this method of lead generation that we have developed involves the design of methods to select small screening sets, that have maximal diversity of molecular properties, from large compound databases. The goals of the project were to provide a rational framework for selecting representative sets of compounds for biological screening, and to provide a mechanism for selecting further compounds to follow up the initial leads. From a statistical analysis of molecular descriptors that can be calculated for each structure, descriptors that are only weakly correlated can be identified. Six such descriptors, used to represent hydrophobicity, electronic properties (polarity), hydrogen bond donor and accepting power, flexibility and shape, were identified and used to distil a corporate compound registry (~ 150 000 compounds) to three sets of about 400 compounds each. Between two and four divisions were made for each descriptor to give 560 combinatorial possibilities. Each compound was classified into one of these 'partitions', and three representatives were selected from each partition wherever possible (using structures from different research sites to maximize diversity); compounds that were excessively large, toxic or reactive were flagged. The same analysis was done for comparison on external databases such as the Standard Drug File. A similar distribution of compounds between partitions was observed, with some partitions always empty, probably corresponding to unfeasible property combinations.

The six descriptors used were all calculated from the SMILES codes: calculated log*P* (cLog*P*; Hansch and Leo, 1979) using the CLOGP3 algorithm (Chou and Jurs, 1979); normalized sum of squares of atom electrotopological indices (Hall *et al*., 1991); hydrogen bond donor and acceptor counts calculated using GENIE (Daylight Chemical Information Systems Inc.); flexibility index from the normalized product of the kappa $\alpha 1$ and $\alpha 2$ molecular shape indices (Kier and Hall, 1986); aromatic density from a division of the number of aromatic rings by the molecular volume. The use of the electrotopological indices was devized to combine information about the electronic interactions and the topological environment of each atom into a single overall molecular value. The standard valence state electronegativity index (including perturbations from neighbouring atoms in the molecule) is computed for each atom in a molecule; the normalized index is the sum of the squares of the atomic indices, divided by the number of atoms.

These six parameters stood out clearly from a statistical analysis of 15 potential molecular descriptors as being only weakly correlated. The final correlation table for a 50 000 compound database is shown in Table 12.4. The largest correlation between any pair of descriptors was 0.5, between clog*P* and the flexibility index. This is perhaps understandable, as rotatable bonds will be composed of saturated groups. Most of the other correlation coeffi-

Table 12.4
Correlation matrix for the molecular descriptors

Descriptor	H-acceptor	H-donor	Flexibility	Electro-topological	clog*P*	Aromatic density
H-acceptor	1.00	0.28	0.22	0.24	−0.16	0.13
H-donor		1.00	0.23	0.00	−0.19	−0.10
Flexibility			1.00	−0.06	0.50	−0.40
Electrotopological				1.00	−0.27	−0.10
clog*P*					1.00	0.04
Aromatic density						1.00

cients were of the order of 0.25, indicating that there is little correlation between the descriptors. This is important to the partitioning strategy, as given these orthogonal descriptors, the data is more likely to be distributed evenly across the descriptor space, producing a representative sampling.

Between two and four divisions were made for each partition value, and a set of partitions was formed by taking all the combinations of all the ranges

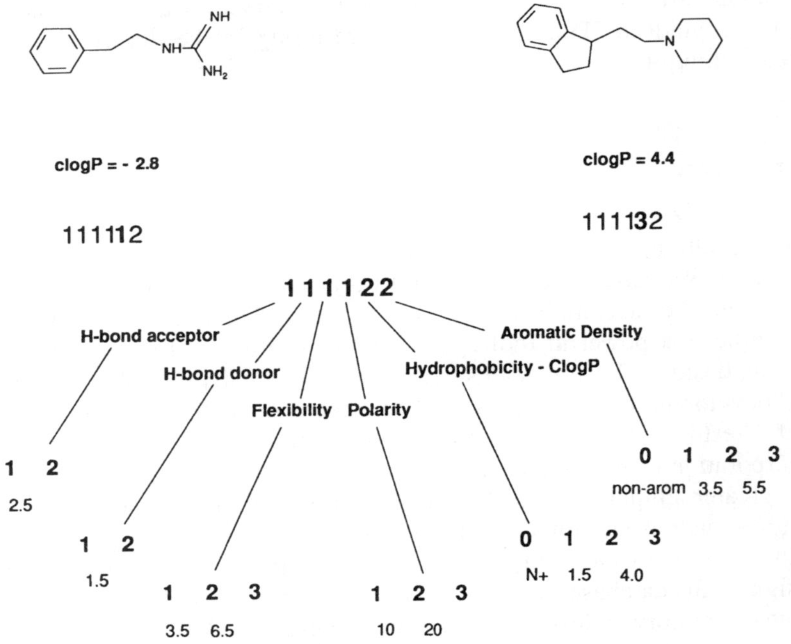

Fig. 12.10 Two examples of property-derived rational screening set codes, showing the properties used, the integer values each component of the code (bin) can take, and the numerical limits used to define the partition between different bins.

into which the molecular descriptors were divided; a number was assigned to each range, to give a final six-digit code for every compound. This is illustrated in Fig. 12.10 for two structures which differ only in their clog*P* range code. A separate class (clog*P* partition 0) was created for compounds containing a quaternary nitrogen, for which the clog*P* could not be calculated. The divisions used gave a total of 576 partitions, of which at least 10% were never filled and 10% had insufficient stock of a suitable compound. Not all the partitions were filled equally, which is expected behavior, as the compounds are not spread evenly over the whole of property space, but are clumped into families.

Screening of this set has produced a number of hits, for example for LDL receptor upregulators, as discussed above. The method groups together compounds with similar properties, so even though the representative compound may have only low affinity, related compounds are already identified and can be rapidly evaluated in follow-up sets; indeed this method can also be used with a lead compound from any source to identify compounds that have similar properties, but which may have little substructure similarity. This can produce a chemically diverse series of leads that assists the production of a pharmacophore model; this was the case in one of our screens, where several hit structures from a partition were used to construct a pharmacophore model to guide a 3D database search, resulting in the discovery of a new potent inhibitor.

Conclusion

The generation of new chemical leads for biological targets is a very challenging task. We have described several CADD techniques that can aid significantly in the accomplishment of this task. Three-dimensional database searching is a powerful tool in the lead generation and optimization stages of drug design. The ability to search conformationally flexible molecules is a key development in this area, and has been found to yield interesting and useful results. The future promises many new possibilities, for instance, the incorporation of flexibility into complementarity-based (DOCK) searching, and the greater emphasis, for distance-based searching, on non-atom centred features such as site interaction points or molecular fields.

In addition to the many new capabilities added to computer-aided drug design by 3D database searching, 3D-QSAR methods are becoming part of the standard armory, whilst the automated site-directed and envelope-directed structure generation techniques are progressing very rapidly; many more developments in these areas are expected. To improve general screening yields, particularly in cases where limited structural information about a biological target or active ligands is known, several methods are being developed including combinatorial and diversomer libraries, and rational screening sets. These latter sets have previously been based on 2D substructure criteria or, as described here, on a partitioning of molecular properties; an exciting future prospect is that selection will be made using various 3D criteria, and techniques to achieve this are currently being developed.

Acknowledgements

The authors thank Dr S.D. Pickett of the Dagenham Research Centre, Drs C. Luttmann and I. Morize of the Centre de Recherches de Vitry-Alfortville and the group of Dr P.M. Dean at the University of Cambridge for their collaboration.

References

Ashton, M.J., Bridge, A.W., Bush, R.C., Dron, D.I., Harris, N.V., Jones, G.D., Lythgoe, D.J., Riddell, D. and Smith, C. (1992). *Bioorg. Med. Chem. Lett.* **2**, 375–380.

Baroni, M., Constantino, G., Cruciani, G., Riganelli, D., Valigi, R. and Clementi, S. (1993). *Quant. Struct.-Act. Relat.* **12**, 9–20.

Blaney, J.M., Crippen, G.M., Dearing, A. and Dixon, J.S. (1990). *DGEOM, QCPE Catalog* **10**(590).

Boyd, D.B. (1994). *In* 'Reviews in Computational Chemistry', vol. 5 (K.B. Lipowitz and D.B. Boyd, eds), pp. 381–428. VCH, New York.

Bures, M.G., Danaher, E., DeLazzer, J. and Martin, Y.C. (1994). *J. Chem. Inf. Comput. Sci.* **34**(1), 218–223.

Chemical Design (1990). *The Chem-X User* **4**, 1, 5, 9.

Chou, J. and Jurs, P.J. (1979). *J. Chem. Inf. Comput. Sci.* **19**, 172–178.

Christie, B.D., Henry, D.R., Wipke, W.T. and Moock, T.E. (1990). *Tetrahedron Comput. Methodol.* **3–6C**, 653–664.

Clark, D.E., Jones, G., Willett, P., Kenny, P.W. and Glen, R.C. (1994). *J. Chem. Inf. Comput. Sci.* **34**(1), 197–206.

Cramer, R.D., Patterson, D.F. and Bunce, J.D. (1988). *J. Am. Chem. Soc.* **110**, 5959–5967.

Dalby, A., Nourse, J.G., Hounshell, W.D., Gushurst, A.K.I., Grier, D.L., Leland, B.A. and Laufer, J. (1992). *J. Chem. Inf. Comput. Sci.* **32**(3), 244–255.

DesJarlais, R.L., Sheridan, R.P., Seibel, G.L., Dixon, J.S., Kuntz, I.D. and Venkataraghavan R. (1988). *J. Med. Chem.* **31**, 722–729.

Golender, V.E. and Vorpagel, E.F. (1993). *In* '3D QSAR in Drug Design: Theory, Methods and Applications', (H. Kubinyi, ed.), pp. 137–149. ESCOM, Leiden.

Good, A.C., So, S.S. and Richards, W.G. (1993). *J. Med. Chem.* **36**, 433–438.

Goodford, P.J. (1985). *J. Med. Chem.* **28**, 849–857.

Hall, L.H., Mohney, B.K. and Kier, L.B. (1991). *J. Chem. Inf. Comput. Sci.* **31**, 76–82.

Hansch, C. and Leo, A. (1979). 'Substituent Constants for Correlation Analysis in Chemistry and Biology', Wiley Interscience, New York.
Haraki, K.S., Sheridan, R.P., Venkataraghavan, R., Dunn, D.A. and McCulloch, D. (1990). *Tetrahedron Comput. Methodol.* **3**, 565–573.
Hurst, T. (1994). *J. Chem. Inf. Comput. Sci.* **34**(1), 190–196.
Jorgensen, W.L. (1991). *Science* **254**, 954–955.
Kellogg, G.E., Semus, S.F. and Abrahams, D.J. (1991). *J. Comput.-Aided Mol. Design* **5**, 545–552.
Kier, L.B. and Hall, L.H. (1986). 'Molecular Connectivity in Structure–Activity Analysis'. Research Studies Press, John Wiley, Chichester.
Kuntz, I.D., Blaney, J.M., Oatley, S.J., Langridge, R. and Ferrin, T.E. (1982). *J. Mol. Biol.* **161**, 269–288.
Lauri, G. and Bartlett, P.A. (1994). *J. Comput.-Aided Mol. Design* **8**(1), 51–66.
Martin, Y.C. (1978). 'Quantitative Drug Design', Marcel Dekker, New York.
Martin, Y.C. (1992). *J. Med. Chem.* **35**, 2145–2154.
Martin, Y.C., Bures, M.G., Danaher, E.A., DeLazzer, J., Lico, I. and Pavlik, P.A. (1993). *J. Comput.-Aided Mol. Design* **7**, 83–102.
Mason, J.S. (1992). *In* 'Trends in QSAR and Molecular Modelling 92: Proceedings of the 9th European Symposium on Structure-Activity Relationships: QSAR and Molecular Modelling, 7–11 September 1992, Strasbourg, France' (C.G. Wermuth, ed.), pp. 252–255. ESCOM, Leiden.
Mason, J.S. (1993). *In* 'Trends in Drug Research', (V. Claassen, ed.), pp. 147–156. Elsevier, Amsterdam.
Moock, T., Henry, D.R., Ozkabak, A.G. and Alamgir, M. (1994). *J. Chem. Inf. Comput. Sci.* **34**(1), 184–189.
Murrall, N.W. and Davies, E.K. (1990). *J. Chem. Inf. Comput. Sci.* **30**, 312–316.
Murrall, N.W. and Davies, E.K. (1993). *In* 'Chemical Structures II', Springer-Verlag, Berlin.
Pearlman, R.S. (1987). *CDA News* **2**, 1–7.
Pearlman, R.S. (1994). *In* '3D QSAR in Drug Design: Theory, Methods and Applications', (H. Kubinyi, ed.), pp. 41–79. ESCOM, Leiden.
Rusinko, A., III, Skell, J.M., Balducci, R., McGarty, C.M. and Pearlman, R.S. (1988). CONCORD, a program for the rapid generation of high quality approximate 3-dimensional molecular structures. Tripos Associates, St. Louis, MO 63144.
Shoichet, B.K., Stroud, R.M., Santi, D.V., Kuntz, I.D. and Perry, K.M. (1993). *Science* **259**, 1445–1450.
Sprague, P.W. (1991). *In* 'Recent Advances in Chemical Information – Proceedings of the 1991 Chemical Information Conference'. (H. Collier, ed.), pp. 107–111. Royal Society of Chemistry, Cambridge, U.K.
Van Drie, J.H., Weininger, D. and Martin, Y.C. (1989). *J. Comput.-Aided Mol. Design* **3**, 225–251.
Weininger, D., Weininger, A. and Weininger, J.L. (1989). *J. Chem. Inf. Comput. Sci.* **29**, 97–101.

Discussion

C. McCarthy

What was the experimental basis for taking just one compound from each box in generating your rational sets – why one, why not ten?

J.S. Mason
It is not one compound, but three. We decided that we could either take the box, do some form of clustering within it and use it to select more than one representative (there is a long-term project to do that by other methods), or to take one compound from each of three corporate libraries. Historically, there is a different structural basis in those libraries. There are thus three compounds chosen from each box, one from each library which will, by historical means, be different in terms of structure – this can of course be verified.

C. McCarthy
When this analysis was done, was it found that many compounds made in one particular research program appeared in the same box?

J.S. Mason
Yes – this can be seen with the low-density lipoprotein example. All those compounds that were made for DHFR came within that box, which is why in using one compound from that box we are able to find a lead. We may have been lucky, but it showed that if enough is taken from the box, a series of compounds should be found that are related by properties. It is not a rule; it just happens that we see a lot of compounds clustered together within the partitions.

C. McCarthy
In the rational sets, a lot of LTB_4 antagonists were found in one box. Were there large variations of activity in the compounds? If there were, on what basis can you cluster them for screening?

J.S. Mason
We are clustering compounds so that we screen as few as possible to find any activity. The idea is that if any activity – weak activity – is found, only a small number of compounds, say, 1000, will have been screened. If weak activity – it could be 5 μM with one compound – is found, we can say this is the only compound that gives any activity. Then the other 100, 200 or 300 compounds in that partition are pulled out and screened. Screening of rational sets is certainly not meant to give the most active compound: that is the idea of 3D searching.

C.G. Wermuth
Now that it is possible to find more rapidly a given molecule for a given target, how can the target endpoint be defined and who will do this? Perhaps substance P has viable clinical targets but what about corticotrophin-releasing factor which has been mentioned. Tomorrow, there may be a molecule which

binds as an antagonist, for example, but what is to be done with it in human clinics and who will decide that?

J.S. Mason

It is important that we always need tools to investigate any new mechanism, so the idea is to find – hopefully, quickly and selectively – a compound that has that mechanism. It would then have to be validated whether it was appropriate for treating human disease. The first thing is to have the compound: no theory can be validated or not validated until there is a compound that can be put into a true model to evaluate. It is necessary to find it.

To answer the question in a different way: how do we decide on what to work? If there is a choice of approaches, we decide on the approach where the most rational design can be done. This is now a deciding factor in selecting new approaches.

A.R. Leach

Clearly, a number of factors come into selecting new approaches. How important would you say that crystal structure is, and would it be a deciding criterion?

J.S. Mason

The quality of the model is important. If we have a molecular model at low resolution, one of the therapeutic programme managers may say: this is wonderful and cannot we do something? and we have to evaluate and look at the quality of the model. If we have a good high-quality structure from crystallography, from NMR, from homology, that is certainly a deciding factor. If we have only a poor model, it would have to be evaluated carefully.

C. McCarthy

What is the role of automated high-throughput screening of the compound libraries in lead generation? Many people seem to turn up their nose at it, but it is very effective – it works.

J.S. Mason

We always need to be sure that a diverse set of leads can be obtained. However good our 3D searching or structure-based design, we should also be passing efficiently compounds through screens to look for a hit on a biological target. Automated high-throughput screening of compounds plays an important part if done sensibly – an important parallel role to any form of structure-based design.

By 'sensibly', I mean not screening two compounds that would be classified by some method as being sufficiently similar such that no more information would be gained by screening both rather than one. It is getting the most diverse set, a sensible library, so that if a hit is found it can be turned into a real drug molecule. I am not so interested in screening anything where, if we get a hit, there is still a long haul to turn it into a drug, but something where the results could be used in a short time-frame to turn it into a drug molecule.

It is open for debate whether compounds should be mixed before screening – if this is what you are alluding to: should we mix every compound that has been made and test them all? If we wish to mix, we should mix everything that we feel is yielding more information – but this can now be rationally analysed. As you have seen, there are rational databases, we have evaluated structures in three dimensions, and I think a fair evaluation can be made now whether two compounds are similar enough for it probably not to be worth screening both.

C. McCarthy

I disagree. I think a methyl group in the wrong position, say, in the endothelin program, can severely reduce activity. A methyl group might be said to be a trivial difference between two molecules, but removing it can diminish activity spectacularly.

J.S. Mason

It is how we focus, and the order in which the screening is done. All these screening sets can be prioritized. We screen 1000 compounds; if they are not active, another group can be screened. We never say *these* compounds will *never* be screened, but decide which to screen first. We want the first 1000 to be the best. Even if the screen is quick, there is no point, and it is a waste of resources, in screening 100 000 if the answer can be obtained from 1000.

My feeling is that this is prioritizing how we screen, but I have always accepted your point. With care, we will not miss suitable compounds, and it is still better to prioritize and rationalize the order in which we screen if diverse screening is being done.

13

'Molecular Mimics' as Approaches For Rational Drug Design: Application to Tachykinin Antagonists

A. LAOUI, C. LUTTMANN, I. MORIZE, G. PANTEL, A. MORGAT, C. RUBIN-CARREZ, V. LAROCHE, J.D. GUITTON, O. GIGONZAC and E. JAMES-SURCOUF

Rhône-Poulenc Rorer Central Research, CRVA, 13, quai Jules Guesde, BP 14, 94403 Vitry-sur-Seine Cedex, France

Introduction

The 'molecular mimic' approach is a rational drug-design concept that deals with logical and efficient design of small molecules based on our knowledge of larger molecular structures. There are a number of interwoven research strategies that are currently under study which have been designed to examine this approach. The general diagram in Fig. 13.1 shows the interplay between these various strategies. These include the receptor mapping approach for new analogue design during the lead optimization process: the 'peptidomimetic' approach which searches for rational principles to convert the information provided by natural peptide ligands into low-molecular-weight non-peptide molecules; 3D database searching techniques which have become efficient in finding new mimetic compounds starting from pharmacophoric or structural queries: and more recently the synthesis of combinatorial libraries which are based on a rational selection of some target molecular scaffolds. This latter

New Perspectives in Drug Design
ISBN 0–12–208070–X

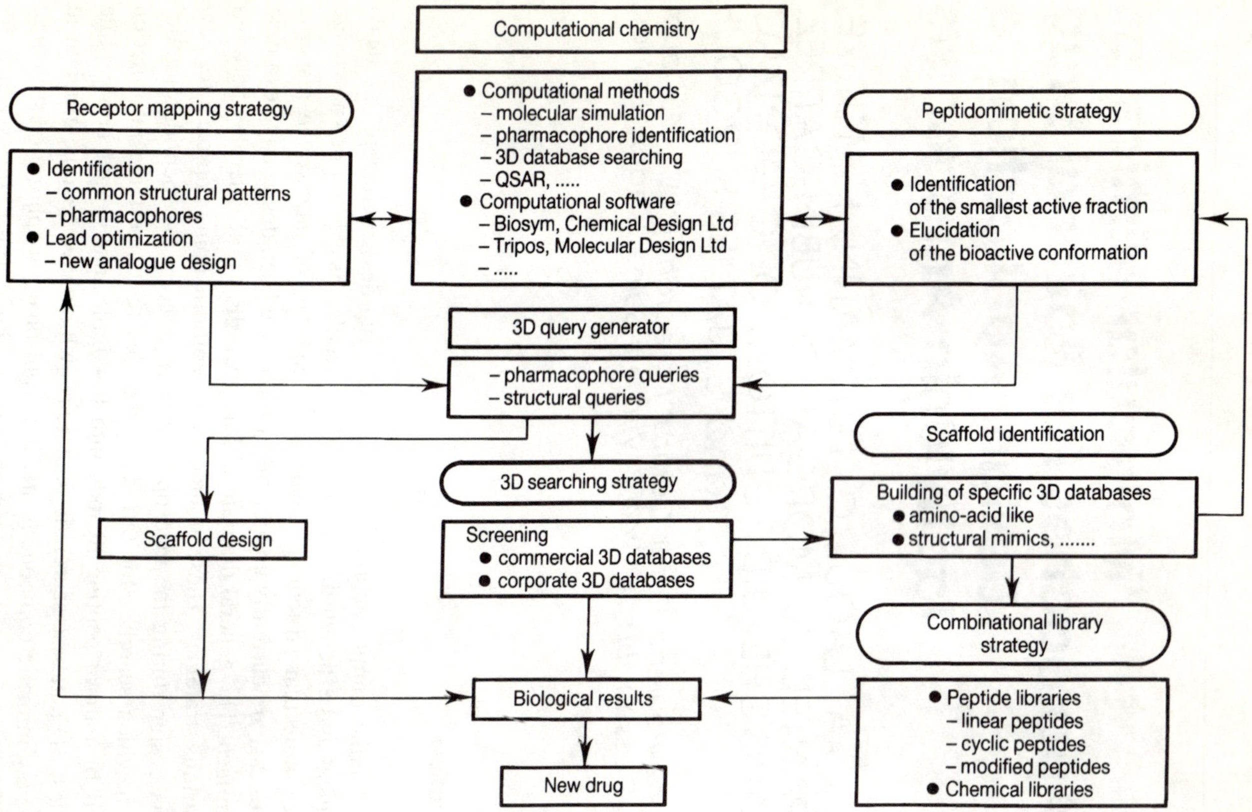

Fig. 13.1 Strategies in rational drug design.

strategy constitutes a promising approach for new lead generation in the drug discovery process.

With the recent advances in the power of computational chemistry the scope of technology available for drug discovery has been expanded. As suggested in Fig. 13.1, future successes in the drug development process will most likely rely upon more collaborative approaches and a successful integration of diverse technologies.

This chapter will focus principally on the peptidomimetic approach cited above. Peptides represent an interesting starting point in drug discovery. First, they influence a multitude of physiological processes often by signal transduction mediated through receptors. Second, there are many peptides whose biological role is well known (Schmidt, 1986; Dutta, 1991). This makes them attractive candidates for drug design; some of these peptides are listed in Table 13.1. Finally, peptides with structural diversity can be prepared in large quantities for use in screening programmes to identify molecules with desired biological properties. However, native peptides are only rarely directly usable as drugs, due to their low bioavailability, rapid metabolism, lack of oral activity, etc. Another limiting problem in peptides is the uncertainty concerning the

Table 13.1,
Examples of some biologically active peptides (neurotransmitters, neuromodulators, hormones)

ACTH	Lipotropin
β-Amyloid	Pentagastrin
Angiotensin[a]	LHRH
Bombesin	α-MSH
Bradykinin	Motilin
Calcitonin	Neurokinin A[a]
Carnosine	Neurokinin B[a]
CGRP	Neuromedin K
Cholecystokinin (CCK)[a]	Neuromedin L
Corticotrophin-releasing factor	Neuropeptide K
Cyclosporin A	Neuropeptide Y
Dynorphin	Neurotensin[a]
β-Endorphin	Oxytocin[a]
Endothelin[a]	Pancreatic polypep
[Met]Enkephalin[a]	Physaleamin
[Leu]Enkephalin[a]	Proctolin
Galanin	Secretin
Glucagon	Somatostatin
Gramicidin S	Substance P[a]
Growth hormone	TRH
Insulin	Vasopressin
Kassinin	VIP
Kyotorphin	Xenopsin

[a] Biomimetic, non-peptide molecules exist for these peptides

three-dimensional structure responsible for their activity. Thus, it is usually necessary to produce highly modified peptides, peptidomimetics, or non-peptide molecules that act through peptide receptors to exploit the use of peptides as first lead molecules.

Development of new drugs based on peptide structures therefore requires a method to extract the conformation and chemical features of the molecules that determine their biological activity, and then to create new or to identify existing molecules with similar properties. The peptidomimetic strategy is a promising approach to rationally design new molecules based on knowledge of peptide structures.

In this chapter, we will address three main points. First, progress in the general strategies of peptidomimetic design will be reviewed. After an introduction to the tachykinin subject, the work that we have performed to design peptidomimetic substance P (SP) antagonists will be summarized. Lastly, we present how 3D searching capabilities may be helpful in generating specific 3D databases of scaffolds which can be exploited in the peptidomimetic approach and for the synthesis of chemical libraries.

Peptidomimetic Approach

The major goal in the transformation of a bioactive peptide into a non-peptide entity is to reproduce, as closely as possible, the relevant 3D topography. This latter is defined as a pharmacophore (a specific spatial arrangement of elements such as charges, lipophilic and hydrophilic groups) that is essential for the recognition and interaction with the complementing domain of the receptor, leading to induction of the biochemical message in the case of agonists, and inhibition in the case of antagonists.

Attachment of the pharmacophores to a molecular template or scaffold which reproduces the bioactive topography offers a rational pathway to the design of non-peptide molecules based on the knowledge of peptide structures. The optimal scaffold could be a polyfunctional small ring (5–7 membered ring, monocyclic or bicyclic) of defined stereochemistry. By limiting the number of structural degrees of freedom, such a ring will allow access only to a restricted space. Thus, reproduction of the bioactive topography becomes a realistic objective.

Strategy

An outline of the general strategy leading to the design of non-peptide molecules is given in Fig. 13.2. As a general approach to drugs based on peptides, the first step is the identification of those residues of the peptide that are critical for biological activity. This is done by truncating the peptide to

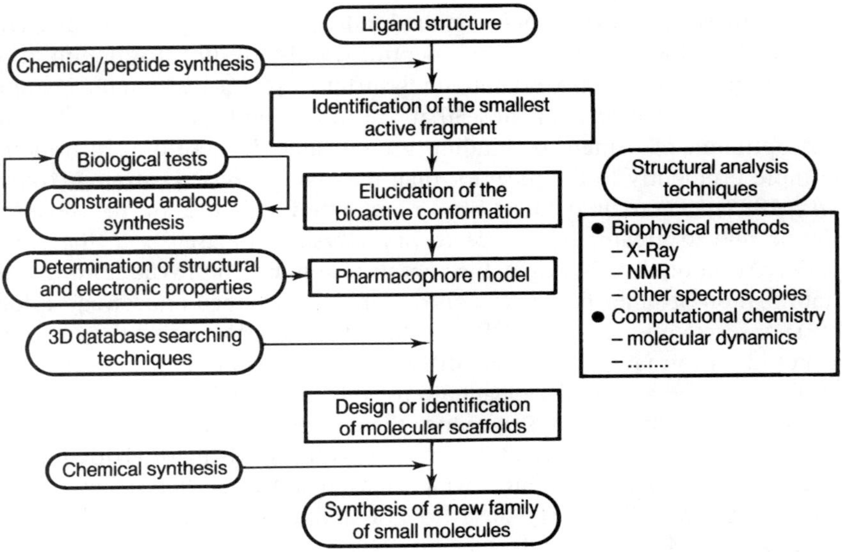

Fig. 13.2 Peptidomimetic strategy.

produce the smallest active fragment. Such studies often reveal that the entire peptide chain is not necessary for full biological activity (Ondetti *et al.*, 1970; Zarandi *et al.*, 1983; Schwyzer, 1985; Boublik *et al.*, 1989; Dutta, 1987). The minimum active fragment is then modified to generate more stable, potent and selective agonist or antagonist analogues. Conformationally restricted analogues are synthetized to provide information on the bioactive conformation of peptides. This information, along with physicochemical and theoretical studies (NMR and molecular dynamics) is used to improve potency and selectivity. The critical interplay of design, synthesis, biological assays and biophysical studies often provide the insights needed for rational design. At this step, from the putative bioactive conformation, it may be possible to deduce a pharmacophore for the peptide ligand of interest. This pharmacophore is then used to design or recognize potential bioactive molecules.

Recently, new 3D searching techniques (Martin, 1992; Borman, 1992) have demonstrated efficiency in finding and designing new biologically active compounds. Three-dimensional searching is used to find all the molecules in a 3D database that contain a specific pharmacophore. It thus can be used to validate such a pharmacophore and to suggest other existing compounds for testing to find a new lead.

Conformational Constraint

Conformational constraint constitutes one of the most promising approaches to the problem of receptor-bound conformation (Fauchere, 1987; Hruby *et al.*,

1990; Smith *et al.*, 1991). The receptor-binding data for a conformationally constrained analogue of a bioactive peptide yields useful information about the parent molecule. Flexible compounds suffer a greater loss in entropy upon binding to the receptor than those that are more rigid. A compound which forces optimum placement of binding groups should, therefore, in principle bind more efficiently to the receptor than the endogenous substrate (Miklavc *et al.*, 1987). There may also be an increased half-life of the resulting analogue due to greater resistance to proteolysis compared with the parent peptide. Additionally, biological selectivity can be improved through the destabilization of other bioactive conformers that produce undesired biological responses (Veber *et al.*, 1979). Furthermore, conformational constraints can provide information about the different requirements that a receptor has for a ligand to be an agonist or antagonist (Hruby, 1987).

There are a number of ways to reduce the conformational space available to peptides (Degrado, 1988). Cyclization is a well-known method for introducing a conformational constraint, which may result in higher selectivity and potency (Kessler, 1982). The insertion of amino acids which reduce conformational space available for the Φ (N_α–C_α bond) and Ψ (C_α–$C_{carbonyl}$ bond) torsional angles may have an impact on the overall conformation of a small peptide. Examples are the insertion of proline residues, C_α methyl amino acid residues (Turk *et al.*, 1975) (in particular, α–amino-isobutyric acid residues), and others. However, the disadvantage of these local conformational constraints is that the resulting overall conformation is not always predictable. Therefore, to obtain conformation–activity relationships, the influence of the restriction on the conformation of the peptide should be investigated using biophysical techniques.

Clearly there is a need for a method to attain a defined conformational constraint in a peptide. Recently, efforts have been devoted to the development of templates that mimic or stabilize several common secondary structures of peptides and proteins. These compounds are called peptide conformation mimetics. A peptide conformation mimetic can be described as a building block which, inserted into a peptide chain, enforces a particular conformation. Therefore, a first requirement for a peptide conformation mimetic should be that the conformation enforced is met with a high degree of accuracy. Second, it is well known that the amino acid side chains of peptides play an important role in molecular recognition. So, an ideal peptide conformation mimetic should therefore be a compound with diverse functional groups (polar, hydrophilic, lipophilic), which could easily be introduced during the synthesis.

Regular peptide secondary structures can be classified into three different types. These are helical structures, pleated sheets and reversed turns (Rose *et al.*, 1985). Whereas only a few compounds are available to mimic an α-helix or a β-sheet, the reverse turns (β-turns or γ turns) are the prime target for peptide conformation mimetics, because they comprise only four (β-turns) or

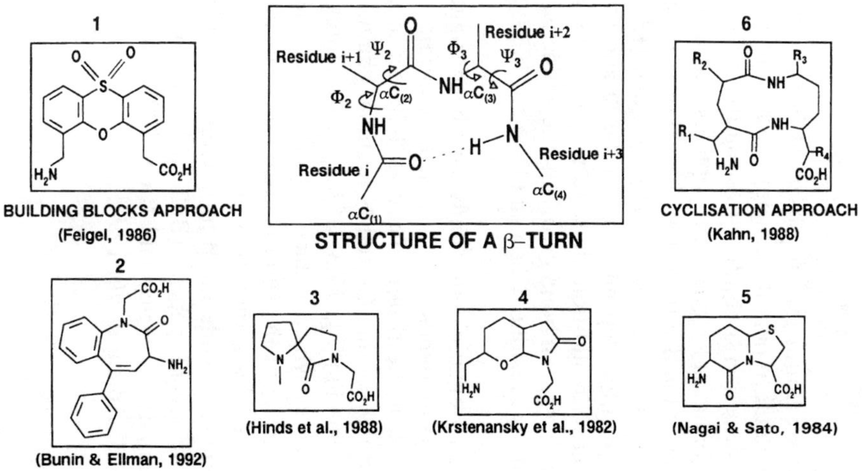

Fig. 13.3 Templates for β-turns. Structures of building blocks having the ability to force or induce a β-turn in peptides.

three (γ-turns) amino acid residues in the turn, and there are many examples where reverse turns are likely to be present in the bioactive conformation of a naturally occurring peptide (Smith and Pease, 1980). It is also widely believed that these reverse turns play an important role in peptide receptor recognition and antigen determination (Dyson *et al.*, 1985).

β-Turn Mimics

As mentioned above, a major structural feature observed in peptides is the reverse turn. Turns are fundamental to peptide structure and occur in regions where the peptide reverses its direction by folding over on itself. There are a number of reverse-turn conformations found in peptides (Milner-White, 1989). One of the most common is the β-turn. Figure 13.3 shows the structure of the β-turn with the four residues designated as *i*, *i*+1, *i*+2, and *i*+3. Several different types of β-turns are possible depending upon the Φ and Ψ torsion angles of the *i*+1 and *i*+2 residues. In addition, these turns may or may not be stabilized by an intramolecular hydrogen bond involving the amide NH of the *i*+3 residue and the carbonyl of the *i* residue (Chou and Fasman, 1977; Wilmot and Thornton, 1988, 1990).

A number of heterocyclic and aromatic compounds have been suggested as surrogates for β-turns. These compounds are designed to mimic the two corner amino acids *i*+1 and *i*+2 of the β-turn. They all have an amino and carboxy substitution to extend the peptide C- and N-terminal chain. Several interesting examples are represented in Fig. 13.3. Of the six structures shown, five (structures **1–5**) are molecules which reduce the conformational flexibility of a peptide with the skeleton of the rigid residue lying outside of the pseudo 10-membered ring formed by a typical β-turn. For structure **6**, the framework of the β-turn mimic lies inside the β-turn. Other examples of β-turn mimics are reviewed in recent papers (Ball and Alewood, 1990; Holzemann, 1991; Hirschmann, 1991; Wiley and Rich, 1993; Olson *et al.*, 1993; Giannis and Kolter, 1993; Adang *et al.*, 1994).

β-Sheet and α-Helix Mimics

Unlike a β-turn, the α-helix and β-sheet incorporate a larger number of amino acid residues to achieve their shape, and their secondary structures are in a more extended conformation. One approach for creating well-defined β-sheets or α-helixes focuses on facilitating rapid intramolecular chain folding. The incorporation of unnatural amino-acids which direct the folding of a polypeptide into a β-sheet or α-helix secondary structure was recently described (Diaz *et al.*, 1992). In the field of this nucleation strategy, some α-helix (structures 1, 2 and 5) and β-sheet (structures 3 and 4) mimetics are represented in Fig. 13.4. In the specific cases where the residues relevant for biological recognition lie along one face of the α-helix or when the helix

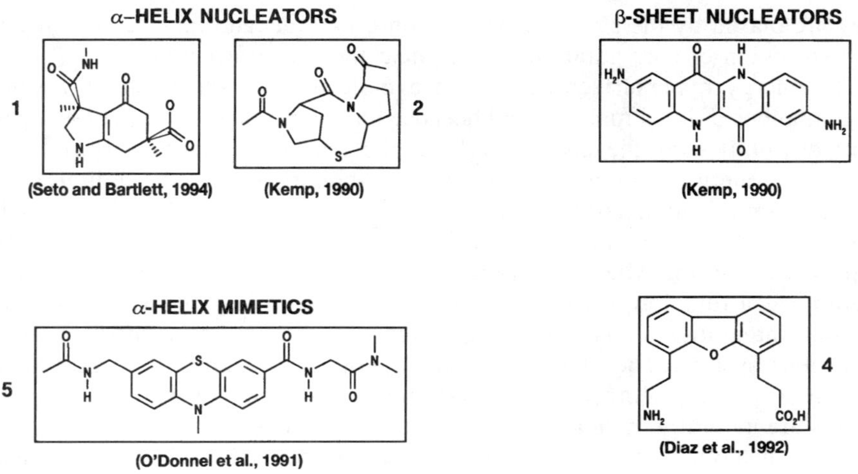

Fig. 13.4 Templates for α-helices and β-sheets.

only plays a spacer role, a small bridging template can be designed as with the β-turn mimics (O'Donnel *et al.*, 1991).

Conformational Analysis

The ability to determine well-defined three-dimensional structures for target compounds is a powerful tool in drug design. A lot of information on the conformation of small polypeptides in solution, and their sensitivity to the environment, can be obtained by two-dimensional NMR spectroscopy (Wuthrich, 1986; Fesik, 1991), and this information can be used in combination with computational techniques such as distance geometry (Crippen, 1981), molecular dynamics (MD) (Karplus and McCammon, 1983; McCammon and Harvey, 1987; van Gunsteren and Berendson, 1990), simulated annealing (Dinola *et al.*, 1984), and variable target function algorithms (Braum and Go, 1985) to yield the desired 3D structures. Molecular dynamics methods have been recently shown to be extremely powerful in a wide variety of applications to biomolecular problems, including drug design, reproduction of structural properties of peptides in solvent environment (Meirovitch *et al.*, 1992) or in crystals (Avbelj *et al.*, 1990), refinement of protein structures (Brunger *et al.*, 1987), and studies on protein dynamics (Elber and Karplus, 1988; Mark and van Gunsteren, 1992) and on protein–ligand interaction (Tilton *et al.*, 1988). To obtain energetically reasonable structures and understand the conformational behaviour under study, in particular when flexibility and conformation equilibria are likely to exist (van Gunsteren and Mark, 1992), MD simulations constitute the most likely method of choice, although they are biased by the choice of initial conformations and may search only a limited region of configurational space near these conformations.

The energy hypersurface describing a molecular system contains a very large number of local minima, and because energy minimization (EM) moves only downhill over the energy surface, the algorithm yields only a local minimum energy configuration in the neighbourhood of the initial one. Energy minimization covers only a small part of the configuration space but is capable of relaxing the strain in a molecule by small local positional adjustments. In the MD simulation method, a trajectory (molecular configurations as a function of time) in a molecular system is generated by simultaneous integration of Newton's equations of motion for all atoms of the molecular system. The state of constant motion of atoms in a molecular system at ordinary temperatures is then mimicked. This means that entropic effects are naturally included. The simulation provides information about the dynamic behaviour of the system, whereas the presence of such motional freedom implies the possibility of overcoming energy barriers of the order of $k_B T$, and a range of molecular conformations is sampled. Therefore, MD searches a larger part of configurational space and generally finds a lower energy minimum than regular EM techniques.

Molecular dynamics simulation protocol

A general diagram of the protocol is shown in Fig. 13.5. One of the major problems in the simulation of the structural and energetic properties of flexible molecules such as peptides arises from the fact that these molecules can adopt a variety of minimum-energy conformations. For simulations at room temperature (300K), the energy available to the molecule is only enough to overcome relatively low-energy barriers in the time scale that currently limits molecular dynamics simulations: about 10 ns. Thus, conformational space is sampled slowly during 300K simulations. One way to overcome this problem is to run dynamics at higher temperatures, on the order of 1000K, to give the molecule enough energy to overcome relatively large energy barriers (and cross low-energy barriers faster) and in this way search conformational space more efficiently. To avoid 'false' high-energy minima, we use a protocol in which a high-temperature snapshot is gradually cooled down and equilibrated at a lower temperature (300K). Then an energy minimization is performed to obtain the 'true' minimum.

When experimental data obtained by NMR studies are available, restrained molecular dynamics (RMD) (van Gunsteren *et al.*, 1991) is used. RMD uses a force field with an additional penalty function constraining the interatomic distances to the experimental NMR data. RMD creates a trajectory which moves the molecule towards conformations satisfying the experimental restraints. Therefore, experimental data provide the necessary restriction of the configuration space which has to be sufficiently sampled in simulation.

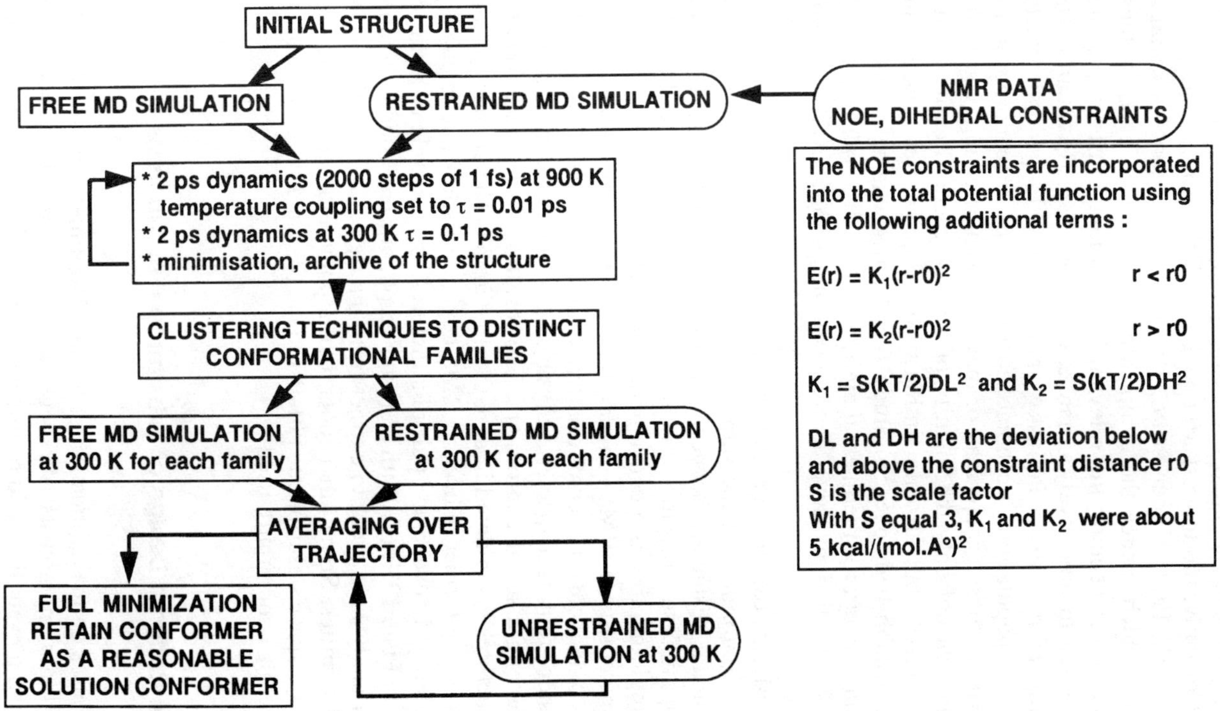

Fig. 13.5 A molecular dynamics protocol.

Analysis tools
As computer technologies advance, increasingly longer molecular dynamics are achieved. Currently, the longest MD have extended into the nanosecond range (Tobias *et al.*, 1991; Soman *et al.*, 1991). It is becoming essential to develop methods which reduce the complexity of data resulting from these long simulations while keeping the relevant information. Clustering techniques are well-suited to objectively organize trajectory data (Rooman *et al.*, 1990; McKelvey *et al.*, 1991; Polinsky *et al.*, 1992). In general, cluster analysis dissects a population into homogeneous groups. Depending on the particular algorithm, these groups may or may not be intersecting. Clustering attempts to establish not only the identity of a new structural entity (is it a β-turn or an α-helix?) but also its similarity to other entities. Once similarity has been established, one can study the detailed characteristics of a single representative family member, thereby reducing the total number of conformers to be studied by several orders of magnitude (Karpen *et al.*, 1993).

Structure similarity can be quantitated easily by a simple superposition analysis. If two conformers of the same molecule are similar, there will be only small residual distances between the corresponding pairs of atoms following an optimal superposition of the conformers. Averaging these distances into a single number is a convenient metric and is commonly referred to as the root mean square (RMS) deviation between two structures.

The central component of a conformational family analysis is the cluster graph. The cluster graph is a special analysis tool which performs a pairwise superposition among a set of conformers. The resulting RMS deviations for each pair of structures is tabulated in a matrix-like graph. The elements of the cluster graph (x, y: conformer indices, z: RMS deviation) allow one to quickly assess the 'similarity' between any pair of structures. An example of a cluster graph is shown in Plate 13.1. (a) With a cluster graph, one can conduct a more rigorous cluster analysis in order to extract from the trajectory data the major conformational families. Some other tools, like a population analysis (histogram (c)), torsion space descriptors (Phi–Psi maps (b)) and potential energy variation (d) are also commonly used.

Application to Rational Design of Substance P Antagonists

This section focuses on the application of the peptidomimetic approach to the design of tachykinin antagonists. We begin with an overview of tachykinin research, and then present the main results we obtained for the rational design of SP antagonists.

The last 3 years have seen the discovery of several tachykinin receptor antagonists (peptidic and non-peptidic) (Watling and Krause, 1993), each possessing high affinity and selectivity for a single tachykinin receptor type, and each belonging to a different chemical class. The stage is set, therefore, for a new era in tachykinin research with the possibility that these promising antagonists will afford pharmacologists and clinicians the opportunity to probe both the physiological consequences and the clinical potential of manipulating mammalian tachykinin neuropeptide systems.

It is of interest that all of the non-peptide tachykinin receptor antagonists described arose, either directly or indirectly, from targeted screening of large compound collections using a radioligand binding assay as the primary screen. Here we present another approach based on peptidomimetic strategy which can produce tachykinin antagonists as a result of rational drug design.

Biology

The naturally occurring neurokinins, substance P (SP), neurokinin A (NKA) and neurokinin B (NKB) have been shown to be present in sensory nerves and involved in the generation of neurogenic inflammation and in pain perception (Pernow, 1983; Logan *et al.*, 1990). When released from the nerves by various stimuli, neurokinins are able to interact with at least three receptor types which have been shown to be widespread and mediate various biological effects, such as vasodilatation, venoconstriction and increase of vascular permeability (the NK-1 receptor) (Lembeck and Holzer, 1979); bronchoconstriction and the activation of sympathetic nervous system (the NK-2 receptor) (Maggi *et al.*, 1993a); and venoconstriction and release of acetylcholine (the NK-3 receptor) (Laneuville *et al.*, 1988). Antagonists are needed for basic pharmacologic characterization of receptors and receptor roles, as well as for clinical use.

Chemistry

It has always seemed likely that the therapeutic potential of manipulating tachykinin-mediated biological effects would not be fully recognized until non-peptide, metabolically stable antagonists became available. During the last 3 years, this has become possible with the discovery of several non-peptide antagonists, each possessing high affinity and high selectivity for tachykinin receptors. We describe herein all the most potent peptide and non-peptide antagonists that have appeared in the literature and patents.

Peptide tachykinin antagonists

Several workers in the field have sought to generate tachykinin receptor antagonists by modifying tachykinin's peptide structure. For SP antagonists, two strategies were ultimately successful: the 'linear' approach used by Folkers' group, which led to spantide II (Folkers *et al.*, 1985) (Fig. 13.6) and the 'conformational constraint' approach, which resulted in the design of

SPANTIDE II

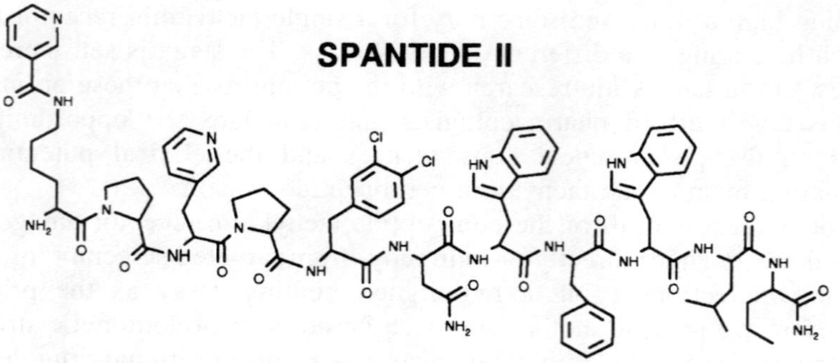

GR-71251

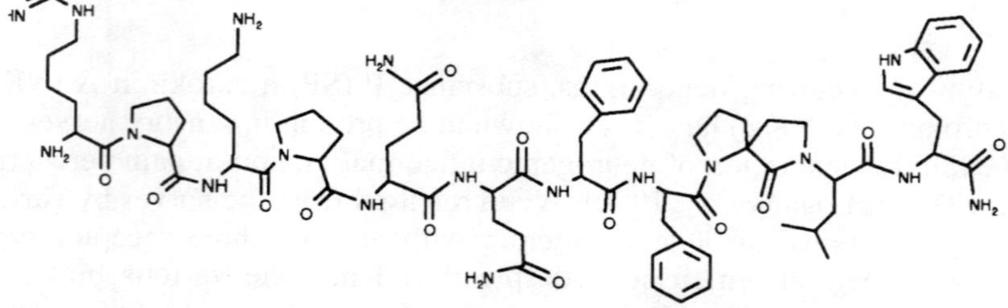

WS-9326A

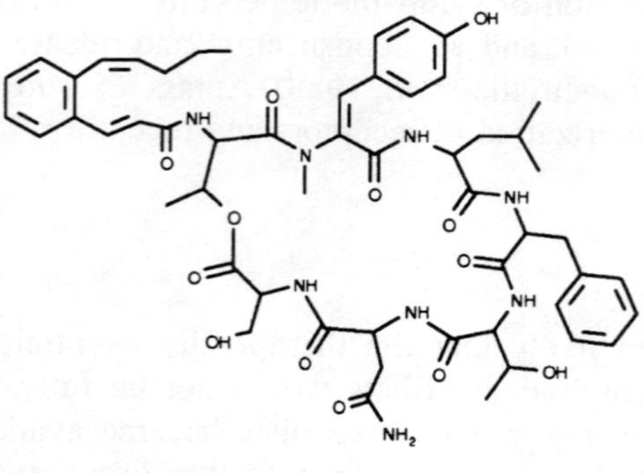

FK888

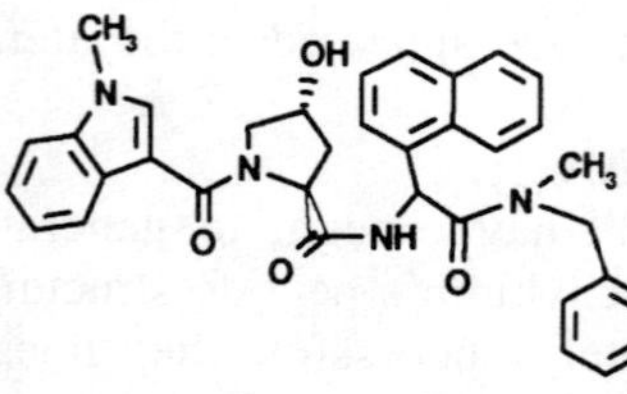

Fig. 13.6 Peptidic substance P antagonists.

Table 13.2
Amino acid sequences of second generation peptidic tachykinin receptor antagonists and their affinities (pA_2) for tachykinin NK-1, NK-2 and NK-3 receptors

Antagonists		Affinities (pA_2) NK-1 GP1	NK-2 RPA	NK-2 HT	NK-3 RPV
Linear peptides					
MEN 10,207	Asp–Tyr–D-Trp–Val–D-Trp–D-Trp–$ArgNH_2$	5.52	7.89	5.94	4.90
R 396	Ac–Leu–Asp–Gln–Trp–Phe–$GlyNH_2$	inactive	5.42	7.63	inactive
GR-94800	PhCO–Ala–Ala–D-Trp–Phe–D-Pro–Pro–$NleNH_2$	–	–	–	–
Cyclic peptides and pseudopeptides					
L 659,877	cyclo(Gln–Trp–Phe–Gly–Leu–Met)	5.60	6.72	7.92	5.40
MDL 29,913	cyclo[Gln–Trp–Phe–Gly–Leu–Psi(CH_2NCH_3)Leu]	5.37	7.77	8.65	inactive

GR-71251 (Ward *et al.*, 1990). This compound is not only a potent NK-1 receptor antagonist, but selective as well, showing no significant binding activity at NK-2 and NK-3 receptors. Two other molecules are described by workers at Fujisawa. These compounds (Fig. 13.6) retain peptidic character while dispensing with most of the sequence of SP itself: WS-9326A (Nishikawa *et al.*, 1991) and FK888 (Fujii *et al.*, 1992). This last compound, although still a tripeptide, represents a considerable simplification of the initial octapeptide lead structure.

In the case of compounds that are selective for the NK-2 receptors, the most potent antagonists (Maggi *et al.*, 1993b) are listed in Table 13.2. These compounds include some linear peptides (the derivatives of the hexapeptide NKA(4–10) MEN 10,207, R 396 and GR 94800), cyclic peptides (L 659,877), and cyclic pseudopeptides (MDL 29,913). The development of high-affinity ligands with high selectivity for the NK-2 receptor has led to the recognition of pharmacological heterogeneity in the NK-2 receptor (Maggi *et al.*, 1990; Vaissade *et al.*, 1992). It now appears obvious that the NK-2 receptors expressed in different systems recognize the above-mentioned antagonists with very different affinities. Prototypical organs which show the greatest ability to discriminate between NK-2 receptor selective antagonists are the endothelium-derived rabbit pulmonary artery (RPA) and the hamster isolated trachea (HT). The NK-2 receptor present in various preparations from various species can be classified according to antagonist affinity for either

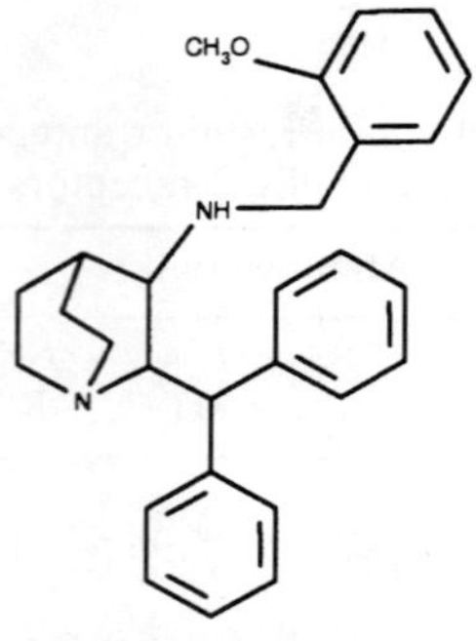

CP96345
PFIZER

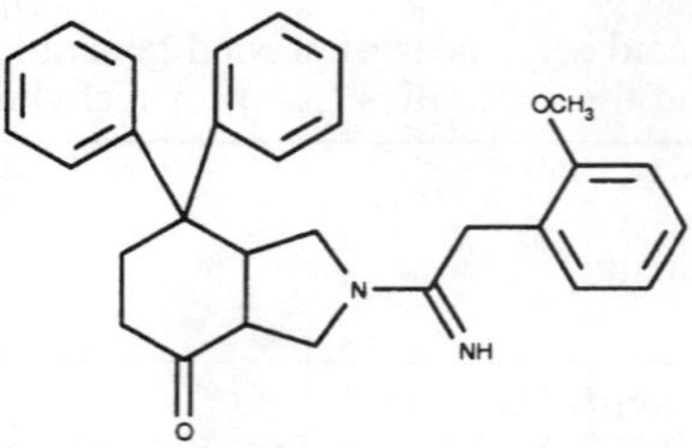

RP67580
RHONE-POULENC RORER

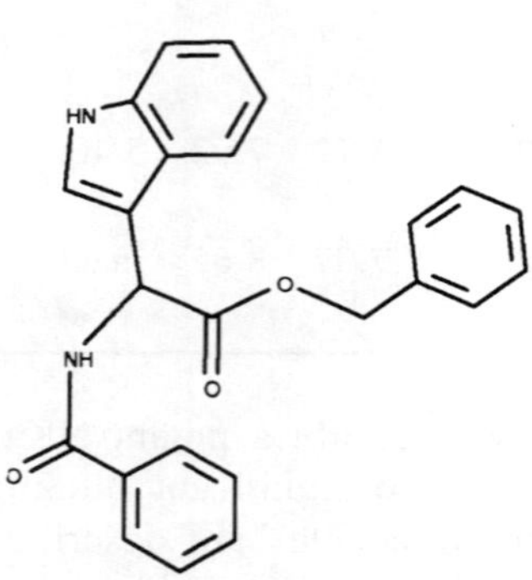

MERCK

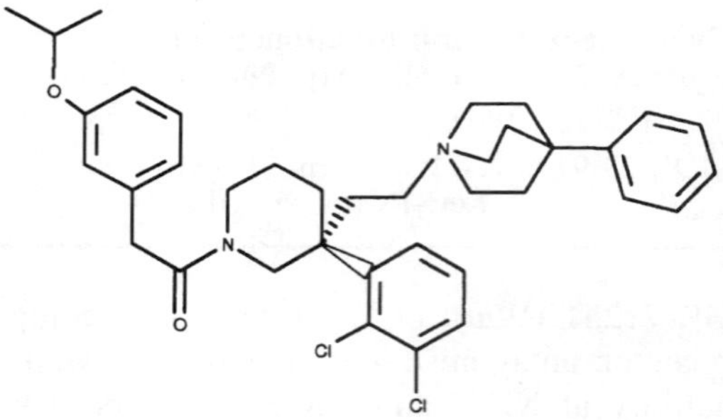

SR140333
SANOFI

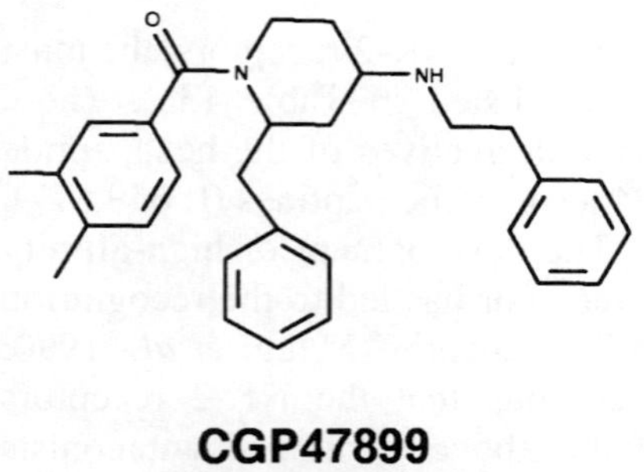

CGP47899
CIBA-GEIGY

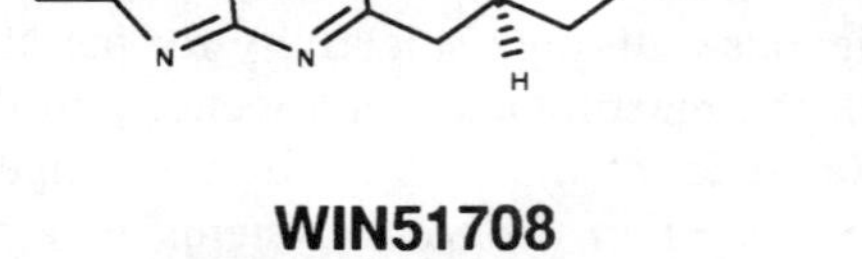

WIN51708
STERLING-WINTROP

Fig. 13.7 Non-peptidic substance P antagonists.

one of two categories which have been provisionally termed NK-2A (RPA-like) or NK-2B (HT-like). At present, it appears that such heterogeneity is largely species-dependent: thus, the pharmacological profile of the human NK-2 receptor is similar to that of bovine, guinea-pig or rabbit NK-2 receptor, but very different in terms of antagonist affinities from that of the rat or hamster NK-2 receptor (Van Giersbergen *et al.*, 1991).

Nonpeptide tachykinin antagonists

The first small molecule, non-peptide SP antagonist, CP-96345, was reported in 1991 by Pfizer (Snider *et al.*, 1991). Since then a large number of patents have appeared and reflect the considerable commercial potential of new agents in this area. Rhône-Poulenc Rorer (Garret *et al.*, 1991), Sterling Winthrop (Venepalli *et al.*, 1992; Appell *et al.*, 1992), Ciba-Geigy (Schilling *et al.*, 1993), Merck (Baker *et al.*, 1993) and Sanofi (Edmonds-Alts *et al.*, 1992) groups have described different chemical classes of non-peptide NK-1 receptor antagonists. The chemical structures are shown in Fig. 13.7. These non-peptide compounds display the profile of specific antagonists of NK-1 receptors (i.e. they are not active on NK-2 and NK-3 receptors). It appears that some antagonists bind preferentially to rat, compared with guinea-pig or human NK-1 receptors (Gitter *et al.*, 1991; Fardin and Garret, 1991; Watling *et al.*, 1991; Beresford *et al.*, 1992). These binding data therefore suggest pharmacologically distinct 'rat/mouse-type' and 'guinea-pig/human-type' NK-1 sites, although the presence of both receptor subtypes within the same species has still to be demonstrated. All these molecules have been claimed to be useful in the management of various clinical pathologies where pain and neurogenic inflammation are involved. Interestingly, in 1993 both Merck and RPR have shown that the non-peptide NK-1 receptor antagonists may have therapeutic use as anti-migraine agents (Shepheard *et al.*, 1993; Moussaoui *et al.*, 1993).

Discovery of non-peptide tachykinin receptor antagonists has not been limited to the NK-1 receptor, and recently two potent non-peptide NK-2 receptor antagonists have been unveiled (Advenier *et al.*, 1992a; Edmonds-Alts *et al.*, 1993) (Fig. 13.8). SR 48968 inhibits the binding of [^{125}I]iodohistidyl-neurokinin A to NK-2 sites present in rat duodenal membranes, with a K_i of 0.5 nM. *In vivo*, SR 48968 shows a dose-dependent inhibition of NKA-induced bronchoconstriction in the anaesthetized guinea-pig (Advenier *et al.*, 1992b; Maggi *et al.*, 1993c). It remains to be seen whether these compounds will have clinical utility in the treatment of asthma. It is also not known whether these compounds cross the blood–brain barrier or induce any CNS effects.

In summary, the efforts of several pharmaceutical companies in the past 5 years have led to the development of a number of novel ligands, either peptidic or non-peptidic, which are highly selective and potent antagonists of tachykinin receptors. It is conceivable that some of these compounds will

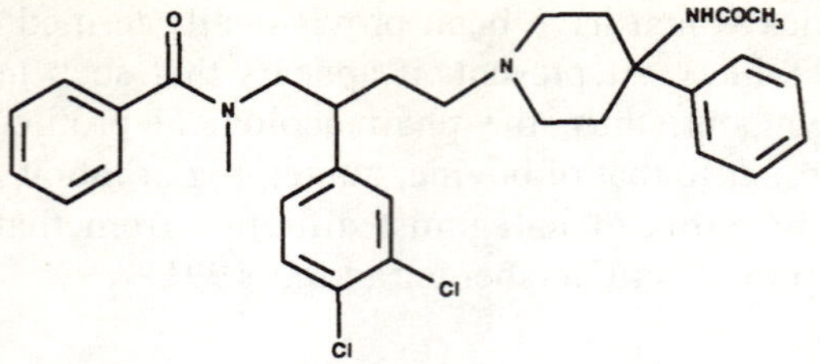

SR48968
SANOFI

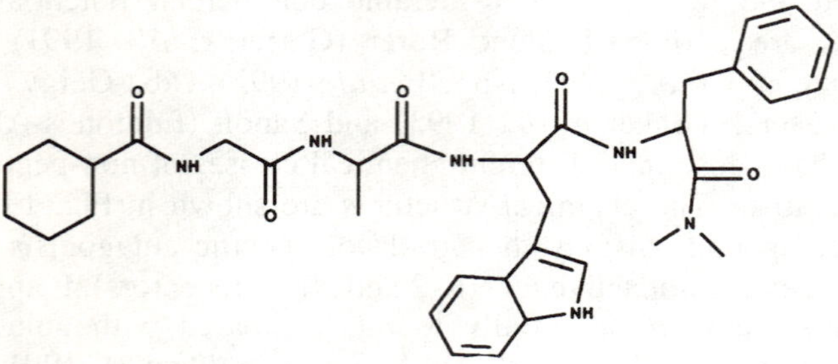

GR100679
GLAXO

Fig. 13.8 Non-peptidic neurokinin A antagonists.

be tested in humans in the near future, hopefully leading to a novel class of spasmolytic, analgesic and anti-migraine agents.

Molecular Modelling

It is widely believed that a peptide agonist might adopt a specific bioactive conformation during the receptor activation process. Conceivably, alternative conformers could bind to the receptor without initiating a response. If so, an antagonist activity might be realized in constrained peptide analogues designed to disfavour the agonist bioactive conformation.

In the following sections we describe and compare the conformational properties of some selected SP analogues (Fig. 13.9). The structural variations might provide key conformational requirements that the receptor NK-1 has for an SP analogue to be an agonist or antagonist.

Methods

Molecular dynamics simulations and other computational procedures were performed with the DISCOVER and INSIGHTII packages (Biosym

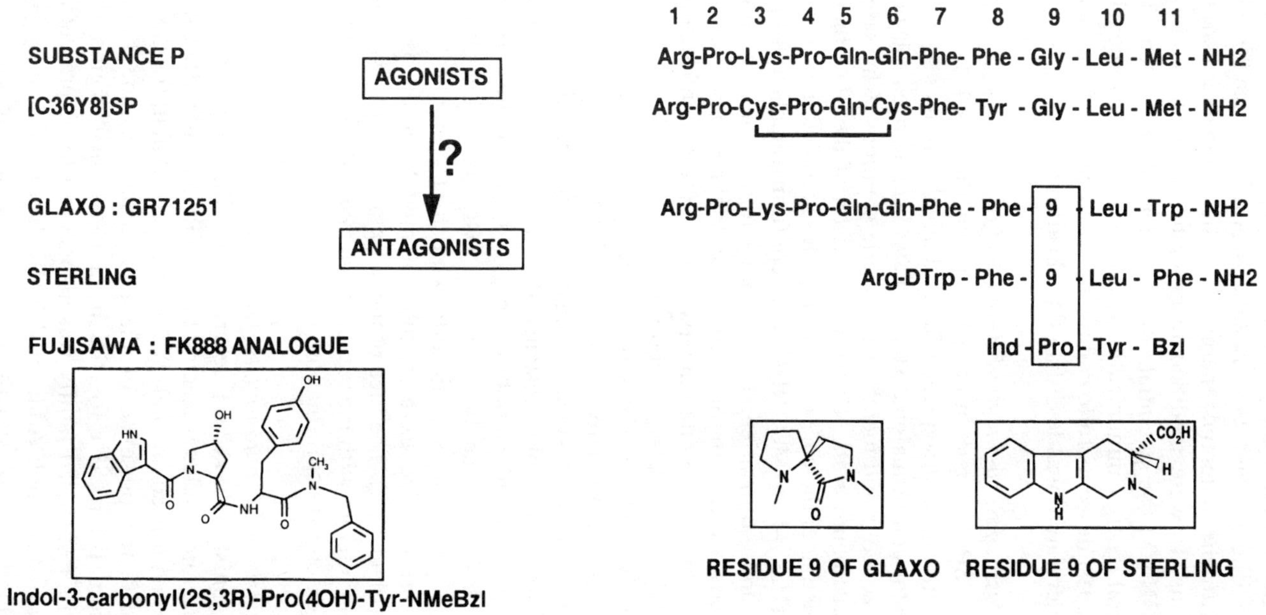

Fig. 13.9 Peptidomimetic strategy to design SP antagonists.

Technologies Inc., 10065 Barnes Canyon Rd, San Diego, CA 92121, USA) and in-house tools on Silicon Graphics workstations. A full valence force field was used to calculate the potential energy. For the simulated annealing protocol, some parameters were modified in order to avoid the amide *cis*/*trans* isomerization. No Morse potentials or cross terms were used in the simulations. In general, energy minimizations carried out *in vacuo* consisted of a few steps of steepest descents followed by the conjugate gradient method until the maximum derivative was less than 0.01 kcal/(mol Å).

Conformational analysis of SP agonists: SP and [C3,6Y8]SP
In the development of SP analogues it became obvious that residues 7–11 of substance P contain the minimal sequence for biological activity.

Various experimental conformational studies have been carried out on SP and its analogues in aqueous and membrane mimetic solutions (Chassaing *et al*., 1986; Levian-Teitelbaum *et al*., 1989). Comparison of the 3D structures have shown that in methanol the core of these peptides is folded in an α-helix. The C-terminal part, Gly–Leu–Met–NH_2 is in conformational equilibrium between α-helix, β- and γ-turn orientations. Taking into account these conformational characteristics and in order to better define these structural features and to have more accurate understanding of the conformational behaviour of the Gly–Leu–Met–NH_2 portion, we have carried out a restrained molecular dynamics analysis of the equipotent cyclic analogue [C3,6Y8]SP. Being conformationally constrained by the disulphide bridge in the central core region, it provides a valuable probe into the bioactive conformation of the linear, flexible substance P. The conformational search yielded two main structural families (poly-C7 and U-shape) for the C-terminal Gly–Leu–Met–NH_2. From the analysis of the NMR data, the measured interproton distances agree more significantly with the C7 than with the U conformation. These results led us to propose a model for the bioactive conformation of SP (Plate 13.2). The face of the helix bearing the two critical phenylalanines should interact with the receptor, whereas Gly–Leu–Met–NH_2 could adopt a more extended conformation.

Conformational analysis of SP antagonists: Glaxo and Fujisawa
The potent SP antagonist (GR-71251) described by Glaxo contains a constrained (*S*)-spiro-γ-lactam residue replacing the SP Gly residue. MD calculations were performed on this compound. We have observed that, for the main conformational family, the presence of the spirolactam residue forces a reverse turn (structure β-turn II′) for the hexa C-terminal region (Plate 13.2). However a minor extended family was also shown to be present even though energetically disfavoured. Additional NMR data published by Glaxo provide us with a better definition of the major orientations of the relevant side chains (Phe7, Phe8 and Trp11). From the constrained MD analysis we can observe that the Phe8 residue near the spirolactam is the least mobile

whereas the other aromatic residues Phe7 and Trp11 adopt distinct orientations with a geometric relationship between the corresponding torsion angles ϕ, ψ and χ_1. The average structure, from constrained MD, with the largest population of the side chain rotamers is shown in Plate 13.3. This structure was used in the superimposition model involving the FK888 analogue antagonist.

The conformation of the smallest fragment SP antagonist (FK888 analogue) has been characterized by 2D-NMR and restrained MD studies. The free MD calculation leads to several families equally populated which are stabilized by different aromatic–aromatic pair interactions (Ind–Tyr, Ind–NMeBzl, Tyr–NMeBzl). In an attempt to discriminate between these conformational families, restrained MD conformational search was used to identify the probable backbone conformations and the spatial orientations of the essential components of the FK888 analogue. We have established that the proline residue induces in almost all conformations a γ-turn characterized by the hydrogen bond CO_{Ind}–NH_{Tyr}. The orientation of the indole group is then precisely defined. The main aromatic–aromatic pair interaction occurs between the Ind and Tyr groups. Two orientations (χ_1 torsion angle) remain possible for the Bzl and Tyr side chains (Plate 13.4).

The two SP antagonists GR-71251 and FK888 analogue, were then compared to elucidate conformational features of the bioactive conformation (Plate 13.5). The overall topology of the two active analogues is very similar in the constrained region. There are small differences in the ϕ and ψ of the side chain rotamers, but the general spatial arrangement of these important side chains is similar. The major difference is the presence of an aromatic substituent in the FK888 analogue fitting on the Leu10 position of GR71251. This may explain the better affinity of the FK888 analogue compound.

Comparison of the agonist and antagonist conformations

From the structure–activity data of spiro-γ-lactam analogues, it has been shown that the conservative modifications of Phe7 and Phe8 substantially reduced antagonist activity. However, considerable structural variation of the C-terminal residues was tolerated with a trend toward increasing activity according to increasing size and lipophilicity. This is in contrast to the marked reductions in agonist activity caused by the same substitutions and suggested that the antagonists adopt a different receptor binding mode.

A comparison between agonist and antagonist conformational families has shown that the antagonist activity may be due to a particular secondary structure of the C-terminal region of the peptide chain. Plate 13.6, which shows ϕ–ψ plots of the 9 and 10 residue conformations generated for the SP agonists and antagonists, illustrates two of the key results of this study. First, for SP agonist analogues the spread of the structures for Gly9 is extremely large. This can clearly be seen in the Ramachandran plots. The ϕ_9 dihedral angle adopts a wide range of values; the ψ_9 angle shows some dispersion although the values are centred about $-60°$ and $+60°$. In the case of the SP antagonist GR-71251 the spirolactam locks the residue 9 backbone in a narrow region of the conformational ϕ,ψ map centred at $+60°$ and $-120°$. The constrained (*S*)-spiro-γ-lactam restricts the ϕ_9 and ψ_9 torsion angles to values which are quite close to those of an ideal type-II′ β-turn ($\phi_2 = -120°$) (Genin *et al.*, 1993). Second, for both SP analogues the greatest range of values are found for residue 10. We can roughly divide the ϕ,ψ values into four different families of conformations.

In summary, the results of the present study show that the constrained residue (*S*)-spiro-γ-lactam of the SP antagonist GR71521 induces a reverse turn (structure β-turn II′) for the hexa C-terminal region and excludes an extended conformation, which seems necessary for agonist activity. This reverse turn seems to be a prerequisite for antagonist activity.

In order to check this assumption, we have looked for β-turn mimics which could enforce this particular conformation.

β-*Turn mimics of SP antagonists*

The ability of a proline residue to define the $i + 1$ position of β-turns is one of the possibilities. Indeed, the principal conformation-determining feature of proline is the pyrrolidine ring restriction of the backbone dihedral angle ϕ to the 50–90° range, the sign being negative for L-proline and positive for D-proline. In most classes of β-turns, the ϕ_{i+1} and the ϕ_{i+2} angles are both in the +/− (50–90°) range. Therefore, two successive prolines of opposite stereochemical configuration ought to be a stronger turn determinant for peptides (Bean *et al.*, 1992). As part of a collaboration between us and A. Marquet (Paris VI University) the turn-determining sequence D-Pro–L-Pro was inserted in the 9–10 position of SP (Chassaing *et al.*, 1992).

At Rhône-Poulenc Rorer (RPR), we have proposed the synthesis of another, proprietary, scaffold devoid of peptidic character and designed to force without ambiguity this secondary structure. It has also been inserted into this critical position. MD calculations have confirmed that the two β-turn mimics induce effectively the expected structure (Plate 13.7). The resulting peptidomimics ([D-Pro9, Pro10, Trp11]SP and RPRPEP1), although less potent in binding on rat brain (RB) and IM9 receptor preparations, were found to be antagonists in the guinea-pig ileum bioassay (Table 13.3). However, these compounds lack a functional group at the key corner residue i+1. As pointed out before, the presence of a hydrophobic group properly oriented in position 10 appears to be important for binding potency. Analogues carrying this hydrophobic group were then synthesized ([D-Pro9, tβ-BPr10, Trp11]SP and RPRPEP2). Such compounds have the potential not only to mimic the change in chain direction of a peptide turn, but also to elicit a response from a receptor that might recognize the side-chain group of the exposed corner residue. Both new analogues present a very significant increase in affinity and in antagonist activity (Table 13.3) (Lavielle *et al.*,

Table 13.3
Antagonist activities and affinities of peptidomimetic SP antagonists

	Antagonists	Antagonist activities IC_{50} (nM)	Affinities IC_{50} (nM)	
		SP	RB	IM9
Peptidomimetic molecules	GR71251	78	7 000	200
	FK888 analogue	30	3 000	40
	[D-Pro9, Pro10, Trp11]SP	10 000	10 000	10 000
	[D-Pro9, tβ-BPr10, Trp11]SP	21[a]	–	20[a]
	RPRPEP1	2 000	7 000	2 500
	RPRPEP2	2.8	18	0.4
Non-peptide molecules	RPR100893	25	2 200	13
	CP96345	0.4	50	0.5

[a] Data from Lavielle *et al.*, 1994
RB = Rat brain; IM9 = Human cell line.

1993, 1994). The conformationally restricted RPR scaffold has given the most potent peptidomimetic SP antagonist described so far [RPRPEP2:IC_{50} = 0.4 nM in a human cell line (IM9)].

From these studies, we can conclude that the structure of agonists could not be used for the elucidation of the bioactive conformation of their corresponding antagonists, since they adopt different conformations and therefore may bind in a different way or to different sites on the receptor.

Building a Specific 3D Database of Amino Acid-like Compounds

During the last 3 years a formidable explosion has occurred in the synthesis of rigid amino acid-like scaffolds. The growing number of successful examples in the peptidomimetic field (Fig. 13.10) and the advances of search techniques in 3D structure databases have led us to develop a rational procedure to select specific molecular templates or building blocks. Substructure search using the available commercial and corporate 2D and 3D databases can be used to select building blocks showing the widest structural and physico-chemical diversities in order to build a specific database. This database will allow the identification of interesting scaffolds for synthesis using 3D queries. Such an approach has been applied to the building of an amino acid-like database which can be exploited in the peptidomimetic approach and in the generation of modified peptide libraries. Using ISIS and MACCS-II system software

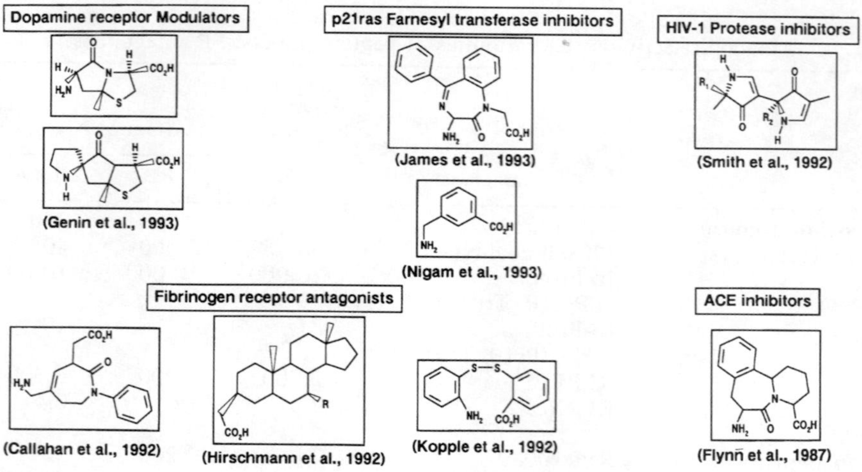

Fig 13.10 Some building blocks used in peptidomimetics.

from Molecular Design Ltd (MDL), a refined query containing a nitrogen and a carboxyl group provided a list of 5525 structures from commercial 3D databases (CMC, FCD and MDDR) and 4758 from the RPR database. Clustering techniques and in-house programs were developed to reduce the size of structural data before visual analysis. The clustering of this database using a similarity index and substructure search has already been performed whilst clustering using a flexibility index is in hand.

This AALIKE database has been used to identify interesting structures for the design of a bradykinin antagonist. These structures could be used to induce the β-turn observed from the molecular dynamics calculations performed on the potent B2 bradykinin antagonist HOE_140::D-Arg–Arg–Pro–Hyp–Gly–Thi–Ser–D-Tic–L-Oic–Arg, (Hyp = 4-hydroxyproline; Thi = Thienyl-2-alanine; D-Tic = tetrahydroisoquinoline carboxylic acid; Oic = octahydroindole carboxylic acid). Some structures have been selected and the synthesis of the corresponding peptidomimetics is planned (Plate 13.8).

Conclusions and Perspectives

In conclusion, this example of design and prediction of a very active compound using a peptidomimetic approach combined with molecular dynamics calculations shows the powerful potential of this strategy. It is expected that such a strategy will have more general application in the logical and efficient design of antagonists at other peptide receptors.

Recently, the conjunction of new approaches has provided tools for improving productivity in the drug discovery process. Advances in robotics, miniaturization and automation make possible simultaneous synthesis to generate libraries of organic compounds. To achieve the synthesis of specific libraries with the widest structural and physico-chemical diversities, the available chemical fragments, or building blocks have to be selected on a rational basis. Scientists can use 3D searching software capabilities and available 3D databases to select the desired building blocks. We have applied such an approach to the building of an amino acid-like database (AALIKE) allowing the identification of exotic residues which can be used in the peptidomimetic methodology and for the generation of modified peptide libraries.

This approach may be extended to build other specific molecular scaffold databases from which selected target compounds could be used for the next generation of chemical libraries.

Acknowledgements

The authors wish to express their thanks to V. Fardin and her group for providing the biological data; to G. Dutruc-Rosset, C. Nemecek and F. Clerc for the chemical and peptide syntheses; to F. Herman, D. Frechet, M. Robin and M. Vuilhorgne for NMR studies; to G. Chassaing and S. Lavielle (Paris VI University) for their valuable collaboration; to J.M. Paris and J.F. Peyronel for fruitful discussions and to Y. Ribeil and C. Burns for their critical reading of the manuscript.

References

Adang, A.E.P, Hermkens, P.H.H, Linders, J.T.M, Ottenheijm, H.C. and van Staveren, C.J. (1994). *Recl. Trav. Chim. Pays-Bas.* **113**, 63–78.

Advenier, C., Edmonds-Alt, X., Vilain, P., Goulaouic, P., Proietto, V., Van Broeck, D., Naline, E., Neliat, G., Le Fur, G. and Brelière, J.C. (1992a). *Br. J. Pharmacol.* **105**, 77P.

Advenier, C., Rouissi, N., Nguyen, Q.T., Edmonds-Alt, X., Brelière, J.-C., Neliat, G. Naline, E. and Regoli, D. (1992b). *Biochem. Biophys. Res. Commun.* **184**, 1418–1424.

Appell, K.C., Fragale, B.J., Lpscig, J., Singh, S. and Tomczuc, B.E. (1992). *Mol. Pharmacol.* **41**, 772–778.

Avbelj, F., Moult, J., Kitson, D.H., James, M.N.G. and Hagler, A.T. (1990). *Biochemistry* **29**, 8658–8676.

Baker, R., Macleod, A., Merchant, K. and Swain, C. (1993). WO Patent 93/01169.

Ball, J.B. and Alewood P.F. (1990). *J. Mol. Recogn.* **3**, 55–64.

Bean, J.W., Kopple, D.K. and Peishoff, C.E. (1992). *J. Am. Chem. Soc.* **114**, 5328–5334.

Beresford, I.J.M., Birch, P.J., Hagan, R.M. and Ireland, S.J. (1992). *Br. J. Pharmacol.* **104**, 292–293.

Borman, S. (1992). *Sci. Technol.* **10**, 18–26.

Boublik, J.H., Scott, N., Taulane, J., Goodman, M., Brown, M. and Rivier, J. (1989). *Int. J. Pept. Protein Res.* **33**, 11–15.

Braun, W. and Go, N. (1985). *J. Mol. Biol.* **186**, 611–626.

Brunger, A.T., Kuriyan, J. and Karplus, M. (1987). *Science,* **235**, 458–460.

Bunin, B.A. and Ellman, J.A. (1992). *J. Am. Chem. Soc.* **114**, 10997–10998.

Callahan, J.F., Bean, J.W., Burgess, J.L., Eggleston, D.S., Hwang, S.M., Kopple, K.D., Koster, P.F., Nichols, A., Peishoff, C.E., Samanen, J.M., Vasko, J.A., Wong, A. and Huffman, W.F. (1992). *J. Med. Chem.* **35**, 3970–3972.

Chassaing, G., Convert, O. and Lavielle, S. (1986). *Eur. J. Biochem.* **154**, 77–85.

Chassaing, G., Brunissen, A., Carruette, A., Garret, C., Petitet, F., Saffroy, M., Beaujouan, J.C., Torrens, Y. and Glowinski, J. (1992). *Neuropeptides.* **23**, 73–79.

Chou, P.Y. and Fasman, G.D. (1977). *J. Mol. Biol.* **115**, 135–175.

Crippen, G.M. (1981). *In* 'Distance Geometry and Conformational Calculations' (D. Bawden, ed.). Research Studies Press, John Wiley, New York.

Degrado, W.F. (1988). *Adv. Protein. Chem.* **39**, 51–124.

Diaz, H., Espina, J.R. and Kelly, F.J.W. (1992). *J. Am. Chem. Soc.* **114**, 8316–8318.

Dinola, A., Berendsen, H.J.C. and Edholm, O. (1984). *Macromolecules.* **17**, 2044–2050.

Dutta, A.S. (1987). *Drugs of the Future,* **12**, 781–792.

Dutta, A.S. (1991). *In* 'Advances in Drug Research' (B. Testa, ed.), vol. 21, pp. 145–286. Academic Press, London.

Dyson, H.J., Cross, K.J., Houghten, R.A., Wilson, I.A., Wright, P.E. and Lerner, R.A. (1985). *Nature.* **318**, 480–483.

Edmonds-Alts, X., Guele, P., Proietto, V. and Van Broeck, D. (1992) FR. Patent 2,696,178.

Edmonds-Alts, X., Proietto, V., Van Broeck, D., Vilain, P., Advenier, C., Neliat, G., Le Fur, G. and Brelière, J.C. (1993). *Biorg. Med. Chem. Lett.* **3**, 925–930.

Elber, R., and Karplus, M. (1988). *Science.* **235**, 318–321.

Fardin, V. and Garret, C. (1991). *Eur. J. Pharmacol.* **201**, 231–234.

Fauchere, J.L. (1987). *In* 'QSAR in Drug Design and Toxicology' (D. Hadzi and B. Jerman-Blazic, eds), pp. 221–230. Elsevier Science Publishers, Amsterdam.

Feigel, M. (1986). *J. Am. Chem. Soc.*, **108**, 181–182.

Fesik, S.W. (1991). *J. Am. Chem. Soc.* **34**, 2937–2945.

Flynn, G.A., Giroux, E.L. and Dage, R.C. (1987). *J. Am. Chem. Soc.* **109**, 7914–7915.

Folkers, K., Rosell, S., Hakanson, R., Chu, J.L., Lu, L.A., Leander, S., Tang, P.F.L. and Ljungqvist, A. (1985). *In* 'Tachykinin Antagonists' (R. Hakanson and F. Sundler, eds), pp. 259–266. Elsevier, Amsterdam.

Fujii, T., Murai, M., Morimoto, H., Maeda, Y., Yamaoka, M., Hagiwara, D., Miyake, H., Ikari, N. and Matsuo, M. (1992). *Br. J. Pharmacol.* **107**, 785–789.

Garret, C., Carruette, A., Fardin, V., Moussaoui, S., Peyronel, J.F., Blanchard, J.C. and Laduron, P.M. (1981). *Proc. Natl Acad. Sci. USA* **88**, 10208–10212.

Genin, M., Ojala, W.H., Gleason, W.B. and Johnson, L.R. (1993). *J. Org. Chem.* **58**, 2334–2337.

Giannis, A. and Kolter, T. (1993). *Angew. Chem. Int. Ed. Engl.* **32**, 1244–1267.

Gitter, B.D., Waters, D.C., Bruns, R.F., Mason, N.R., Nixon, J.A. and Howbert, J.J. (1991). *Eur. J. Pharmacol.* **191**, 237–238.

Hinds, M.G., Richards, N.G.J. and Robinson, J.A. (1988). *J. Chem. Soc. Chem. Commun.*, 1447–1449.
Hirschmann, R. (1991). *Angew. Chem. Int. Ed. Engl.* **30**, 1278–1301.
Hirschmann, R., Sprengeler, P.A., Kawasaki, T., Leahy, J.W., Shakespeare, W.C. and Smith, A.B. (1992). *J. Am. Chem. Soc.* **114**, 9699–9701.
Holzemann, G. (1991). *Kontakte.* **1**, 3–12.
Hruby, V.J. (1987). *Trends Pharmacol. Sci.* **8**, 336–339.
Hruby, V.J., Al-Obeidi, F. and Kazmierski, W. (1990). *Biochem. J.* **268**, 249–262.
James, G.L., Goldstein, J.L., Brown, M.S., Rawson, T.E., Somers, T.C., McDowell, M.S., Crowley, C.W., Lucas, B.K., Levinson, A.D. and Marsters, J.C. (1993). *Science* **260**, 1937–1942.
Kahn, M. and Chen, B. (1987). *Tetrahedron Lett.* **28**, 1623–1626.
Karpen, E.M., Tobias, J.D. and Brooks, C.L. (1993). *Biochemistry* **32**, 412–420.
Karplus, M. and McCammon, J.A. (1983). *Annu. Rev. Biochem.* **52**, 263–300.
Kemp, D.S. (1990). *Tibtech.* **8**, 249–255.
Kessler, H., (1982). *Angew. Chem.* **94**, 509–520.
Kopple, K.D., Baures, P.W., Bean, J.W., D'Ambrosio, C.A., Peishoff, C.E. and Eggleston, D.S. (1992). *J. Am. Chem. Soc.* **114**, 9615–9623.
Krstenansky, J.L., Baranowsky, R.L. and Currie, B.L. (1982). *Biochem. Biophys. Res. Commun.* **109**, 1368–1374.
Laneuville, O., Dorais, J. and Couture, R. (1988). *Life. Sci.* **42**, 1295–1305.
Lavielle, S., Brunissen, A., Rodriguez, M., Martinez, J., Convert, O., Carruette, A., Garret, C. Petitet, F., Saffroy, M., Torrens, Y., Beaujouan, J.-C. and Glowinski, J. (1993). *Int. J. Peptide. Protein Res.* **42**, 270–277.
Lavielle, S., Brunissen, A., Carruette, A., Garret, C. and Chassaing, G. (1994). 'Neuropeptides Fourth Meeting of the European Neuropeptide Club', vol. **26**, suppl. 1, p. 31, 13–15 April, Strasbourg, France.
Lembeck, F. and Holzer, P. (1979). *Naunyn-Schmiedeberg's Arch. Pharamacol.* **310**, 155–183.
Levian-Teitelbaum, D., Kolodny, N., Chorev, M., Selinger, Z., Gilon, C. (1989). *Biopolymers.* **28**, 51–64.
Logan, E.M., Goswami, R., Tomczuc, B.E., and Venepalli, B.R. (1990). *Annu. Report. Med. Chem.* **26**, 43–51.
Maggi, C.A., Patacchini, R., Giuliani, S. (1990). *Brit. J. Pharmacol.* **100**, 588–664.
Maggi, C.A., Patacchini, R., Rovero, P., Giachetti, A. (1993a). *J. Autonom. Pharmacol.* **13**, 1–70.
Maggi, C.A., Quartara, L., Giuliani, S. and Patacchini, R. (1993b). *Drugs of the Future.* **18**, 155–158.
Maggi, C.A., Patacchini, R., Giuliani, S. and Giachetti, A. (1993c). *Eur. J. Pharmacol.* **234**, 83–90.
Mark, A.E., and van Gunsteren, W.F. (1992). *Biochemistry* **31**, 7745–7748.
Martin, Y.C. (1992). *J. Med. Chem.* **35**, 2147–2154.
McCammon, J.A. and Harvey, S.C. (1987). 'Dynamics of Proteins and Nucleic Acids'. Cambridge University Press, Cambridge.
McKelvey, D.R., Brooks, C.L. and Mokotoff, M. (1991). *J. Protein. Chem.* **10**, 265–271.
Meirovitch, H., Kitson, H.D. and Hagler, T.D. (1992). *J. Am. Chem. Soc.* **114**, 5386–5399.
Miklavc, A., Kocjan, D., Avbelj, F., Hadzi, D. (1987). *In* 'QSAR in Drug Design and Toxicology' (D. Hadzi and B. Jerman-Blazic, eds), pp. 185–190. Elsevier Science Publishers, Amsterdam.
Milner-White, E.J. (1989). *Trends Pharmacol. Sci.* **10**, 70–74.

Moussaoui, S.M., Phillipe, L., Le Prado, N. and Garret, C. (1993). *Eur. J. Pharmacol.* **238**, 421–424.

Nagai, U. and Sato. K. (1984). *Tetrahedron Lett.* **26**, 647–650.

Nigam, M., Seong, C.-M., Qian, Y., Hamilton, A.D. and Sebti, S.M. (1993). *J. Biol. Chem.* **268**, 20695–20698.

Nishikawa, L.M., Kino, T., Yamashita, M., Esaki, M., Kiyoto, S., Fujii, T., Okuhara, M., Kohsaka, M., and Imanaka, H. (1991). '*Annual Meeting of the Society for Industrial Microbiology*' p. 14, 4–9 August, Philadelphia.

O'Donnell, M., Garippa, R.J., O'Neill, N.C. and Bolin, D.R. (1991). *J. Biol. Chem.* **266**, 6389–6392.

Olson, G.L., Bolin, D.R., Bonner, D.R., Bos, M., Cook, M.C., Fry, D.C., Graves, B.J., Hatada, M., Hill, D.E., Kahn, M., Madison, V.S., Rusiecki, V.K., Sarabu, R., Sepinwall, J., Vincent, G.P. and Voss, M.E. (1993). *J. Med. Chem.* **36**, 3040–3049.

Ondetti, M.A., Pluscec, J., Sabo, E.F., Sheehan, J.T. and Williams, N. (1970). *J. Am. Chem. Soc.* **92**, 195–199.

Pernow, B. (1983). *Pharmacol. Rev.* **35**, 85–141.

Polinsky, A., Goodman, M., Williams, K.A. and Deber, C.M. (1992). *Biopolymers.* **32**, 399–406.

Rooman, M.J., Rodriguez, J. and Wodak, S.J. (1990). *J. Mol. Biol.* **213**, 327–336.

Rose, G.D., Gierasch, L.M. and Smith, J.A. (1985). *Adv. Protein. Chem.* **37**, 1–109.

Schilling, W., Bittiger, H., Brugger, F., Criscione, L., Hauser, K., Ofner, S., Olpe, H.-R., Vassout, A. and Veenstra, S. (1993). *In* 'Perspectives in Medicinal Chemistry' (B. Testa, E. Kyburz, W. Fuhrer and R. Giger, eds). pp. 207–220, VHCA, Basel.

Schmidt, G. (1986). *Top. Curr. Chem.* **136**, 109–159.

Schwyzer, R. (1985). *Ann. N.Y. Acad. Sci.* **297**, 3–26.

Seto, C.T. and Bartlett, P.A. (1994). *In* 'New Advances in Peptidomimetics and Small Molecule Design', Meeting 23–25 March, vol. 1, Philadelphia, USA.

Shepheard, S.L., Williamson, D.J., Hill, R.G. and Hargreaves, R.J. (1993). *Brit. J. Pharmacol.* **108**, 11–12.

Shigematsu, N., Hayashi, K., Kayakiri, N., Takase, S., Hashimoto, M. and Tanaka, H.J. (1993). *Org. Chem.* **58**, 170–175.

Smith, J.A. and Pease, L.G. (1980). *Crit. Rev. Biochem.* **8**, 315–399.

Smith, P.E., Al-Obeidi, F. and Pettitt, M.B. (1991). *Methods Enzymol.* **202**, 411–437.

Smith, A.B., Keenan, T.P., Holcomb, R.C., Sprengeler, P.A., Guzman, M.C., Wood, J.L., Carroll, P.J. and Hirschmann, R. (1992). *J. Am. Chem. Soc.* **114**, 10672–10674.

Snider, R.M., Constantine, J.W., Lowe III, J.A., Longo, K.P., Lebel, W.S., Woody, H.A., Drozda, S.E., Desai, M.C., Vinick, F.J., Spencer, R.W. and Hess, H.J. (1991). *Science.* **251**, 435–437.

Soman, K.V., Karimi, A. and Case, D.A. (1991). *Biopolymers.* **31**, 1351–1361.

Tilton, R.F., Singh, U.C., Kuntz, I.D. and Kollman, P.A. (1988). *J. Mol. Biol.* **199**, 195–211.

Tobias, D.J., Mertz, J.E. and Brooks, C.L. (1991). *Biochemistry* **30**, 6054–6058.

Turk, J., Panse, G.T. and Marshall, G.R. (1975). *J. Org. Chem.* **40**, 953–955.

Vaissade, F., Jolly, A., Fallourd, A., Boniface, O., Mercken, L., Crespo, A. and Fardin, V. (1992). *Fund. Clin. Pharmacol.* **6**, p209.

Van Giersbergen, P.L.M., Shtazer, S.A. and Henderson, A.K. (1991). *Proc. Natl Acad. Sci. USA* **88**, 1661–1665.

van Gunsteren, W.F. and Berendsen, H.J.C. (1990). *Angew. Chem. Int. Ed. Engl.* **29**, 992–1023.

van Gunsteren, W.F. and Mark, A. (1992). *Eur. J. Biochem.* **204**, 947–961.

van Gunsteren, W.F., Gros, P., Torda, A.E., Berendsen, H.J.C. and van Schaik, R.C.

(1991). *In* 'Protein conformation' (F.M. Richards, ed.), pp. 150–166, Wiley-Interscience, London.
Veber, D.F., Holly, F.W., Paleveda, W.J., Nutt, R.F., Bergstrand, S.J., Tochiana, M., Giltzer, M.S. and Saperstein, R. (1979). *Nature.* **280**, 512–514.
Venepalli, B.R., Bell, M.R. and Yanni, J.M. (1992). *J. Med. Chem.* **35**, 374–378.
Ward, P., Ewan, G.B., Jordan, C.C., Ireland, S.J., Hagan, R.M. and Brown, J.R. (1990). *J. Med. Chem.* **33**, 1848–1851.
Watling, K.J. and Krause, J.E. (1993). *Trends Pharmacol. Sci.* **14**, 81–84.
Watling, K.J., Guard, S., Howson, W. and Walton, L. (1991). *Brit. J. Pharmacol.* **104**, p27.
Wiley, A.R. and Rich, D.H. (1993). *Medicinal Research Reviews.* **13**, 327–384.
Wilmot, C.M. and Thornton, J.M. (1988). *J. Mol. Biol.* **203**, 221–232.
Wilmot, C.M. and Thornton, J.M. (1990). *Protein Eng.* **3**, 479–493.
Wuthrich, K. (1986). *In* 'NMR of Proteins and Nucleic Acids', John Wiley, New York.
Zarandi, M., Penke, B., Varga, J. and Kovacs, K. (1983). *In* 'Peptides 1982' (K. Blaha and P. Malon, eds), pp. 577–581. Walter de Gruyter, Berlin.

Discussion

A.R. Leach
Was the database searching that was used to find alternatives to these peptidomimetics a 3D flexible database search?

A. Laoui
Yes, ultimately. It is important to distinguish two different steps in this work. First, we generated the 3D AALIKE database, considering a query with the amino and carboxy groups which identified the requisite amino acids present in the commercial and corporate databases. Second, according to a pharmacophore query including the amino and carboxy groups, we performed a classical 3D search in the 3D AALIKE database to seek the right building blocks.

A.R. Leach
It could perhaps be envisaged that if we are looking for conformationally rigid building blocks, we might want not only to be able to do a flexible search but also to take into account the number of range of conformations of flexibility of that particular molecule.

A. Laoui
Yes, of course. As I showed in the bradykinin example, to identify mimetics of the Tic and Oic residues we have performed a flexible 3D search to take into account the problem of flexibility.

J.S. Mason
That is important, and it is why we need to have flexibility – so we know that if something is found, it can fit in other ways. It is why we like to have the multiple conformational answer, because then we know whether it is just a single or multiple hits.

A.R. Leach
My point was more that in these cases, as I understand it, you seem to be looking for molecules that fit the particular turn or whatever it might be, but ideally that would be the only conformation that was adopted. Is this something you can do, or have done, or have you any comment?

J.S. Mason
It is something that is in the design process.

S. Clementi
I was involved in a study on the agonist and antagonist activity of peptides to the NK-2 receptor. In this case, chemometrically speaking, we were trying to have a discriminant plot between activity and inactivity. Apparently, the main factor was a change at the 5-position, changing serine to tyrosine. Do you think such a small change in structure can explain such a change in activity, for example in terms of change between an extended and a turned conformation?

A. Laoui
Yes, I think so. D.H. Rich has described an interesting theory called 'hydrophobic collapse'. Introduction of such hydrophobic groups as aromatic rings can cause 'collapse' of protein structures, changing markedly the backbone conformations. In the case of SP, the antagonist character is clearly dependent on the presence of aromatic residues in some critical positions. So, I do believe that even a small change, like the replacement of serine by tyrosine, could be responsible for a switch between agonist and antagonist activity.

14

Modelling and Chemometrics in Medicinal Chemistry

S. CLEMENTI, G. CRUCIANI, D. RIGANELLI and R. VALIGI

Laboratorio di Chemiometria, Dipartimento di Chimica, Università di Perugia, Via Elce di Sotto, 10; 06123 Perugia, Italy

Introduction

Chemometrics and molecular modelling were used, until a few years ago, as separate tools for drug design (Jolles and Wooldridge, 1982), both aimed at providing a better understanding of the structural features affecting the biological response. On the one hand, chemometrics represents the statistical support for quantitative structure–activity relationship (QSAR) studies, along the tradition opened by Hansch, by means of analogy constants, some 30 years ago (Hansch and Leo, 1979; Kubinyi, 1993a): QSARs derive information, encoded in numbers, by empirical models comparing the properties of a number of molecules. On the other hand, molecular modelling techniques, based on theoretical grounds, allow us to study individual molecules in 3D space by several different approaches, in order to identify sites and types of favourable interactions.

It was only in recent years that these two approaches have been brought together in a unique procedure, called comparative molecular field analysis (CoMFA) (Cramer *et al.*, 1988a), which made available to the scientific community the rapidly moving field of 3D-QSAR (Kubinyi, 1993b). In this chapter, we will briefly cover some notable aspects of chemometrics in the traditional QSAR area, the merits of its developments for handling 3D-QSAR

New Perspectives in Drug Design
ISBN 0–12–208070–X

models and the latest efforts presently carried out to solve new problems continuously appearing.

Chemometric Strategies in Traditional QSAR

Developing a QSAR for a given problem is useful since it gives us information on how changes in the structure of the actual compounds influence their biological activity, which allows us to modify the structure in order to improve the biological response (Wold, 1991). Therefore, there are two main objectives in QSAR studies: (1) interpretation, i.e., understanding the actual biological mechanism and what structural features affect the response, and (2) prediction, i.e. estimating the activity of new compounds before they become available.

The requirements of a chemometric tool aimed at these objectives have been described several times (Wold and Dunn, 1983; Dunn and Wold, 1990; Wold, 1991, 1993; Wold *et al.*, 1991, 1993a; Clementi *et al.*, 1991). A correct problem formulation and the fact that data contain information relevant to the problem are usually more important than the chemometric method selected to carry out the statistical computations. For handling QSAR problems 'expert systems' seem to be less suitable than general tools aimed at extracting and visualizing the hidden information, according to the user's needs.

Chemometrics in QSAR was derived from a physical organic chemistry background, since the traditional QSAR approach uses parameters for small chemical groups called substituents. They are analogy parameters and their use implies the assumption that the substituent effect in a reference reaction is somehow proportional to that in the investigated system.

Similarly, the philosophy of the Soft Independent Modelling of Class Analogy (SIMCA) method and package is based on a physical organic chemistry background (Wold and Sjöström, 1977). At present, it constitutes a unique framework where interpretation and understanding of new problems is based on three main tools: principal component analysis (PCA), partial least squares (PLS) and design. They suggest an overall chemometric strategy for drug design studies, which relies on design in latent variables and PLS modelling (Clementi *et al.*, 1989a; Wold *et al.*, 1986).

Principal component analysis (PCA) and partial least squares (or projections to latent structures, PLS) are statistical multivariate techniques for extracting and rationalizing the maximum common amount of information from a multivariate description of a biological system. PCA is a projection method that provides an approximation of a matrix **X**, here termed the descriptors matrix, in terms of the product of two smaller matrices: **T** and **P′** (equation (1)). The matrices **T** and **P′** extract the essential information and patterns from **X**. By plotting the columns in **T**, a picture of the dominant 'object pattern' of **X** is obtained and, analogously, plotting the rows of **P′** shows the complementary 'variable pattern'. The number of statistically significant dimensions for the PCA model is determined by cross-validation by means of the NIPALS algorithm (Wold *et al.*, 1984). The principal components (PCs) are linear combinations of the original variables, that are orthogonal to each other, so that they represent independent effects.

$$\mathbf{X} = \bar{\mathrm{x}} + \mathbf{TP}' + \mathbf{E} \tag{1}$$

$$\mathbf{Y} = \bar{\mathrm{y}} + \mathbf{UQ}' + \mathbf{F} \tag{2}$$

$$\mathbf{U} = \mathbf{BT} + \mathbf{H} \tag{3}$$

$$\mathbf{Y} = \bar{\mathrm{y}} + \mathbf{BTQ}' + \mathbf{F}' \tag{4}$$

The two-blocks PLS model relates a matrix **X** (chemical descriptors) to a matrix **Y** (biological activities) with the purpose of predicting **Y** from **X**. The **X**-block model is the same as in PCA (equation (1)). The **Y**-block matrix is modelled in a similar manner (equation (2)), and the maximum correlation between the **X** and **Y** block models is obtained using a PLS-weight matrix **W′** (Wold *et al.*, 1984). The relation between **U** and **T**, the inner relation, can therefore be modelled by equation (3), where **B** is a diagonal matrix and **H** is a residual matrix. In the case of a single biological response, equations (2) and (3) are substituted by equation (4). Similarly to PCA, the statistical significance for each model dimension is determined by cross-validation (Wold *et al.*, 1984, 1993a). Predictions of y values for new compounds are obtained from the x data of these compounds inserted into the PLS model in the sequence: $x \rightarrow t \rightarrow u \rightarrow y$. As for the principal components in PCA, the PLS latent variables are linear combinations of all the original variables.

The pair of methods PCA/PLS seems to be particularly appropriate in QSAR both for the exploratory analysis of the structural data and for establishing the quantitative relationship under the same descriptor space. The selection of a designed set of informative molecules to explore at best the structural variation in the series ensures the reliability of the derived model.

The PLS algorithm appears to be the most appropriate tool for establishing quantitative relationships between a biological activity vector and a matrix of structural descriptors, especially in detecting the structural features affecting the biological activity and in providing reliable predictions (Dunn and Wold, 1990; Cruciani *et al.*, 1990). A recent statistical report claimed that another method, ridge regression, gives slightly better predictions (Frank and Friedman, 1993). However, it was shown that the assumptions underlying PLS are much closer to the requirements of a real problem formulation of the QSAR area (Wold, 1993). Accordingly, since PLS has no limitations about the number of variables to be used from the beginning, we suggest that all possible variables should be taken into account and then let the chemometric method select only the important ones.

Two main requirements should be met in order to derive sound chemometric models which permit reliable predictions of the activity of new structures. The first is the selection of a few informative structures by means of design criteria, so that the database is well balanced and gives reliable models (Clementi *et al.*, 1993a; Clementi and Wold, 1995). The second is to use validated models (Wold, 1991).

The Design Approach

Optimization strategies in organic chemistry can be applied not only to process optimization but also to product optimization, where the goal is to find out the structural features which optimize the desired response in terms of biological properties.

In all such cases optimization means keeping under control a number of factors affecting the response in order to find out the best combination of them, i.e. the values that each factor should simultaneously assume to produce the optimal response. Usually, the examination of the effect of each factor on the response is made in a very inefficient way, studying one variable at a time (OVAT). The inefficiency of this approach is shown in Fig. 14.1: OVAT requires a large number of experiments, but the maximum response found depends exclusively upon the starting value examined, and the way the data are collected cannot give any information whatsoever about the pair of factors which would have given the real optimum.

In contrast, using the strategy suggested by statistical experimental designs (Box *et al.*, 1978; Box and Draper, 1987) permits us to gain information on how to reach the coordinates of the optimum, with the lowest possible number of experiments. The merit of this approach is twofold: it not only allows us to save a lot of resources by dramatically diminishing the number of required experiments, but it also furnishes greater information on the process, which in turn allows us to identify the combination of factors producing the optimal result.

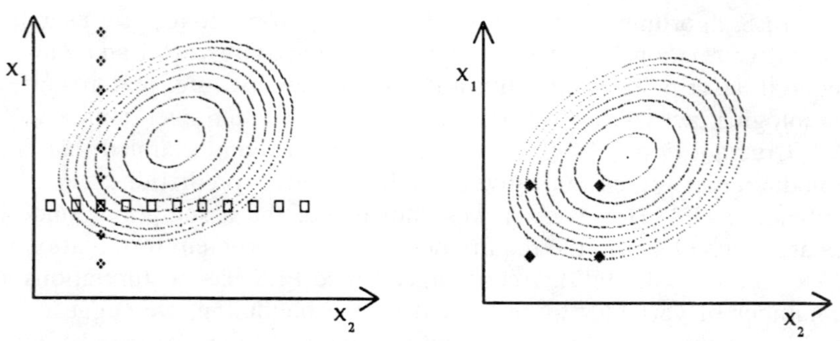

Fig. 14.1 OVAT and factorial design strategies for collecting experimental data.

Thus, design means a computer-assisted strategy able to span the operational space in the best possible way. The operational space is that containing the objects under control, described by numerical values. These descriptors define the operational space, which is usually called variable or factor space.

Chemometrics provides methods and tools to interpret experimental data collected by varying simultaneously all factors under investigation: the information contained in such data is more complete and better suited for a thorough understanding of the process under study, and, consequently, for identifying the combination of factors giving the optimal response.

In QSAR, unfortunately, new structures are usually derived by changing one substituent at a time for each substitution site. Sets of molecules obtained in this way do not contain enough information for ranking the importance of individual features in affecting biological activity and for providing stable models to be used in predictions.

The use of design strategies to select a test series in QSAR studies is particularly valuable, as it permits us to select only a few molecules to be synthesized and tested, but in such a way that they contain the widest information, and therefore they allow us to derive the most reliable QSAR models, while saving a lot of the resources presently required for a single study (Clementi *et al.*, 1993a; Clementi and Wold, 1995).

The preliminary idea of multivariate design in latent variables was developed by Wold and co-workers some 10 years ago (Wold *et al.*, 1986). The chemometric strategy for QSAR problems relies on three major phases: (a) multivariate characterization, giving the latent variables; (b) a design in these latent variables and (c) modelling by PLS. In fact, experimental design provides a strategy for selecting the few most informative molecular structures in a series of homologues. It is also possible to apply design criteria with discrete systems, provided these are multivariately characterized by a representative number of available data.

Although traditional descriptors are many, PCA provides a tool for collecting systematic patterns of their behavior into a few orthogonal scales (phase a). The latent variables obtained as statistical scores are often called principal properties (PPs) and represent in an appropriate way each system by a few (usually two or three) constants, which condense the systematic behaviour of the original data. It has been applied for describing amino acids in peptides (Hellberg *et al.*, 1987; Jonsson *et al.*, 1989; Eriksson *et al.*, 1990) or aromatic substituents in general organic series (van de Waterbeemd *et al.*, 1989; Skagerberg *et al.*, 1989).

A QSAR table can be prepared describing each amino acid in a peptide sequence, or each substituent in a polysubstituted organic skeleton by their PPs, in pairs or triplets: the descriptor matrix. This is the matrix that will be analysed by PLS in phase (c) in order to find out its relationship with the y vector, or the **Y**-matrix, measuring the biological activity.

How do we apply design criteria to select the molecules needed to form the

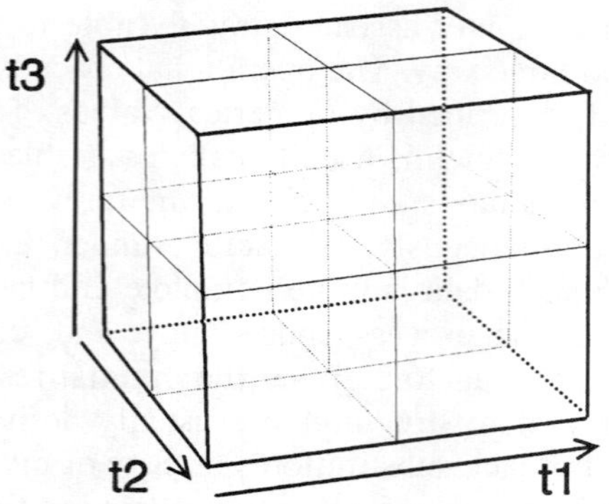

Fig. 14.2 Graphical representation of the PP space showing its division in octants.

QSAR table in phase (b)? The set of possible substituents is divided into subsets according to their relative position in the PPs space (as in Fig. 14.2). A substituent representing each subspace (quadrants or octants) is selected thereafter, and labelled by the pair or triplet of signs corresponding to that subspace. Any design strategy can be applied by using blocks of PPs to define each item at each varying site and by selecting a representative item for each position of the PPs space. Factorial designs (FDs) and fractional factorial designs (FFDs) are simple, and therefore good in helping to understand the concept of design: spanning the variable space.

Each experiment of a factorial design matrix can be transformed into a molecule if we assign pairs or triplets of columns of the signs matrix to define the substituent corresponding to each site. The substituents selected as representative for each octant of the resulting three-dimensional PP space for organic substituents are NO_2, Br, Me, CO_2Et, COPh, OPr, Ph and H (or OH) (Skagerberg *et al.*, 1989). More recently we have suggested (van de Waterbeemd *et al.*, 1995) the use of a set of disjoint principal properties (DPPs), which requires the use of 12 representative substituents. These include, besides Br, Me, COPh, OPr, Ph and both H and OH, also CN, ^{t}Bu, $COCH_3$ or COOH, NMe_2 or NHMe and SO_2Me, as reported in Clementi *et al.* (1993a).

In the case of polysubstitution, we can always consider pairs or triplets of variables as representing a single substitution site: a trisubstituted skeleton with substituents controlled by two PPs is a problem in six variables (Fig. 14.3). However, within the FD strategy a molecule should bear as many substituents at as many sites as one wishes to control. Therefore, the FDs approach might not be easy to apply when a synthetic chemist wants to control, at the same time, a number of different substitution sites. It is clear that FDs give plans in which the most informative compounds are difficult to synthesize because they contain too many substituents.

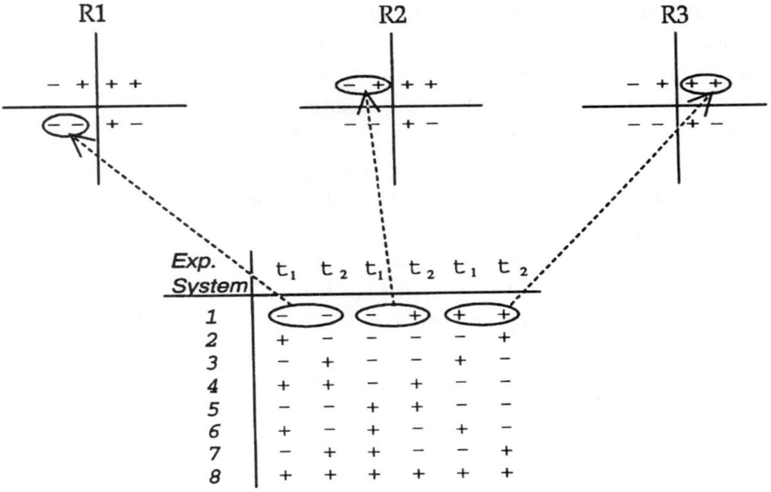

R1
R2
R3
Exp. System
t1 t2 t1 t2 t1 t2
1 − − − + + +
2 + − − − − +
3 − + − − + −
4 + + − + − −
5 − − + + − −
6 + − + − + −
7 − + + − − +
8 + + + + + +

Fig. 14.3 Construction of a design matrix for a three-substituted series.

Because of these reasons we have recently investigated (Clementi *et al.*, 1991; Baroni *et al.*, 1993a) the effect of using D-optimal designs instead of FDs with PPs in QSAR, since D-optimal designs can be used as an alternative to FDs in constrained situations, e.g. when some regions of the variable space are excluded or when the data set is discrete, as with molecular structures.

The D-optimality criterion consists of determining the n experiments in the accessible domain which contain together the maximum amount of information. In other words the D-optimal algorithm selects a few points optimally spanning the domain. The dimensionality of the domain is equal to the number of factors to vary and it contains as many candidates as there are combinations of such factors. FDs are D-optimal when each substitution site is controlled by a single parameter. However, on increasing the number of PPs for describing each substitution site the efficiency of D-optimal designs becomes far better.

In fact, if the problem formulation is that of six variables generated by controlling three sites by pairs of PPs, the total number of possible molecules, allowing our eight selected substituents for each site, is $8^3 = 512$. The FFD approach would first generate a design matrix with 8 rows and 6 columns and then would assign substituents to the three pairs of signs according to the subspace codes. In contrast, the D-optimality approach works in a six-dimensional space with the actual values of the PPs. The D-optimality criterion then provides the selection of the seven points out of the 512 which meet the requirement of maximizing the quoted determinant, i.e. roughly spanning in the best way the domain in the six-dimensional space.

The advantages of using D-optimal designs instead of fractional factorial designs in principal properties can be summarized as follows. It is possible: (a) to reduce the number of required structures; (b) to reduce polysubstitution even when controlling several sites; (c) to exclude molecules too difficult to synthesize; (d) to include molecules already available and/or tested. In particular, D-optimal designs are favourable when the number of sites under control is three or larger. The D-optimality algorithm was implemented in a program, called DESDOP, aimed at determining D-optimal designs in principal properties for QSAR studies (Baroni *et al.*, 1993a).

Over the last few years we used twice the strategy of FFD in PPs for QSAR studies. In particular, using the PPs for amino acids we studied a series of peptides behaving as highly selective NK-2 antagonists (Clementi *et al.*, 1990) and using the PPs for substituents we studied the toxicity of monosubstituted benzenes on algae and daphnids (Tosato *et al.*, 1988), within the framework of developing a general strategy for priority ranking of molecules in toxicological studies (Tosato *et al.*, 1991). More recently we preferred using D-optimal designs for handling polysubstitution (Baroni *et al.*, 1993a). D-optimal designs were used for selecting solvents to be used in a study of water–organic solvent mixtures (Cipiciani *et al.*, 1990), and to study the binding of nonapeptides to major histocompatibility complex (MHC) class I proteins (Rovero *et al.*, 1994), stimulating the interest of immunologists in this chemometric strategy.

The CARSO Procedure

The final phase of an optimization problem is usually formulated as a response surface study. However, the coefficients of the polynomial which describes the surface are usually computed by multiple linear regression, which is possible only if the data have been collected according to a rotatable design. Because of this, it was extremely valuable to develop a procedure where the response surface could also be developed in cases when the data could not be properly designed, as in QSAR studies, when all factors vary simultaneously.

This procedure, called CARSO (Clementi *et al.*, 1989b), consists of modelling the response by PLS instead of by ordinary multiple regression. The PLS loadings are transformed thereafter into the coefficients of the polynomial, and the response surface is then studied by canonical analysis and by Lagrange analysis: for the point of the surface with the highest y-value it is possible to find out analytically the ranges allowed for reaching a certain response level. In our experience the CARSO procedure was found to be the most efficient chemometric tool for solving real QSAR problems (Fig. 14.4).

The importance of deriving a QSAR model by the CARSO response surface on a well-balanced set of structures even in the presence of a much larger number of available data for the same series was shown in two studies

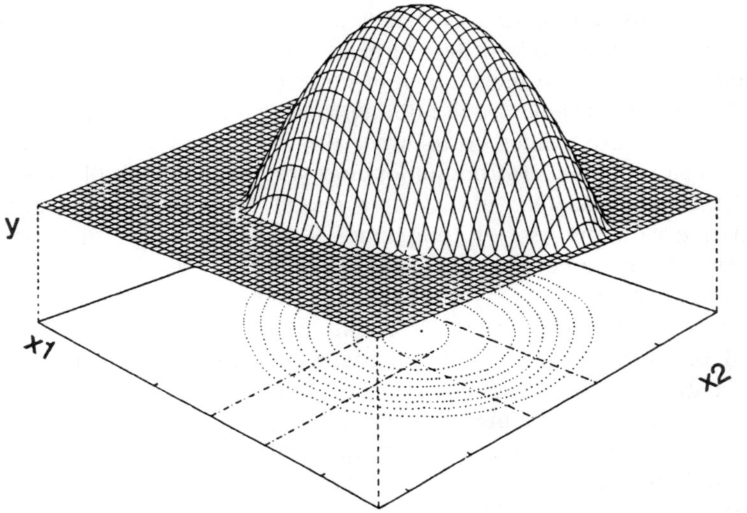

Fig. 14.4 Response surface and its corresponding isoresponse plot.

regarding the antibacterial and antimycotic activity of benzofused heteroaromatic derivatives (De Meo *et al.*, 1990) and of quinolones (Bonelli *et al.*, 1991, 1993).

In the former case, the activity of 16 informative molecules, analysed by a linear PLS model, permitted us to optimize three structural features out of four. The fourth feature, an aromatic substituent, was finally optimized by the CARSO procedure in terms of the substituents PPs, predicting as optimal structures two new compounds which were shown later to be true (Pedini *et al.*, 1994). In the second case we took into account over 400 quinolones reported in the literature. A chemometric approach based on multivariate characterization and design in the resulting latent variables permitted us to select a set of 32 molecules with a well-balanced structural variation on which to derive the QSAR models; by the CARSO analysis it was possible to predict a new class of compounds, the lead of which was tested and shown to be active as expected. This preliminary lead has been modified to give a molecule undergoing further development.

Validation

The usual measures of the goodness of fit for a QSAR model are the size of the residuals (given by the standard deviation: s or RSD) and R^2, the multiple correlation coefficient, which gives the explained y-variance. However, a large R^2 and small s are not sufficient for model validity, because regression models give a closer fit the larger the number of parameters and terms in the model. With many descriptor variables to select from, a model can fit almost all data very closely even with few terms, provided that descriptor variables are selected according to their apparent contribution to the fit. This is true even if the chosen variables have nothing to do with the current problem. In the presence of these chance correlations the model may fit the training set data well but it is useless for prediction and understanding (Wold, 1991).

In order to evaluate the validity of a model the best thing would be a representative validation set of compounds, for which the predicted activity values can be compared with the actual values. In the absence of a real validation set we can use a simulated one, since recent developments in statistics provide us with a new interesting set of measures of validity that are based on simulating the self-consistent predictive power of a model. Cross-validation and bootstrapping constitute the basis of the modern statistical philosophy of 'replacing standard assumptions about the data with massive calculations', for assessing the generality of a relationship found from a sample data set (Cramer *et al.*, 1988b).

In cross-validation, the data set is divided into a number of groups. The model, with a given complexity, is fitted to the data set reduced by one of the groups at a time. Predictions are calculated by the fitted model for the deleted data, and the sum of squares of observed minus predicted values for the deleted data is formed. The total sum of squares of observed minus predicted values, which contains one term for each point, abbreviated PRESS (equation (5)), is a measure of predictive power of the model with the given complexity for the given data set.

$$\text{PRESS} = \Sigma\,(y_{\text{OBS}}\text{-}y_{\text{PRED}})^2 \tag{5}$$

$$Q^2 = 1 - \text{PRESS/SSY} \tag{6}$$

$$\text{SDEP} = (\text{PRESS}/N)^{1/2} \tag{7}$$

PRESS is a good estimate of the real prediction error of the model, provided that the observations (compounds) are independent. If PRESS is smaller than the sum of squares of the response values (SSY), the model predicts better than chance and can be considered statistically significant. To be a reasonable QSAR model, PRESS/SSY should be smaller than 0.4. If the PRESS value is transformed into a dimensionless term by relating it to the initial sum of squares, one obtains Q^2 (equation (6)), also called cross-validated R^2.

PRESS and Q^2 have good properties which render them appropriate for statistical testing with critical distributions. However, the use of the square root of PRESS/N (equation (7)) seems to be more directly related to the uncertainty of the predictions, since it has the same units as the actual y-values. Accordingly, we suggested (Cruciani *et al.*, 1990, 1992) using the term SDEP (standard deviation of error of predictions).

Either PRESS, Q^2 or SDEP can be used to check the predictivity of regression models, including PLS. These equations, however, do not yet define a unique way of computing the parameters, since the way the predictions are obtained should also be selected. For example, in defining the cross-validation procedure, the data set should be divided into a number of groups, which can be increased until it equals the number of data points, thus obtaining the leave-one-out (LOO) procedure. The LOO procedure should be theoretically best, provided data are randomly distributed or carefully designed, but LOO gives SDEP values lower than the groups approach when data are clustered. Since, in QSAR, the descriptor variables usually generate grouped data, the predictive ability of a model should be evaluated in a non-favourable cross-validation technique, i.e. by the formation of the lowest reasonable number of groups.

Moreover, one should not be satisfied by using a cross-validation technique that forms groups in a unique way, and thus we have computed SDEP several times on groups formed in a random way (Cruciani *et al.*, 1992). This definition of SDEP makes it somewhat halfway between cross-validation and bootstrapping. Accordingly, the SDEP parameter can be logically associated with the uncertainty of any new prediction made by that model. However, being parameter scale dependent, it is obvious that the 'absolute' prediction ability of the model should be evaluated by Q^2.

Variable Selection

Procedures for variable selection have long been used with ordinary least squares regression methods (Draper and Smith, 1981). However, almost all previous work in variable selection has been done exclusively for describing data sets, and, in order to evaluate the relevance of individual variables in validated regression models, the model predictivity should be checked.

By means of the SDEP parameter it is possible to select the groups of variables capable of giving the best predictive ability of a single model (Baroni *et al.*, 1992). In this latter report we suggested a preliminary outline of a procedure, called GOLPE (Generating Optimal Linear PLS Estimations) aimed at obtaining the best predictive PLS models. The procedure was based on statistical designs, as the design matrices used in FFDs provide a suitable tool for finding an efficient way of selecting the most representative combinations of variables (Box *et al.*, 1978). The strategy was developed by using combinations of variables according to an FFD where each of the two levels (1, −1) corresponds to the presence and absence of the variable. The design matrix, including only the 'plus' and excluding the 'minus' variables, suggested that we test the predictive ability of these reduced models only, each involving a different combination of variables, that altogether constitute a good representation of all possible combinations. For each such combination the prediction ability of the corresponding PLS model can be evaluated by means of SDEP. Accordingly, one obtains a response vector indicating the model predictivity for each combination of variables as the lowest SDEP value corresponding to the dimensionality for which SDEP assumes the minimum value.

In order to estimate more precisely the significance of a single variable effect on predictivity, the GOLPE procedure was later refined (Baroni *et al.*, 1993b) by introducing a number of dummy variables in the design matrix. These dummy variables are not involved in the variable combinations evaluating the predictivity of each row of the design matrix: they are only used to compute, by means of the Yates algorithm, the apparent effects on predictivity given by a non-existent variable, so that the decision on the positive or the negative effects of individual true variables can be taken on the basis of a Student *t* tailoring. Variables with a positive effect on predictivity can be fixed within the variables combinations, while variables with a negative effect on predictivity can always be excluded from the variable combinations. If variable selection works in an iterative manner it increases at each iteration the stability of the results, thus furnishing the complete list of selected variables.

The GOLPE procedure appears therefore to be a powerful and efficient tool for variable selection. However, we should remark that it can be properly applied only provided the regression model on the whole data set has at least some initial predictive ability ($Q^2 > 0.3$). GOLPE allowed us to show that: (a) in PLS modelling all variables are relevant for fitting but some of them may be detrimental to predictivity; (b) the GOLPE procedure provides a method for detecting variables increasing predictivity; (c) the PLS models obtained by using only variables selected by GOLPE are more predictive than the PLS model on all variables; and (d) PLS models with variable selection are more predictive than similar models obtained by ordinary least squares.

An independent measure of the relative importance of the *x*-variables can be calculated as VIP (variable influence on the prediction). VIP is derived from the PLS weights, taking into account the fraction of variance explained in each model dimension (Wold *et al.*, 1993b). In addition to VIP, the regression coefficients are also useful for assessing the importance of *x*-variables: only those with *b*-values larger than about half the maximum *b*-value are indicated as important. A comparison between the selection of important *x*-variables by GOLPE and by VIP and *b*-values is presently being investigated jointly by our research teams also extended to the IVS procedure (Rännar *et al.*, 1994). In fact, selecting variables is difficult and risky. In order to avoid pruning, the elimination of variables should be done to simplify the model, and not be guided by the degree of fit or the prediction error; the latter usually leads to partly spurious models that seriously overfit the data, especially if cross-validation is made in leave-one-out.

Molecular Modelling Techniques and 3D-QSAR

Molecular modelling techniques have become widely used for drug design problems. At first, modelling was used only to look at molecules individually, in order to understand the 3D requirements underlying their biological activities. Later on a number of procedures were developed for pharmacophoric searching, by which the 3D structure of the putative receptor could be mapped on a complementarity basis: Crippen suggested the distance geometry approach (Crippen, 1977); Hopfinger proposed the molecular shape analysis concept (Hopfinger, 1980); and the active analogue approach, based on constrained minimization of different molecules to examine the existence of pharmacophoric patterns, was eventually formulated by Marshall (Marshall *et al.*, 1979). However, the 3D descriptors produced by modelling techniques can also be used as a precise description of 3D structures.

The GRID and CoMFA Approaches

When a probe is moved in a rectangular box of grid points around and through a target molecule it produces a 3D box of interaction fields. According to the different computational procedure used, these fields may represent total interaction energies (GRID) (Goodford, 1985), steric or electrostatic fields (CoMFA) (Cramer *et al.*, 1988a), etc. These fields may be used as precise descriptors of the 3D molecular structure and physico-chemical behaviour of the target molecule. Moreover, a graphical analysis allows a simple interpretation of the fields such as the visualization of the regions where the probe interacts strongly with the target in an attractive or repulsive way.

However, when a number of molecules are studied at the same time, this simple graphic analysis is not sufficient to provide the necessary information for us to understand the observed variation of the biological properties of the series. In such a case chemometric tools are appropriate for condensing and extracting the hidden information.

Ordinary PCA and PLS methods require a two-way table of objects and variables. An object is often a physically distinguishable entity, like a target molecule, while a variable represents the results of a computation made on this object. However 3D-QSAR methods produce 3D matrices of molecular descriptors where the rows, the columns and the sheets are variables; the table itself representing the object and this 3D array can be easily rearranged as a one-dimensional vector. In the presence of several molecules, the procedures should be repeated for all the molecules and the vectors of variables assembled together in a 2-way table in order to obtain a target matrix (Cruciani and Goodford, 1994). Target matrices can be combined, thus obtaining one single larger matrix. In the CoMFA procedure two probes are used as blocks of descriptors and the resulting two target matrices combined in a single one containing the same number of objects and a double number of variables.

3D-QSAR: The CoMFA Procedure

3D-QSAR modelling is totally within the QSAR tradition, where the contribution of the chemometricians was to suggest how to update the chemometric tools to be used: namely, to use PLS, design criteria, validated models and to avoid using indicator variables. However, the traditional approach may be considered to have some limitations: conformational equilibria are not taken into account and no information on the 3D structure is used.

On the other hand, molecular modelling techniques have become extremely popular because of the increasing use of computer facilities. These methods, based on some theoretical grounds at different levels of approximation, are aimed at calculating the energy of the accessible conformations for each molecule, and then studying the possible interactions between the molecule and its binding site. From this approach it became possible to describe each molecule/conformation item by a series of theoretically computed parameters, some of which have a 3D nature.

A 3D-QSAR is therefore, strictly speaking, a QSAR relationship where the structural descriptors have a 3D nature: several molecules are studied at the same time within the framework of a regression model, with the objective of finding out what structural features significantly affect the biological response. These 3D-descriptors are usually derived by the different modelling techniques.

The CoMFA procedure (Cramer *et al.*, 1988a) is generally accepted as the most complete and advanced method for handling the whole problem; it is also recognized that the GRID method (Goodford, 1985) gives accurate estimations of the interaction energies with a wide variety of different probes. Our research group, because of the experience in problem solving by chemometric methods (namely PLS and design), suggested procedures to use that would improve this new research instrument (Baroni *et al.*, 1993b; Clementi *et al.*, 1993b).

Therefore, 3D-QSARs represent the logical update of the analogy QSAR studies based upon the Hansch tradition, putting together chemometrics and modelling techniques in order to develop a unique procedure: $(mc)^2$, the acronym for Modelling and Chemometrics in Medicinal Chemistry. Handling 3D-QSAR problems needs a good balance of suitable chemometric tools and information derived by molecular modelling techniques.

In the CoMFA procedure, molecules are first represented by a long vector of interaction energies, with a probe at regular intervals in the three dimensions, which are subsequently aligned according to some fitting criterion. The chemometric method used is PLS, because of the higher number of variables (descriptors) over the number of objects (molecules). The PLS models are usually validated by the leave-one-out (LOO) cross-validation technique. The results are shown in terms of coefficients of a pseudo-regression equation in the original variables, here locations in the 3D space, and represented by 3D graphics.

The GOLPE Procedure

GOLPE is a chemometric procedure, based on an advanced PLS method, aimed at obtaining models for highly reliable predictions by means of variable selection criteria. The procedure was developed over 5 years, and is now implemented in a computer program, which complements methods like SIMCA and CoMFA.

Since data matrices in 3D-QSAR are characterized by thousands of variables and tens of molecules, the requirements of an appropriate chemometric tool should involve a sound validation method and a reliable variable selection procedure. We have shown that the SDEP parameter decreases on increasing the number of cross-validation groups (Cruciani *et al.*, 1993). Consequently, using the maximum possible number of groups, i.e. LOO, will always give a better result (a higher predictivity) than using a small number of groups. Therefore, although LOO is computationally simpler and faster, we should be aware that it gives the most optimistic estimation of predictivity, based both on simple numerical grounds and because of the clusters of QSAR structures. The use of groups was recently claimed to be better than LOO also on theoretical bases (Shao, 1993).

The GOLPE procedure is designed to improve as much as possible the reliability of future predictions. Clearly, the way statistics are computed depends upon how one wishes to present results. Reliable estimates of model parameters should be given, so that uncertainties on future predictions are equally reliable. Quite often, however, the objective seems to be in showing how good models are, just in terms of R^2 or Q^2.

Consequently, in principle one should not expect GOLPE to give Q^2 values higher than those derived by other chemometric techniques. If it does so, eventually, it is because of variable selection. In principle, the statistics suggested by GOLPE are less favourable in showing how good the model is, and therefore seem to be closer to real cases in QSAR studies. Accordingly, GOLPE suggests using a small number of groups (say five) instead of LOO, but the group formations should be repeated several times (say 100) in a random way, in order to avoid the possibility that the results depend on a single, casual, computational grouping.

The variable selection used in GOLPE according to FFD on variable combinations is illustrated in Figure 14.5. The method implemented in GOLPE is aimed at evaluating the effect of each individual variable on the model predictivity; other methods select variables on the basis of their importance on the validated models.

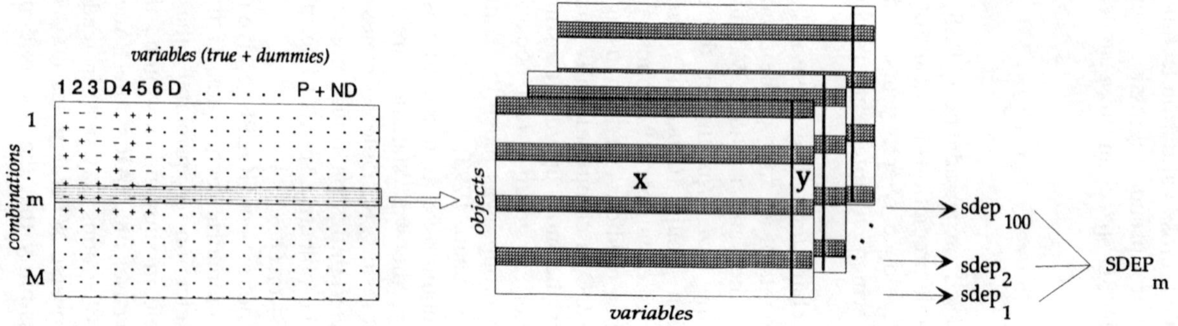

Fig. 14.5 GOLPE procedure: for each variable combination suggested by the design matrix the model validation is made by dividing the data set into (usually five) groups and repeating the group formation several times (usually 100) to give the mean SDEP value.

However, the FFD strategy is impractical in 3D-QSAR problems, and therefore we have developed an alternative method which provides from the beginning a reduced number of variables. For the purpose of this preliminary selection the most efficient way is to select variables in the loading space according to a D-optimal design. In fact, with so many variables the information is largely redundant and D-optimality appears to be an appropriate criterion to select variables in such a way that almost all the information is retained by a much smaller number of variables, spread as much as possible in principal component space. This preselection ends with taking away redundancy without destroying colinearities, since it is recommended that the D-optimality criterion is used to keep not less than a half of the variables each time in an iterative manner, and stops as soon as the model predictivity begins to change. Of course this may not be the only, or the best, way of reducing redundancy. Furthermore, the D-optimal preselection might not be needed (Clementi *et al.*, 1995c).

The results of 3D-QSAR analyses, based on projection methods, depend upon the way chosen for data pretreatment, and this matter has already been thoroughly discussed (Cramer *et al.*, 1993; Wold *et al.*, 1993a). Results recently reported on an appropriate data set of small molecules embedded in their receptor cavity showed that, in an investigation by GOLPE, variable preselection should be done on non-scaled data, whilst the FFD selection should be carried out on autoscaled data (Cruciani and Watson, 1994).

In conclusion, the GOLPE procedure appears to be a powerful and efficient tool for 3D-QSAR. In fact, it works by a very fast algorithm, it uses a suitable validation criterion and it relies on a unique philosophy of variable selection, based on design criteria, which permits a sound evaluation of the predictivity of each individual variable, here grid location. This procedure is presumably sounder than other methods based on a stepwise reduction of variables by means of their chemometric results, or by means of neural networks, genetic algorithms or simulated annealing, which may induce some unwarranted pruning.

GOLPE has been successfully applied to a number of problems over the last 2 years. These include molecular descriptions by CoMFA in polychlorodibenzofurans (PCDFs) (Baroni *et al.*, 1993b), benzodiazepine analogues (Allen *et al.*, 1992), and monosubstituted benzenes (van de Waterbeemd *et al.*, 1993b), by GRID in prazosine analogues (Cocchi *et al.*, 1993), glucose analogues (Cruciani and Watson, 1994), triazines (Riganelli *et al.*, 1995a), dioxins (Valigi *et al.*, 1995), xanthines (Clementi *et al.*, 1995a), ACE inhibitors (Davis *et al.*, 1995), and similarity matrices (Good *et al.*, 1993a,b).

The best way of checking the reliability of a regression model is by permuting a large number of times the elements of the *y*-vector; in no instance can one obtain high Q^2 values, unless one proceeds to 'prune' the variables according to the chemometric results. So far we have published only illustrative examples of such a procedure (Baroni *et al.*, 1993b, Clark and

Cramer, 1993) but we have used it successfully in several other data sets quoted above. Significantly, in one of these studies (Riganelli *et al.*, 1995a), we have found that GOLPE gave a positive Q^2 value in one case only, out of the 32 possible combinations of aligning five triazines, three of which could be superimposed in two alternative ways.

The ACC Transforms

The drawbacks in 3D-QSAR are strictly linked to the continuity and congruency requirements of such models. The main problem in 3D-QSAR is alignment, which is a consequence of the dependence of the 3D-description upon the position of each molecule within the 3D-grid. Indeed, at present, 3D-QSAR models depend almost exclusively on the alignment criterion used, so that it is customary to realign molecules after the first analysis in order to improve the model. Only when the scientific community will be able to derive a 3D-description which is independent of shifting or bending a molecule within the grid, will a 3D-QSAR table contain variables which are really congruent and therefore appropriate for chemometric modelling.

We have suggested (Clementi *et al.*, 1993a,b) a promising perspective on the problem of congruency of the 3D-description: the auto- and cross-covariance (ACC) transforms. There are two main drawbacks with the present use of CoMFA in 3D-QSAR: (a) doubts about the congruency of the descriptor matrix and (b) the absence of continuity constraints between the fields computed at neighbouring grid nodes. Both these problems may be solved by the ACC-based description, proposed by Wold and co-workers to handle biopolymers (Wold *et al.*, 1993b; Riganelli *et al.*, 1994a). ACC transforms have been developed, together with Fourier transforms, to account for dependencies between consecutive observations. We have extended this concept into three dimensions and applied it to molecules described by their CoMFA fields (Clementi *et al.*, 1993b) or GRID energies (Valigi *et al.*, 1994).

The basic idea was to consider the two fields calculated by CoMFA for each grid point as the two descriptors to be used for the ACC transforms as the auto-covariance and cross-covariance between the fields at grid points defined by 3D distances (3D lags). The 3D-ACC transforms were used to describe a series of PCDFs by CoMFA and a series of PCDDs by GRID: the results showed that the problem of having a unique and congruent description of 'degenerate' numbering of molecules is solved. We are now able to obtain the same ACC vector, at least for planar molecules, independently of their nomenclature and their direction along any of the three coordinate axes.

ACC transforms are suitable tools to enable us to recognize the information contained in the 3D fields generated by CoMFA in such a way that they appear to be more appropriate for 3D-QSAR. This rearrangement provides new data that have two nice properties: they take into account neighbour effects, and therefore the required continuity between grid nodes, and they are independent of alignment within the grid lattice (Clementi *et al.*, 1993b). Data descriptions derived by CoMFA or GRID after ACC transformation can be modelled by PLS without any need for alignment, thus meeting both the congruency and continuity requirement.

However, the 3D-ACC transforms developed so far permit us to have a unique and congruent description of 'degenerate' numbering of molecules (Clementi *et al.*, 1993b). At present we can deal satisfactorily with planar molecules but cannot yet describe properly flexible molecules. Moreover, ACC transforms cannot describe different conformers in a unique way, since different conformers give different ACC transforms due to the different relative positions of atoms in 3D-space. An overall strategy for handling all of them needs to be developed, possibly similar to that suggested by the research team in Milan (Belvisi *et al.*, 1991; Cosentino *et al.*, 1992). If 3D-QSAR is based on PLS modelling of the activity vector against the ACC matrix by means of GOLPE, the results would determine interactions between locations that affect the biological response and this would constitute a new tool for mapping unknown receptors.

Conclusions and Perspectives

One obvious conclusion of this presentation would have been the proposal of a strategy for design in 3D, merging both chemometric philosophy and the 3D information being used in 3D-QSAR. However, on developing 3D principal properties for organic substituents by analogy with that explored by other authors (van de Waterbeemd *et al.*, 1993a; Cocchi and Johansson, 1993; Norinder, 1991, 1993) it has been possible to compare the 3D PPs derived from monosubstituted benzenes with those obtained for the corresponding aliphatic compounds where the partner of the substituent is a methyl group instead of phenyl group. It is noteworthy that, whereas the steric PPs parallel each other, the electrostatic PPs do not (van de Waterbeemd *et al.*, 1993b).

In other words, whilst analogy models in traditional QSAR allowed us to use PPs derived from aromatic systems for modelling any structural variation, the finer insight furnished by 3D descriptors will not allow us to do this any more. Furthermore, in generating 3D PPs for aromatic substituents by using the ACC transforms, the tricky question is how to superimpose the substituents. The results of a study (van de Waterbeemd *et al.*, 1993b) indicated that the PCA on the CoMFA fields shows mainly the expected groupings of conformations, but some incongruencies were found. In contrast the PCA on the ACC matrix showed better defined clusters. Accordingly, we found that the ACC matrix can give PC results which limit greatly the dependency upon molecule orientation, but cannot get rid of the problem of dealing with different conformers (Clementi *et al.*, 1993b) and, therefore, different orientations. Consequently, using ACC transforms is much better than using the starting CoMFA fields, but we still need some self-consistency rule for letting the substituents assume a congruent orientation that may have nothing to do with that suggested by the optimal geometry (van de Waterbeemd, 1993b). To sum up, this study has pointed out that field or energy descriptions really seem inappropriate for deriving substituent scales which can be used for information retrieval. Consequently, it is perhaps more appropriate to avoid thinking in terms of 3D PPs and to develop a totally different strategy to work with 3D-QSARs.

Another important statement to make is that the way conformational freedom should be dealt with in the framework of 3D-QSARs depends upon problem formulation and cannot be solved numerically. At present, it seems to us that it might be appropriate to evaluate, for each flexible molecule, all the conformations accessible within an appropriate energy window. A PCA carried out thereafter can show the existence of clusters of conformations (Wold *et al.*, 1993b; Riganelli *et al.*, 1995a). It is our feeling that regression models should be looked for within each of these clusters. Our experience in the quoted studies on triazines (Riganelli *et al.*, 1995a), confirmed later on a series of xanthines, which were shown to be superposed only by their lone pairs (Clementi *et al.*, 1995a), encourages this point of view.

A possible solution of the problem might be that design and alignment should be done on ACC transforms. Design should take into account the whole molecules in the 3D grid and not fragments (substituents defined by their PPs) although some substituents representative of their ACC database may help a lot in designing candidate molecules. The selection of a balanced set of molecules could be properly made by an appropriate D-optimal design in the ACC transform space.

Besides the exploration of the suitability of 3D ACC transforms to deal with 3D problems in medicinal chemistry, we have investigated several alternative transformations of the 3D data produced by CoMFA or GRID, potentially embedding information easier to handle. One of the nice aspects of ACC transforms is that each element of the ACC vector can be interpreted as the amount of interaction between descriptors at different lag values, and therefore at different distances. With description of this kind, a chemometric model derived thereby might be readable as a map of the receptor, provided that the ACC elements really describe the level of each possible interaction for each molecule. In this connection summing over all possible pairs of grid nodes belonging to the same lag value does not appear to be appropriate. It seems that, for each element of the ACC vector, using the maximum value (instead of the sum of all values) identifies better the capability of each molecule to give the interaction defined by the pair type/distance.

In consequence, we developed a variation of the ACC transform, that we called MACC-1 (Riganelli *et al.*, 1995b), containing only the maximum value of the ACC descriptors, coded between -1 and $+1$, to be used for one-dimensional problems, e.g. peptides. Accordingly, we decided to label amino acids by three descriptors: the first two principal properties (Jonsson *et al.*, 1989) and a new scale that we developed to describe the capability of each amino acid to accept/donate hydrogen bonds.

These three descriptors were used to compute the MACC-1 transforms in three case studies: (1) the bradykinin potentiating activity of pentapeptides (Hellberg *et al.*, 1987), (2) the NK-2 receptor antagonist heptapeptides (Clementi *et al.*, 1990), and (3) the MHC nonapeptides (Rovero *et al.*, 1994). These examples have shown that it is possible: (a) to interpret the QSAR model derived from MACC-1 in terms of the interaction between amino acids, e.g. the presence of two amino acids, one capable of donating hydrogen-bonds and the other with an aromatic side chain separated by three other spacer amino acids, (b) to describe in a congruent way linear peptides of different length in the same data set, and (c) to predict new peptides with enhanced activity.

Another alternative procedure for producing a unique molecular description, independent of the position of the molecule within the 3D grid, is presently under investigation (Clementi *et al.*, 1995b). The method, tentatively called 3WD (3D-grid Whim Description), uses the WHIM (weighted holistic invariant molecular) indices, recently defined as new molecular indices containing information about the whole molecular structure, in terms of size, shape, symmetry and atom distribution (Todeschini *et al.*, 1994). These theoretical indices are calculated from *x-y-z* coordinates of a molecule, within different weighting schemes, in a straightforward manner that works in a unitary conceptual framework, representing a holistic view of the molecule.

The engine of the calculation is PCA, which projects the weighted original coordinates on to three new principal axes, thus producing ten theoretical molecular descriptors. They are the three eigenvalues which represent the variance of atoms along each component, and therefore are related to molecular size, two of the eigenvalue proportions which represent molecular shape, three third-order moments of the scores, which represent the molecular symmetry along each component, and two of the kurtosis, calculated from the fourth-order moments of the scores, which are related to the atom distribution and density. These ten molecular descriptors are invariant to rotation and translation and differ for each molecular geometry.

The idea presently under development is to use the WHIM indices in the framework of a GRID or CoMFA molecular description, in order to render it independent of its position within the grid. The general WHIM procedure is therefore modified in these points: (a) the indices are calculated, after centring the molecule, from the grid nodes instead of from molecular coordinates and (b) the field or energy values at each node are taken as its weight, but positive and negative fields are to be treated separately, thus generating a double number of indices.

Preliminary results obtained on a few dioxins, rotated and shifted in a number of ways, seem to indicate that 3WD indices really do represent each molecule by the same vector, independently of the position within the grid. However, we should still be very careful in interpreting these encouraging results, since the description depends heavily upon the grid characteristics and/or the centring procedure. Furthermore, we should fully clarify the present difficulty in interpreting the molecular meaning of these descriptors, especially backwards in an information retrieval context.

Acknowledgements

Thanks are due to the funding agencies (MURST and CNR) which made it possible to develop expertise in the field by research grants for chemometrics as such or for its development on specific themes, and to a number of colleagues who contributed to this development by continuous discussion, advice and encouragement.

References

Allen, M.S., La Loggia, A.J., Dorn, L.J., Martin, M.J., Costantino, G., Hagen, T.J., Koehler, K.K., Skolnick, P. and Cook, J.M. (1992). *J. Med. Chem.* **35**, 4001–4010.

Baroni, M., Clementi, S., Cruciani, G., Costantino, G., Riganelli, D. and Oberrauch, E. (1992). *J. Chemometrics* **6**, 347–356.

Baroni, M., Clementi, S., Cruciani, G., Kettaneh-Wold, N. and Wold, S. (1993a). *Quant. Struct.-Act. Relat.* **12**, 225–231.

Baroni, M., Costantino, G., Cruciani, G., Riganelli, D., Valigi, R. and Clementi, S. (1993b). *Quant. Struct.-Act. Relat.* **12**, 9–20.

Belvisi, L., Brossa, S., Salimbeni, A., Scolastico, C. and Todeschini, R. (1991). *J. Comput.-Aided Mol. Design* **5**, 571–584.

Bonelli, D., Cecchetti, V., Clementi, S., Cruciani, G., Fravolini, A. and Savino, A. (1991). *Quant. Struct.-Act. Relat.* **10**, 333–343.

Bonelli, D., Cecchetti, V., Clementi, S., Cruciani, G., Fravolini, A. and Savino, A. (1993). *Pharm. Pharmacol. Lett.* **3**, 13–16.

Box, G.E.P. and Draper, N.R. (1987). 'Empirical Model Building and Response Surfaces'. John Wiley & Sons, New York.

Box, G.E.P., Hunter, W.G. and Hunter, J.S. (1978). 'Statistics for Experimenters' John Wiley & Sons, New York.

Cipiciani, A., Cruciani, G. and Primieri, S. (1990). *Gazz. Chim. Ital.* **120**, 757–763.

Clark, M. and Cramer III, R.D. (1993). *Quant. Struct.-Act. Relat.,* **12**, 137–145.

Clementi, S. and Wold, S. (1995). *In* 'Chemometric Methods in Molecular Design' (H. van de Waterbeemd, ed.). VCH, Weinheim.

Clementi, S., Bonelli, D., Cruciani, G., Skagerberg, B., Ebert, C., Linda, P. and Tosato, M.L. (1989a). *Chimica oggi,* **7**, 19–22.

Clementi, S., Cruciani, G., Curti, G. and Skagerberg, B. (1989b). *J. Chemometrics.* **3**, 499–509.

Clementi, S., Cruciani, G., Riganelli, D., Rovero, P., Pestellini, V., Maggi, C.A. and Baroni, M. (1990). *Tetrahedron Comput. Methodol.* **3**, 379–387.

Clementi, S., Cruciani, G., Baroni, M. and Skagerberg, B. (1991). *Pharmacochem. Lib.* **16**, 217–226.

Clementi, S., Cruciani, G., Baroni, M. and Costantino, G. (1993a). *In* '3D QSAR in Drug Design: Theory, Methods and Applications' (H. Kubinyi, ed.), pp. 567–582. ESCOM, Leiden.

Clementi, S., Cruciani, G., Riganelli, D., Valigi, R., Costantino, G., Baroni, M. and Wold, S. (1993b). *Pharm. Pharmacol. Lett.* **3**, 5–8.

Clementi, S., Cruciani, G., Fifi, P., Riganelli, D. and Bonacchi, G. (1995a). *J. Med. Chem.* (to be submitted).

Clementi, S., Cruciani, G., Fifi, P., Riganelli, D. and Todeschini, R., (1995b). *J. Chemometrics* (to be submitted).

Clementi, S., Cruciani, G., Riganelli, D. and Valigi, R. (1995c). *In* 'Trends in QSAR and Molecular Modelling '94' (Sanz, F., ed.). Prous Sci, Barcelona (in press).

Cocchi, M. and Johansson, E. (1993). *Quant. Struct.-Act. Relat.* **12**, 1–8.

Cocchi, M., Cruciani, G., Menziani, M.C. and De Benedetti, P.G. (1993). *In* 'Trends in QSAR and Molecular Modeling '92' (C.G. Wermuth, ed.), pp. 527–529. ESCOM, Leiden.

Cosentino, U., Moro, G., Pitea, D., Scolastico, S. Todeschini, R. and Scolastico, C. (1992). *J. Comput.-Aided Mol. Design* **6**, 47–60.

Cramer, R.D. III, Patterson, D.E. and Bunce, J.D. (1988a). *J. Am. Chem. Soc.* **110**, 5959–5967.

Cramer III, R.D., Bunce, J.D., Patterson, D.E. and Frank, I. (1988b). *Quant. Struct.-Act. Relat.* **7**, 18–25.

Cramer III, R.D., DePriest, S.A., Patterson, D.E. and Hecht, P. (1993). *In* '3D QSAR in Drug Design: Theory, Methods and Applications' (H. Kubinyi, ed.), pp. 443–485. ESCOM, Leiden.

Crippen, G.M. (1977). *J. Comp. Phys.* **24**, 96–107.

Cruciani, G. and Goodford, P.J. (1994). *J. Mol. Graph.* **12**, 116–129.

Cruciani, G. and Watson, K.A. (1994). *J. Med. Chem.* **37**, 2589–2601.

Cruciani, G., Baroni, M., Bonelli, D., Clementi, S., Ebert, C. and Skagerberg, B. (1990). *Quant. Struct.-Act. Relat.* **9**, 101–107.

Cruciani, G., Baroni, M., Clementi, S., Costantino, G., Riganelli, D. and Skagerberg, B. (1992). *J. Chemometrics,* **6**, 335–346.

Cruciani, G., Clementi, S. and Baroni, M. (1993). *In* '3D-QSAR in Drug Design: Theory Methods and Applications' (H. Kubinyi, ed.), pp. 551–566. ESCOM, Leiden.

Davis, A., Baxter, A., Cruciani, G. and Filipponi, E. (1995). *J. Med. Chem.* (to be submitted).

De Meo, G., Pedini, M., Ricci, A., Bastianini, L., Jacquignon, P.C., Bonelli, D., Clementi, S. and Cruciani, G. (1990). *Il Farmaco* **45**, 313–330.

Draper, N.R. and Smith, H. (1981). 'Applied Regression Analysis'. John Wiley, New York.

Dunn, W.J. III and Wold, S. (1990). *In* 'Comprehensive Medicinal Chemistry' (C. Hansch, P.G. Sammes, and J.B. Taylor, eds, vol. 4 (C.A. Ramsden, ed.) pp. 691–714. Pergamon Press, Oxford.

Eriksson, L., Jonsson, J., Hellberg, S., Lindgren, F., Skagerberg, B., Sjöström, M. and Wold, S. (1990). *Acta Chem. Scand.* **44**, 50–56.

Frank, I.E. and Friedman, J.H. (1993). *Technometrics* **35**, 109–148.

Good, A.C., So, S.S. and Richards, W.G. (1993a). *J. Med. Chem.*, **36**, 433–438.
Good, A.C., Peterson, S.J. and Richards, W.G. (1993b). *J. Med. Chem.*, **36**, 2929–2937.
Goodford, P.J. (1985). *J. Med. Chem.* **28**, 849–857.
Hansch, C. and Leo, A.J. (1979). 'Substituent Constants for Correlation Analysis in Chemistry and Biology'. John Wiley & Sons, New York.
Hellberg, S., Sjöström, M., Skagerberg, B. and Wold, S. (1987). *J. Med. Chem.* **30**, 1127–1135.
Hopfinger, A.J. (1980). *J. Am. Chem. Soc.*, **102**, 7196–7206.
Jolles, G. and Wooldridge K.R.H. (eds.) (1982). 'Drug Design: Fact or Fantasy?' Academic Press, London.
Jonsson, J., Eriksson, L., Hellberg, S., Sjöström, M. and Wold, S. (1989). *Quant. Struct.-Act. Relat.*, **8**, 204–209.
Kubinyi, H. (1993a). 'QSAR: Hansoh Analysis and Related Approaches'. VCH, Weinheim.
Kubinyi, H. (ed.) (1993b). '3D QSAR in Drug Design: Theory Methods and Applications'. ESCOM, Leiden.
Marshall, G.R., Barry, C.D., Bosshard, H.E., Dammkoehler, R.A. and Dunn, D.A. (1979). *In* 'Computer-Assisted Drug Design' (E.C. Olsen and R.E. Christoffersen, eds), pp. 205–226. American Chemical Society, Washington.
Norinder, U. (1991). *Peptides* **12**, 1223–1227.
Norinder, U. (1993). *J. Comput.-Aided Mol. Design* **7**, 671–682.
Pedini, M., DeMeo, G. and Ricci, A. (1994). *Il Farmaco* **49**, 671–674.
Rännar, S., Lindgren, F., Geladi, P. and Wold, S. (1994). *J. Chemometrics* **8** 111–126.
Riganelli, D., Clementi, S., Cruciani, G., Mabilia, M. (1995a). *J. Comput.-Aided Mol. Design* (submitted).
Riganelli, D., Cruciani, G., Clementi, S., Costantino, G. and Baroni, M. (1995b). *Quant. Struct.-Act. Relat.* (to be submitted).
Rovero, P., Riganelli, D., Viganò, S., Pegaro, S., Revoltella, R., Fruci, D., Greco, G., Butler, R., Clementi, S. and Tanigaki, N. (1994). *Mol. Immunol.* **31**, 549–554.
Shao, J. (1993). *J. Am. Stat. Assoc.* **88**, 486–494.
Skagerberg, B., Bonelli, D., Clementi, S., Cruciani, G. and Ebert, C. (1989). *Quant. Struct.-Act. Relat.* **8**, 32–38.
Todeschini, R., Lasagni, M. and Marengo, E. (1994). *J. Chemometrics* **8**, 263–272.
Tosato, M.L., Cesareo, D., Galassi, S., Viganò, L., Cruciani, G., Clementi, S., Skagerberg, B. (1988). *Chimica oggi* **6**, 41–45.
Tosato, M.L., Viganò, L., Skagerberg, B. and Clementi, S. (1991). *Environ. Sci. Technol.* **25**, 695–702.
Valigi, R., Clementi, S., Cruciani, G., Riganelli, D. and Wold, S. (1995). *Quant. Struct.-Act. Relat.* (submitted).
van de Waterbeemd, H., El Tayar, N., Carrupt, P.A. and Testa, B. (1989). *J. Comput.-Aided Mol. Design* **3**, 111–132.
van de Waterbeemd, H., Carrupt, P.A., El Tayar, N, Testa, B. and Kier, L.B. (1993a). *In* 'Trends in QSAR and Molecular Modeling '92' (C.G. Wermuth, ed.), pp. 69–75. ESCOM; Leiden.
van de Waterbeemd, H., Clementi, S., Cruciani, G., Costantino, G., Carrupt, P.A. and Testa, B. (1993b). *In* '3D-QSAR in Drug Design: Theory Methods and Applications (H. Kubinyi, ed.), pp. 697–707. ESCOM, Leiden.
van de Waterbeemd, H., Clementi, S., Costantino, G., Cruciani, G. and Valigi, R. (1995). *In* 'Chemometric Methods in Molecular Design' (H. van de Waterbeemd, ed.), vol. 2 'Methods and Principles in Medicinal Chemistry' (R. Mannhold, P. Krogsgaard-Larsen and H. Timmerman, eds). VCH, Weinheim.

Wold, S. (1991). *Quant. Struct.-Act. Relat.* **10**, 191–193.
Wold, S. (1993). *Technometrics* **35**, 136–139.
Wold, S. and Sjöström, M. (1977). *In* 'Chemometrics: Theory and Application' (B.R. Kowalski, ed.), pp. 243–282. ACS Symposium Series, Washington.
Wold, S. and Dunn, W.J. III (1983). *J. Chem. Inf. Comput. Sci.* **23**, 6–13.
Wold, S., Albano, C., Dunn, W.J. III, Edlund, U., Esbensen, K., Geladi, P., Hellberg, S., Johansson, E., Lindberg, W. and Sjöström M. (1984). *In* 'Chemometrics' (B.R. Kowalski, ed.), pp. 17–94. Reidel, Dordrecht.
Wold, S., Sjöström, M., Carlson, R. Lundstedt, T., Hellberg, S., Skagerberg, B., Wikström, C. and Öhman, J. (1986). *Anal. Chim. Acta* **191**, 17–32.
Wold, S., Berntsson, P., Eriksson, L., Geladi, P., Hellberg, S., Johansson, E., Jonsson, J., Kettaneh-Wold, N., Lindgren, F., Rännar, S., Sandberg, M. and Sjöström, M. (1991). *Pharmacochem. Lib.* **16**, 15–24.
Wold, S., Johansson, E. and Cocchi, M. (1993a). *In* '3D QSAR in Drug Design: *Theory, Methods and Applications*' (H. Kubinyi, ed.) pp. 523–550. ESCOM: Leiden.
Wold, S., Jonsson, J., Sjöström, M., Sandberg, M., Rännar, S. (1993b). *Anal. Chim. Acta* **277**, 239–254.

Discussion

A. Laoui
You said that the auto- and cross-correlation and covariance (ACC) transforms are available at present only for planar molecules. Can you give some details about the problems with non-planar molecules?

S. Clementi
There are two different kinds of problems. First, that even planar molecules, when bent out of the coordinate plane, give a different representation in the ACC transform. Second, there is also a cultural problem on how to handle different conformers. Each conformer, because it has different spatial positions of the atoms, should give different ACC transforms. My view is that some sort of principal component analysis has to be used on the conformer population, followed by working on the clusters of the conformers using some strategy which is still to be developed.

K. Zakrzewska
Is there any way of forseeing the toxicity of new drugs, any expert system or anything else, or is it only accumulated experience?

S. Clementi
Very few data are available on the possibility of predicting toxicity. It is extremely difficult to obtain good toxicity data on the several thousand chemicals that have been evaluated. There may, however, be a chemometric strategy here, in the sense that the appropriate collecting of data could be

concentrated on a very few compounds which are representative of a series of chemicals according to some statistical design criteria. By means of these few compounds for which good toxicity data have been collected and shared, the toxicity of almost all the others could easily be predicted. Such a proposal was put forward by the Italian member of the OECD Committee a few years ago but, as far as I know, this has not progressed.

I.D. Kuntz

There are quite a lot of toxicity data, at least in America, but all the data are at the Food and Drug Administration – all locked up as proprietary data because of company policies. I strongly advise people here who can make decisions about this sort of thing to think through the consequences of those proprietary data. If the data were to be released in appropriate forms, this could make an enormous leap forward in our knowledge of toxicology, particularly human toxicology.

Index